26.50

Shielia Hughes
457 Lowe
Danville, Il 61832
217/3-2223

Practical Approaches
to
Alcoholism Psychotherapy
SECOND EDITION

Practical Approaches
to
Alcoholism Psychotherapy
SECOND EDITION

Edited by

Sheldon Zimberg, M.D.
Director of Psychiatry
Joint Diseases, North General Hospital
Associate Professor of Psychiatry
Mount Sinai School of Medicine
New York, New York

John Wallace, Ph.D.
Director of Treatment
Edgehill Newport
Newport, Rhode Island

and

Sheila B. Blume, M.D.
Medical Director
Alcoholism and Compulsive Gambling Program
South Oaks Hospital
Amityville, New York

Plenum Press · New York and London

Library of Congress Cataloging in Publication Data

Main entry under title:

Practical approaches to alcoholism psychotherapy.

Includes bibliographies and index.
1. Alcoholism—Treatment. 2. Psychotherapy. I. Zimberg, Sheldon. II. Wallace, John,
1931–   . III. Blume, Sheila B. [DNLM: 1. Alcoholism—therapy. 2. Psychotherapy.
WM 274 P895]
RC565.P715   1985   616.8′61′06   84-24922
ISBN 0-306-41762-6

First Printing—August 1982
Second Printing—July 1987

© 1985 Sheldon Zimberg, John Wallace, and Sheila B. Blume

Plenum Press is a division of Plenum Publishing Corporation
233 Spring Street, New York, N.Y. 10013

Printed in the United States of America

Contributors

L. A. ALIBRANDI, PH.D. • Director, Genesis II Outpatient Dependency Treatment, South Coast Medical Center, South Laguna, California

SHEILA B. BLUME, M.D. • Medical Director, Alcoholism and Compulsive Gambling Programs, South Oaks Hospital, Amityville, New York

DOUGLAS K. CHALMERS, PH.D. • Associate Professor of Psychology, School of Social Sciences, University of California, Irvine, California

JUNE JACKSON CHRISTMAS, M.D. • Medical Professor and Director, Behavioral Science Program, City College of the City University of New York

SIDNEY COHEN, M.D. • Clinical Professor of Psychiatry, Neuro-Psychiatric Institute, UCLA, Los Angeles, California

CELIA DULFANO, M.S.W. • Private Consultant, Family Therapy and Alcoholism, Newton, Massachusettes

JAY FISCHER, PH.D. • Assistant Director for Management and Administration, The Door-Center of Alternatives, New York, New York

MARC GALANTER, M.D. • Professor of Psychiatry, Albert Einstein College of Medicine, Bronx, New York

DONALD M. GALLANT, M.D. • Professor of Psychiatry and Adjunct Professor of Psychopharmacology, Tulane University School of Medicine, New Orleans, Louisiana

DONALD P. HOWARD, M.ED. • The Howard Institute Family Counseling Center, Columbia, Missouri

NANCY T. HOWARD, B.S. • The Howard Institute Family Counseling Center, Columbia, Missouri

JOSEPH C. KERN, PH.D. • Director, Alcohol Treatment Services for Nassau County Department of Drug and Alcohol Addiction, Hempstead, New York

DAVID B. MALLOTT, M.D. • Assistant Professor of Psychiatry, Tulane University School of Medicine, New Orleans, Louisiana

DAVID J. POWELL, PH.D. • President, Education and Training Programs, Inc., Granby, Connecticut

JOHN S. TAMERIN, M.D. • Clinical Associate Professor of Psychiatry, Cornell University College of Medicine, New York, New York

JOHN WALLACE, PH.D. • Director of Treatment, Edgehill Newport, Newport, Rhode Island

SHELDON ZIMBERG, M.D. • Director of Psychiatry, Joint Diseases, North General Hospital, New York, New York; Associate Professor of Psychiatry, Mount Sinai School of Medicine, New York, New York

Foreword to Second Edition

What is less interesting than writing a foreword for a second edition of a book whose first edition I had already read? I thought. As it turned out, it was an interesting and rewarding exercise.

Practical Approaches to Alcoholism Psychotherapy is a complete compendium of psychotherapy, not only of the alcoholic, but also of his or her children and spouse. It discusses in good detail and with case examples all the psychotherapies. In fact, it goes beyond psychotherapy into sociotherapy and even pays attention to the biological therapies. So it is wide-ranging and unusually even handed. It can almost be called a wise book, but that adjective has an alien sound to the ear these days.

There are so many important points made in the text, but only one or two can be mentioned here.

1. Treat the alcohol disorder first. Then treat the depression, the schizophrenia, the borderline state or the attention-deficit disorder if it exists. Little can be accomplished before detoxification and abstinence. Diagnosis becomes more precise after the ethanol has been eliminated from the picture.

2. At stage I the patient says, "I can't drink" meaning that further imbibing will lead to external threats becoming realities. The alcoholic stops because someone out there sees the behavior as a problem. Directive psychotherapy is indicated.

As he learns where he has been, the alcoholic says, "I won't drink," (stage II). Controls have been internalized and decisions about whether to drink or not are more easily made. Directive and supportive psychotherapy has made this possible.

The end of the process is stage III. The alcoholic says, "I don't have to drink," because he or she has insight into why drinking to excess occurred. Uncovering psychotherapy has helped provide the understanding of the underlying conflicts and has resolved them. Stage III is

not often achieved, but when it is, it leads to a better ordered life. At
no stage is social drinking an option.

This second edition is a worthwhile revision of the first.

SIDNEY COHEN, M.D.

Neuropsychiatric Institute
U. C. L. A. School of Medicine
Los Angeles, California

Foreword to First Edition

Societal attitudes toward alcoholism are characterized by several types of denial, with disastrous personal and social consequences. Refusal to admit the extent of alcoholism as a major national health problem leads to a public policy which allocates relatively few resources to research, prevention, treatment, or rehabilitation. On an individual basis, the combination of socially approved drinking and the stigma assigned to the chronic alcoholic results in individuals blinding themselves to the existence of the problem in family, friend, and self until it has reached such an advanced or obvious degree that denial is no longer possible.

There is the third kind of denial, exemplified by therapeutic despair, which proclaims that gaps in knowledge of the cause of alcoholism are so great and failures to treat alcoholics successfully so dramatic that there is no assurance that efforts will lead to a positive outcome. This denial is perhaps the most troublesome because it reflects an attitude of therapeutic helplessness. It discourages families from seeking help, and it reinforces the tendency of physicians and other human-services workers to overlook the presence of alcoholism as they treat its physical, social, and economic consequences. Denial frequently surrounds those who treat alcoholics with an aura of hopelessness, which itself is a negative therapeutic force.

Indeed, even within programs that provide alcoholism services, a limited conception of the possibility of therapeutic effectiveness is sometimes based on the underlying assumption that there are no interpersonal skills essential to treating alcoholism which can be clearly defined, written about, or taught to others. This assertion frequently goes hand in hand with the belief that only those who have themselves experienced the pain and anguish of alcoholism can be helpers of others and that even this experiential knowledge is something intuitive over which there can be no intellectual mastery.

This book puts the lie to these views. Written by practitioners from various fields, each with years of experience in the provision of alcoholism services, this book is based on the assumption that there *is* knowledge of what works, and that this knowledge can be delineated with justice to both theoretical underpinnings and practical guidance. At the same time, this volume recognizes the need for alcoholism services to stand the test of evaluation as well as of conviction and of time.

Therapeutic techniques discussed, based on a psychosocial philosophy, are considered from a wide perspective. Yet the book does not attempt to deal with all types of alcoholism services. Instead, it focuses on a range of psychotherapeutic approaches, including individual, group, and family therapies, along with the folk psychotherapy intrinsic to the most successful approach, Alcoholics Anonymous. As we look at these techniques, the basic theoretical knowledge that operates is underlined and the usefulness of understanding psychodynamics in applying general principles of psychotherapy to treatment of alcoholism is pointed out.

Moreover, we recognize that social status, income, ethnic background, sex, and age are not merely entries on an intake record, as they are too often considered to be. They are, instead, significant factors that have to be addressed in the provision of services to those who abuse alcohol and to their families. The need for socioculturally syntonic services is sometimes underemphasized as if "the case" existed outside of the social environment or "the disease," outside of the human being.

While the holistic sociopsychological approach does not accept singular causality and recognizes that much more information is needed about determinants, it nevertheless addresses the significant factors of adolescent task accomplishments and emotional development, of the pressures of being poor in an affluent society, of sexism, of discrimination against racial minorities, and of rejection of the elderly. These critical forces have to be reckoned with as part of the therapeutic plan if alcoholism services are to relate to the individual in a social context as, indeed, they should.

To plan and implement services that may be effective in treating alcoholism requires an orientation that relates to these factors as they contribute to human personality, growth, and social behavior. This is far different from the traditional psychiatric approach, which focused (when psychiatrists were willing to accept alcoholics as patients) on individual psychopathology, or the medical approach, which resulted in only repeated detoxifications and trips through the revolving hospital door. This orientation does not espouse a single rigid response to what could be incorrectly described as a unilaterally determined disorder. Although the focus is on psychotherapeutic approaches, it does not reflect the view that alcoholism can be helped solely through the resolution of intrapsychic conflicts, nor the moralistic approach which speaks to defects of will. Even though the sections on social disadvantage reflect recognition of the interaction of the individual and society, the approach is not restricted to the social-environmental view sometimes espoused by those who deeply feel the effects of deprivation—that alcoholism would no longer exist if social and economic inequities were to be removed. Instead, several possible rehabilitative and treatment approaches are addressed and clearly defined, and significant questions are raised about the need to evaluate the effectiveness of each.

The very practical approach that is taken by Sheldon Zimberg, John Wallace, Sheila Blume, and their collaborators is a significant addition to the armamentarium of writings on alcoholism. More than a "how to" book, this volume raises questions about the course of recovery and the factors that are in operation at every stage of health and disease.

For those who are already involved in the provision of alcoholism services, these writings should provide a stimulating and provocative addition to the literature that has erred in the past by being too general and impressionistic. To those who have recognized the need for skillful, well-trained professional and paraprofessional practitioners, this book should be an encouraging beacon.

June Jackson Christmas, M.D.
Former Commissioner of Mental Health
Mental Retardation and Alcoholism Services
City of New York

Medical Professor and Director
Behavioral Science Program
City College of the City University of New York

Preface to Second Edition

Why publish a second edition of *Practical Approaches to Alcoholism Psychotherapy*? Well, the first edition was designed as a text to offer theoretical and clinical guidelines for verbally oriented therapies in the treatment of alcoholism, and this second edition follows the same orientation. However, since 1978, when the first edition was published, new knowledge and experience in the treatment of alcoholism have been developed. The second edition seeks to incorporate this recent knowledge and experience by updating many of the previous chapters and by adding new case histories. There is also an awareness of the greater need of specific treatments for specific subpopulations of alcoholics. The importance of differential diagnosis in delineating subpopulations and biological factors that contribute to alcoholism is stressed. Newer and effective treatment techniques, including early intervention, family couples therapy, social and family network therapy, and treatment of sexual dysfunction in alcoholics, are also presented. The increasing concern with the consequences of alcoholism in the family, and especially with the children, is addressed in a chapter on the treatment of children of alcoholics.

The analysis of relapse and recovery and an approach to outcome evaluation research indicate the concern of clinicians in dealing with the long-term chronic illness of alcoholism. Outcome evaluation is essential in order to generalize our clinical experience with selected populations because alcoholism is a disease of very high prevalence and of a great variety of manifestations. It is hoped that this volume will offer practical help in the treatment of alcoholism and stimulate further reading of the burgeoning clinical and research literature.

The editors would like to acknowledge the assistance of Althea Bass in the preparation and editing of the second edition.

SHELDON ZIMBERG, M.D.
JOHN WALLACE, PH.D.
SHEILA B. BLUME, M.D.

Preface to First Edition

This book is designed to provide theoretical and practical guidelines for practitioners and students in alcoholism psychotherapy. It is based on the knowledge of clinicians who have had considerable experience and success in the treatment of alcoholism. A variety of psychotherapeutic methods which have been applied effectively are described.

Modified approaches for the treatment of various subpopulations of alcoholics, including adolescents, women, the elderly, and the socioeconomically deprived, are presented to highlight the fact that alcoholism is a complex illness that manifests itself in differing patterns among particular populations.

The volume generally can be viewed as a text on applications of verbally oriented therapies in the treatment of alcoholism. The final chapter discusses the evaluation of patient progress and can serve as a guide to assessing clinical effectiveness.

The editors would like to acknowledge the assistance of Doris Borakove in the preparation and editing of this book.

SHELDON ZIMBERG, M.D.
JOHN WALLACE, PH.D.
SHEILA B. BLUME, M.D.

Contents

Chapter 3

CRITICAL ISSUES IN ALCOHOLISM THERAPY

JOHN WALLACE

TECHNIQUES OF TREATMENT

Chapter 4

PSYCHIATRIC OFFICE TREATMENT OF ALCOHOLISM

SHELDON ZIMBERG

Chapter 5

GROUP PSYCHOTHERAPY IN THE TREATMENT OF ALCOHOLISM

Sheila B. Blume

Chapter 6

PSYCHODRAMA AND THE TREATMENT OF ALCOHOLISM

Sheila B. Blume

Chapter 7

BEHAVIORAL MODIFICATION METHODS AS ADJUNCTS TO PSYCHOTHERAPY

JOHN WALLACE

Chapter 8

FAMILY THERAPY OF ALCOHOLISM

CELIA DULFANO

Chapter 9

INTERVENTION TECHNIQUES AND MARRIED COUPLES GROUP THERAPY

Donald M. Gallant and David B. Mallott

Chapter 10

USE OF THE SOCIAL AND FAMILY NETWORK IN INDIVIDUAL THERAPY

Marc Galanter

Chapter 11

TREATMENT OF THE SIGNIFICANT OTHER

DONALD P. HOWARD AND NANCY T. HOWARD

Chapter 12

MANAGEMENT OF SEXUAL DYSFUNCTIONS IN ALCOHOLICS

DAVID J. POWELL

Chapter 13

THE FOLK PSYCHOTHERAPY OF ALCOHOLICS ANONYMOUS

L. A. ALIBRANDI

TREATMENT OF SPECIFIC POPULATIONS OF ALCOHOLICS

Chapter 14

THE PSYCHOTHERAPY OF ALCOHOLIC WOMEN

JOHN S. TAMERIN

Chapter 15

TREATMENT OF SOCIOECONOMICALLY DEPRIVED ALCOHOLICS

SHELDON ZIMBERG

Chapter 16

PSYCHOTHERAPY OF ADOLESCENT ALCOHOL ABUSERS

JAY FISCHER

Chapter 17

MANAGEMENT OF CHILDREN OF ALCOHOLICS

JOSEPH C. KERN

Chapter 18

PSYCHOSOCIAL TREATMENT OF ELDERLY ALCOHOLICS

SHELDON ZIMBERG

CLINICAL EVALUATION OF PATIENT PROGRESS

Chapter 19

EVALUATION OF PATIENT PROGRESS

DOUGLAS K. CHALMERS AND JOHN WALLACE

I

THEORETICAL
CONSIDERATIONS

Principles of Alcoholism Psychotherapy

SHELDON ZIMBERG

INTRODUCTION

An article in the *New York State Journal of Medicine* indicated that many physicians had problems in the diagnosis and management of alcoholics (Douglas, 1976). The author suggested that Alcoholics Anonymous was the only effective treatment for alcoholics. Most professionals in the field of alcoholism consider AA an effective method of treatment for many, but by no means all, alcoholics. The experience has been that a variety of treatment approaches, often including AA, is needed for the various subpopulations of alcoholics that are to be found in a community (Zimberg, 1975).

Physicians, psychiatrists, and other mental health professionals have been ineffective in the treatment of alcoholics and have lost interest in attempting to treat them. Such a situation is not unexpected since physicians and other health personnel are exposed only to the medical and psychiatric complications of alcoholism and not the diagnosis and treatment of the disorder itself. This lack of training in alcoholism, as well as the lack of awareness of successful treatment outcomes, supports the myth that this illness is untreatable.

Psychiatry and other behavioral-science disciplines, with their understanding of physiology, pharmacology, psychodynamics, and so-

SHELDON ZIMBERG • Director of Psychiatry, Joint Diseases, North General Hospital, New York, New York; Associate Professor of Psychiatry, Mount Sinai School of Medicine, New York, New York.

ciopsychological factors relating to human behavior, can make important contributions to the field of alcoholism and provide a substantial amount of effective treatment. Health care professionals should not abdicate their responsibility toward the treatment of alcoholics. Education about effective techniques can make it possible for psychiatrists, nonpsychiatric physicians, and other mental health professionals to treat alcoholics in their offices and in institutional settings. The experiential knowledge of recovering alcoholics working as alcoholism counselors and using basic knowledge of the psychodynamics and interpersonal aspects of alcoholism can also be very effective in the treatment of alcoholism.

It is generally accepted that psychological factors alone are not sufficient to produce alcoholism in an individual. Sociocultural and physiological factors (possibly of genetic origin) along with psychological mechanisms contribute to alcoholism.

This chapter will present a psychiatrist's understanding of the sociopsychological factors relating to alcoholism and the approaches for successful psychotherapy of this condition in a significant number of alcoholics. The experience and views presented are based on the author's work with many alcoholics in urban ghetto alcoholism programs, in a suburban community mental health center, and in private psychiatric practice.

PSYCHODYNAMICS OF THE ALCOHOLIC

Blum (1966) reviewed the literature on psychoanalytic theories of alcoholism and concluded that psychoanalytic concepts can be applied to the psychodynamic understanding of alcoholism. Oral fixation is thought to be the arrested stage of development in the alcoholic. This fixation accounts for infantile and dependent characteristics such as narcissism, demanding behavior, passivity, and dependence. The fixation occurs after a significant degree of deprivation during early childhood development. Much evidence supports the view that alcoholics were exposed to rejection by one or both parents and that dependency needs are among the major psychological factors that contribute to the development of alcoholism (Knight, 1937; McCord and McCord, 1960; Bacon, Barry, and Child, 1965; Tahlka, 1966; Blane, 1968). Other developmental factors that have been noted to contribute to a conflict with dependency have been overprotection and the forcing of premature responsibility on a child.

The dependency needs of many of the alcoholics the author has treated have been profoundly repressed, with little evidence of overt passivity or dependent traits when the patients were sober. These traits became apparent, however, under the influence of alcohol. In many cases, alcoholics, while sober, had obsessive-compulsive personality traits. They were often perfectionistic, had the need to maintain control over their lives, and were completely unaware of even the most intense feelings, particularly anger. These observations were confirmed by an experimental study of drinking to intoxication among a group of alcoholics conducted by Tamerin and Mendelson (1969). Therefore, it is not appropriate to look for or to characterize an "alcoholic personality." The conflict discussed below forms a psychodynamic constellation which is the key psychological factor in alcoholism and is the core conflict that must be recognized in therapy. This psychodynamic constellation is a common problem among alcoholics, but it does not produce a common personality.

The conflict consists of a lack of self-esteem along with feelings of worthlessness and inadequacy. These feelings are denied and repressed and lead to unconscious needs to be taken care of and accepted (dependent needs). Since these dependent needs cannot be met in reality, they lead to anxiety and compensatory needs for control, power, and achievement. Alcohol tranquilizes the anxiety and, more important, creates pharmacologically induced feelings of power, omnipotence, and invulnerability. When the alcoholic wakes up after a drinking episode, he experiences guilt and despair because he has not achieved anything more than before he drank and his problems still remain. Thus, his feelings of worthlessness are intensified and the conflict continues in a vicious circle that often has a progressive downward spiral.

Alcohol provides an artificial feeling-state of power and control that cannot be achieved in reality. The very act of producing this feeling of power at will feeds the alcoholic's grandiose self-image. This intense need for grandiosity can be called *reactive grandiosity*.

These observations are supported by the work of McClelland, Davis, Kalin, and Wanner (1972), which indicated that alcohol produces in alcoholics "ego enhancing" effects and thoughts of power and strength. McCord and McCord (1960, 1962) conducted longitudinal studies of families in which some of the boys later became alcoholics. They noted that the alcoholics had evidence of heightened unacceptable dependency needs and had feelings of being victimized by society with compensatory grandiosity.

Wilsnack (1976) conducted similar studies among women and found that alcohol enhances feelingness of womanliness. McClelland's *et al.* (1972) and Wilsnack's work suggest that male alcoholics strive for power and control consciously and female alcoholics strive for womanliness as compensation for unconscious feelings of worthlessness, low self-esteem, and the need to be nurtured. The pharmacological effect of alcohol produces an artificial feeling-state of power and control in men and enhanced feelings of feminity in women that can not be achieved in reality. Thus, the use of alcohol can be viewed as a reinforcement of unconscious needs that lead to habitual use and eventually physiological addiction.

Vaillant (1983) reported on *The Natural History of Alcoholism* based on a prospective study of 200 college men, 400 socially underprivileged men in a core city sample, and 100 hospitalized alcoholics that had been followed for eight years. He found that alcoholics did not have more psychopathology and were not more dependent than non-alcoholics prior to their becoming alcoholic. This conclusion differed from McCord and McCord's (1962) longitudinal study. However, Vaillant found that "compared to asymptomatic drinkers, alcoholics are more likely to be premorbidly antisocial" during adolescence. He also noted that there was a substantial rate of spontaneous remission not accounted for by treatment efforts in the course of alcoholism. The remission resulted from the development of a "substitute dependency" that included AA involvement, increased religious affiliation, or a new love relationship. It is not clear whether the methodology used in this major study could pick-up evidence of unconscious dependent conflicts as was done by McCord and McCord (1962). However, the questions arise as to why alcoholics seemed to be more antisocial during adolescence and why was a "substitute dependency" likely to produce recovery? The "substitute dependency" was a substitute for what? As indicated, a large number of studies and clinical observations suggest that the unconscious conflict with dependency can lead to antisocial behavior and alcoholism and that the "substitute dependency" is in fact a substitute for unresolved dependent needs.

These observations are summarized in Figure 1, which illustrates the psychodynamics of alcoholism. Childhood rejection, overprotection, or premature responsibility leads to an unconscious need for nurturance that cannot be met in reality and results in rejection. The rejection leads to anxiety, which in turn leads to the development of a number of defense mechanisms, particularly denial and a compensatory need for grandiosity. The grandiosity causes such individuals to try harder and results in inevitable failure. The failures lead to more anxiety, depression, anger, and guilt. These unpleasant affects can be reduced by alcohol, at least for a time, and lead to the pharmacologically induced feelings of power and omnipotence in men and enhanced womanliness in women, thus reinforcing the denial and reactive grandiosity.

An individual with such a psychological conflict will become an

Know for Test

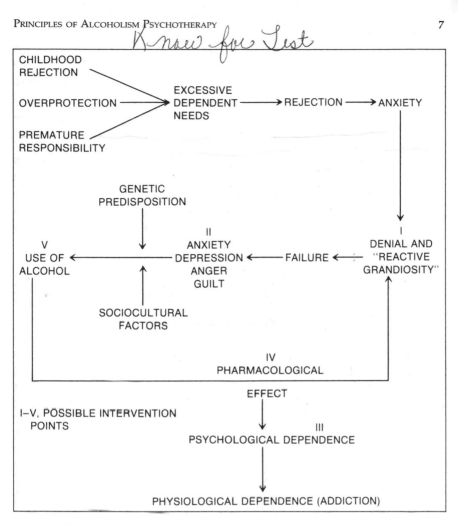

Figure 1. Paradigm of the Psychodynamics of Alcoholism.

alcoholic if there is a genetic predisposition to alcoholism and if he lives in a society in which the use of alcohol is sanctioned as a way to feel better or in which there is considerable ambivalence regarding the use of alcohol. In any particular individual, one or more of these etiological factors may predominate and lead to alcoholism.

TREATMENT OF ALCOHOLISM

Alcoholics Anonymous. Alcoholics Anonymous has been one of the most successful treatment approaches for alcoholism; it is also the model for other successful self-help movements. How does the effectiveness of AA relate to the psychodynamic understanding of alcoholism just presented?

Tiebout (1961) described a similar psychodynamic understanding of alcoholism in his paper discussing the process by which an alcoholic becomes involved in Alcoholics Anonymous. The process occurs in four steps: (1) the need to hit bottom; (2) the need to be humble; (3) the need to surrender; and (4) the need for ego reduction. These steps were based on Tiebout's observation of an excessive amount of narcissism in the alcoholic's ego that gives rise to feelings of omnipotence. The steps in the conversion process are necessary to produce a reduction in the narcissism which has perpetuated the self-destructive drinking behavior and the coexisting denial. Tiebout did not indicate in his paper, however, what happens to the excessive narcissism of the alcoholic's ego. Clearly, the narcissism is sublimated toward the goal of AA to rescue other alcoholics. Thus, the grandiosity becomes fulfilled and socially useful and much of their dependent needs are met by the group. AA members recognize that their support of other alcoholics helps themselves maintain sobriety. Therefore the successful development of AA was based on an intuitive understanding of the alcoholic's psychological conflict and needs.

Other Treatment Approaches.   Other treatment approaches can be understood by looking at Figure 1 in relation to possible intervention points on this paradigm. Intervention point I represents the traditional psychoanalytic approach to treating alcoholism. In this case, the therapist attempts to work backwards from the defenses so as to uncover the underlying psychological conflicts. This approach has failed simply because the pharmacological effects of alcohol are too strong to be altered through insight alone and the very technique of uncovering-therapy produces anxiety that results in the need to drink.

Intervention point II represents an area in which mood-altering drugs might reduce the need to use alcohol in order to reduce dysphoric feelings. After many studies there is not evidence to suggest that the major tranquilizers, the anti-depressants, or the minor tranquilizers (anti-anxiety drugs) are beneficial in the treatment of chronic alcoholism. Subpopulations of alcoholics who were clinically depressed were noted in a study as having benefited from lithium treatment (Merry, Reynolds, Bailey, and Coppen, 1976). Most likely, such patients represent secondary alcoholism rather than primary alcoholism.

Intervention point III represents the use of drugs or other modalities that would alter the effect of alcohol on the brain and result in a reduced craving for alcohol, a lessening of the pleasant effect of alcohol, and/or a reduction in the degree of physiological dependence. With our understanding of the mechanisms of how alcohol affects the brain, we may be able to alter the adverse effects selectively. This area probably represents the future for alcoholism treatment. Considerable research effort is underway to determine the acute and chronic effects of alcohol on the opiate and benzodiazepine receptors and neurotransmitters that include norepinephrine, serotonin, GABA, endorphins, and enkephalins.

Intervention at point IV can interrupt the pleasurable feelings associated with alcohol consumption that become reinforced by the repetitive drinking that leads to alcoholism. Lovibond and Caddy (1970) applied aversive conditioning with electric shocks to enable alcoholics to discriminate their blood alcohol levels and to maintain low levels that were characterized by controlled social drinking. They reported considerable success with this approach. Ewing and Rouse (1976) utilized a similar approach in an attempt to replicate Lovibond and Caddy's work. Ewing and Rouse reported that although the alcoholic patients were able to learn to recognize their levels of blood alcohol and develop controlled drinking patterns while in the program, all relapsed into loss-of-control drinking during the 27 to 55 month follow-up period. Sobell and Sobell (1976) reported high rates of success with electric aversion therapy that led to controlled drinking in addicted alcoholics. However, a recent study by Pendery, Maltzman, and West (1982) on the same patients studied by the Sobells found that none of the patients were able to maintain controlled drinking. All the patient's either had relapsed into alcoholic drinking, died, or recovered with the maintanence of abstinence. The literature is replete with such equivocal results in various controlled drinking conditioning approaches. Aversive conditioning that leads to abstinence with the nausea producing drug Emetine has been used in a number of European countries and in the United States. A recent paper by Neubeurger, Miller et al. (1982) reported high rates of abstinence for one year with this aversive conditioning approach. This approach remains an important area for treatment research.

The fifth point of possible intervention represents our current approach to alcoholism psychotherapy and is the basis of the material in this chapter. This method involves eliminating the use of alcohol by directive approaches and helping the alcoholic learn to live without alcohol when confronted with stress and unpleasant feelings.

The central problem in the psychotherapy of the alcoholic is breaking through the reactive grandiosity. This grandiosity produces the massive denial of profound feelings of inferiority and dependency that permit the pattern of self-destructive drinking to continue. The alcoholic destroys not only himself but also his loved ones without perceiving his lack of control of his behavior pattern. The typical response of an alcoholic without insight into this behavior is, "I can stop drinking any time I want to," despite overwhelming evidence to the contrary. This self-deception must be penetrated if rehabilitation is to succeed.

SOCIOPSYCHOLOGICAL FACTORS AFFECTING PSYCHOTHERAPY

During the initial evaluation of the alcoholic, one not only must look for areas of psychological conflict and psychopathology, but must also try to understand the patient's social circumstances. It is necessary to evaluate the family and marital relationships that exist or existed and the employment situation. Information should also be obtained regarding the cultural attitudes toward drinking and drunkenness in the individual's family while he was growing up and how he integrated these attitudes into his drinking behavior.

There must be a determination as to how the individual has handled crises and stress, and whether he has been able to modify or stop destructive drinking behavior spontaneously in the past, and for how long. One must determine the individual's psychological, social, and developmental levels and how he reached them.

The social, family, and cultural contexts in which problem drinking occurs are significant in determining the most effective treatment and what influences can be brought to bear to convince the alcoholic of his need for help. Coercion is often necessary because of the massive denial and self-deception. Industrial alcoholism programs often use the implied threat of losing one's job unless the individual enters treatment. Such programs report relatively high rates of success in rehabilitating their alcoholic employees. Such coercion can be viewed as *therapeutic leverage* in which a small degree of self-awareness is forced upon the alcoholic. Such therapeutic leverage can be useful; however, it cannot in and of itself produce recovery, which can occur only in the treatment process described below. Therapeutic leverage should be sought in the initial evaluation of an alcoholic as a source of increasing motivation for treatment.

All alcoholics are not the same, even though most share the common psychodynamic conflict of dependency and the need for compensatory power and control. Alcoholics exist in differing age groups, socioeconomic circumstances, and cultural groups (Pattison, Coe, and Rhodes, 1969; Kissin, Platz, and Su, 1970; Mindlin, 1959; Zimberg, 1974a). Approaches with the skid-row homeless alcoholic cannot be the same as with the so-called high-bottom executive, or with the individual living in poverty in an urban ghetto.

It should be noted that alcoholism does not occur as an all-or-none phenomenon but has varying degrees in the same individual. Figure 2

Know test

LEVEL	CHARACTERISTICS
1. None	Drinks only on occasion, if at all.
2. Minimal	Drinking is not conspicuous, occasional intoxications (up to four per year). No social, family, occupational, health, or legal problems related to drinking.
3. Mild	Intoxication occurring up to once a month, although generally limited to evening or weekends, and/or some impairment in social, family relations, or occupational functioning related to drinking. No physical or legal problems related to drinking.
4. Moderate	Frequent intoxications, up to one or two times per week and/or significant impairment in social, family, or occupational functioning. Some suggestive evidence of physical impairment related to drinking such as tremors, frequent accidents, epigastric distress, loss of appetite at times. No history of delirium tremens, cirrhosis, nutritional deficiency, hospitalizations related to drinking, or arrests related to drinking.
5. Severe	Almost constantly drinking (practically every day). History of delirium tremens, liver cirrhosis, chronic brain syndrome, neuritis, nutritional deficiency, or severe disruption In social or family relations. Unable to hold a steady job but able to maintain himself on public assistance. One or more arrests related to drinking (drunk and disorderly). Two or more drunk driving citations. One or more hospitalizations related to drinking.
6. Extreme	All the characteristics of severe impairment plus homelessness and/or inability to maintain himself on public assistance.

Figure 2. Alcohol Abuse Scale.

shows a scale (Zimberg, Lipscomb, and Davis, 1971) that defines the degrees of alcohol abuse from no problem to the skid-row alcoholic at level 6. Improvement in treatment can be measured by movement upward from level 6 to level 1 in this scale.

THE TREATMENT PROCESS

Principles of Treatment. Alcoholism is a chronic illness with a high potential for relapse. As in other chronic disorders, continuous care for life is required in some cases. Alcoholics Anonymous is particularly well-suited to provide this supportive treatment for an indefinite duration. However, professional intervention is necessary during the early stages of treatment to provide detoxification from alcohol, a thorough psychosocial evaluation, and to continue support for alcoholics unwilling or unable to make effective use of AA. After detoxification, alcoholics should not be maintained on minor tranquilizers since these may be readily abused. Detoxification can be carried out in many cases on an ambulatory basis. Some patients with more severe manifestations of alcoholism may require inpatient detoxification.

Directive counseling during the process of detoxification can enhance an alcoholic's motivation to continue the treatment. Counseling, or more intensive psychotherapeutic approaches, is necessary after detoxification. Acquainting the alcoholic with the physical effects of alcohol on his body and on his ability to perform necessary functions should be part of this effort. The deterrent use of disulfiram (Antabuse) is also effective.

Patients with serious depression, anxiety, or psychoses, along with alcoholism, should have these conditions treated first. At times, it has been found that alcoholism is secondary to these major psychiatric disorders and clears up when the primary disorder is effectively treated. With such patients, a period of observation in a hospital setting or office when the patient has been alcohol-free for three to four weeks may be required to make such a differential diagnosis.

Differential Diagnosis. It is essential to realize that alcoholics are not a homogeneous population. They can present with a variety of acute and chronic behavioral problems, mood and thought disorders, and age related developmental problems as well as with alcoholism. In order to effectively treat the alcoholic person, these coexisting problems must be evaluated and the coexisting problem elucidated as to whether the drinking came before or after the other coexisting problem. Primary alcoholics, once alcohol-free, have intact egos, function well, and do not have disabling psychiatric symptoms. When psychiatric symptoms persist four to six weeks beyond detoxification, one must consider the disorders discussed below.

The complicating problems found in alcoholics include the acute and chronic organic mental syndromes associated with alcoholism. Other conditions found to coexist with alcoholism include attention deficit disorder (residual type), schizophrenia, borderline syndrome, and other personality and neurotic disorders such as anxiety, and affective disorders.

The alcohol withdrawal syndrome includes tremulousness, withdrawal seizures, hallucinosis, and alcohol withdrawal delirium (D.T.s).

Tremulousness can, in most cases, be managed with ambulatory detoxification (see Chapter 4). The other more serious withdrawal manifestations should be treated in a hospital with the use of benzodiazepines in a detoxification regimen. Alcohol idiosyncratic intoxication (pathological intoxication), an acute organic mental syndrome in certain susceptible individuals, is due to the ingestion of small amounts of alcohol and is generally not seen among alcoholics since such individuals can consume only small amounts of alcohol before they become disorganized.

memory

Alcohol amnestic disorder (Korsakoff's psychosis), an acute and chronic organic mental disorder with neurological disorders, is due to thiamine deficiency and is seen rarely today. Such patients should be hospitalized and treated with parenteral thiamine.

Dementia associated with alcoholism is a chronic organic mental disorder with memory impairment and intellectual and cognitive defects. This disorder results from a relatively long history of excessive alcohol consumption. Cerebral atrophy, found with a CAT scan of alcoholics' brains, is not generally correlated with the presence of this disorder. Diagnosis has to be established by a precise mental status examination and neuropsychological testing. Individuals with this disorder should be hospitalized or treated in long-term residential treatment so as to improve their mental functioning to some degree.

Protracted withdrawal syndrome, although not an official diagnosis, has been noted in many alcoholics. This is a disorder characterized by irritability, emotional lability, insomnia, and anxiety that persists for weeks to months after alcohol withdrawal. It is due to the residual effects of alcohol toxicity on the central nervous system. It generally clears spontaneously after prolonged abstinence. In AA it is called a "dry drunk." Many alcoholics return to drinking because of the persistence of these unpleasant symptoms. Patients should be warned about this condition and be told that it will pass in time. Small doses of thioridazine (Mellaril) may be helpful.

It is possible that a number of psychiatric disorders have existed in individuals prior to their becoming alcoholic. Therefore, a complete psychiatric history and mental status examination is important in evaluating all alcoholic patients. Some alcoholics have been found to have a history of attention deficit disorder from childhood with the disorder continuing into adulthood. As adults they developed alcoholism but retained the disorder in a modified form characterized by defects in attention and impulsivity. The diagnosis can be established by taking a careful history that includes a developmental history and determining if hyperactivity, as well as attention defects and impulsivity, was present in the individuals as children. The diagnosis is established by history and observation of the alcohol-free patient for six to eight weeks. Such patients must be treated for their alcoholism but the addition of stimulating drugs such as imipramine or magnesium pemoline can be helpful in reducing the symptoms of the residual attention deficit disorder and facilitate recovery.

Patients with schizophrenia have been noted to use and abuse alcohol as self-medication. Such patients when observed alcohol-free for three to four weeks can be noted to have persistent functional psychotic symptoms and usually give a history of prolonged duration of these symptoms and psychiatric hospitalization prior to their drinking problem. The schizophrenia should be treated with injectable, long-acting phenothiazines and the involvement of the patients in social and vocational rehabilitation programs. When the schizophrenia is effectively treated, the alcohol abuse clears up. Such patients generally do not do well at AA meetings.

A significant number of patients with borderline syndrome abuse alcohol and become alcoholics. The borderline patients give a history of mood and behavioral disturbances that exist prior to the alcoholism. Such disturbances include impulsive behavior, very poor interpersonal relationships, inappropriate and intense anger, poor self-identity, physical self-mutilation, and having long-term feelings of depression, emptiness, boredom, loneliness and intense anxiety. Such patients should be specifically treated for their alcoholism and involved in AA. Supportive psychotherapy is necessary, as well as small doses of thioridazine (Mellaril) at 50 mg a day for the serious depression and anxiety. AA can supply many of the dependency needs for these patients and reduce their severe feelings of social isolation and loneliness. A period of four to six weeks of alcohol-free observation, plus the history of these symptoms, is necessary to establish the diagnosis.

Anxiety is a common symptom among alcoholics. However, in primary alcoholics, it generally clears up within four weeks of detoxification with the maintenance of abstinence. In some alcoholics, it will persist longer as part of the protracted withdrawal syndrome. Some alcoholic patients will present themselves with a long history of episodic bouts of intense anxiety characterized as panic reactions. Such patients have panic–anxiety disorder and are secondary alcoholics. The patient should be maintained alcohol-free and treated with imipramine for the panic disorder. Once the panic disorder is effectively treated, the alcoholism lessens and clears up.

Alcoholism can coexist with other neurotic or personality disorders. In such situations, the alcoholism must be initially addressed until sobriety is well established for six months to one year before any uncovering therapy is attempted for the existing neurotic or personality disorder.

Depression is a common symptom in alcoholics. In most cases, the feelings of depression will lessen or disappear with four weeks of abstinence. However, in a small number of male alcoholics (less than 5%) and in a substantial number of female alcoholics (25% to 50%), the depression will persist in the alcohol-free state. Such individuals have a major affective disorder and should be treated with lithium carbonate if there is a history of recurrent depression or episodes of mania. Antidepressants should be used if the current depression is the first episode. It should be pointed out to the patient that this medication is used for the mood disorder and not the alcoholism. There is no current drug treatment for alcoholism itself.

One must be able to provide an effective differential diagnosis and appropriate treatment for coexisting major psychiatric disorders. Most alcoholics are primary alcoholics and do not require psychiatric treatment. However, for those that do, such a multitreatment approach is essential if the alcoholic is to recover. A more detailed discussion of the diagnosis and differential diagnosis of alcoholism can be found in the author's book *The Clinical Management of Alcoholism* (Zimberg, 1982).

Principles of Alcoholism Psychotherapy. Several principles are important in the treatment of an alcoholic individual. These principles apply whether the alcoholic individual is involved in a therapeutic relationship with a physician, with a mental health professional, or with a paraprofessional alcoholism counselor. First, the drinking itself must be terminated if therapy is to be effective in achieving rehabilitation. A common mistake mental health professionals have made is to consider alcoholism as a symptom of underlying personality disorder and attempt to treat this underlying disorder. Psychological conflict does exist as indicated, but the first principle is that efforts must initially be directed to achieve sobriety for the patient through detoxification and the maintenance of sobriety. This may be achieved through intensive directive counseling or psychotherapy and the use of disulfiram. A patient who continues to drink will not respond to counseling or psychotherapeutic approaches with the result that a power struggle will develop between the therapist and the drinking patient.

The second principle is that alcoholics are not a homogeneous group and that a thorough differential diagnosis must be made to exclude coexisting major psychiatric disorders. If a major psychiatric disorder coexists with the alcoholism, it must be effectively treated as well as the alcoholism.

3The third principle is the understanding of the transference that the alcoholic will establish with the therapist. This transference is very intensive and is characterized by a considerable amount of dependence coupled with hostile, manipulative, and testing behavior. Thus, a great deal of ambivalence will be noted in the transference relationship. The alcoholic will be dependent but at other times be grandiose since he believes he can control his drinking, as well as his life, when the evidence is obviously to the contrary.

The fourth principle is understanding the countertransference that may develop in a therapist as a response to the provocative behavior and drinking of the patient who is testing the therapist's continued interest. Because of this type of testing behavior, the treatment of an alcoholic can be felt as frustrating and unrewarding. The therapist must recognize, however, that he is not omnipotent in regard to the alcoholic's drinking. He cannot, and no one can, stop an alcoholic determined to drink. A therapist can only provide the means to assist the alcoholic in achieving sobriety but cannot force him into refraining from drinking for long. Only the patient's conscious efforts can achieve this. The therapist who recognizes this reality must impose limits on the behavior of the patient and on the conditions under which treatment can continue. If the patient cannot meet these conditions, treatment should be discontinued. The door, however, should be left open to renew the efforts to achieve sobriety as the first step in the treatment process. Figure 3 summarizes the basic principles that should be observed in the psychotherapy of alcoholism.

In Chapter 2 of this book (concerning the defense structure of the alcoholic), John Wallace describes the defensive pattern alcoholics have built up to protect their drinking. Wallace believes that this defensive structure should not be exposed, uncovered, or modified, but rather it should be swung into the service of achieving and maintaining sobriety. Therefore, it is important to recognize that some defenses utilized by alcoholics may be helpful in achieving sobriety if redirected rather than removed (as was the case with the sublimation of the reactive grandiosity). Insight should not be the goal of psychotherapy during the early stages of recovery with alcoholics; sobriety is the necessary goal. Understanding what aspects of the alcoholic's personality structure should *not* be tampered with is probably the most difficult part of the therapeutic process and can be learned only with experience. The effort to redirect defenses has the risk of being incorrectly applied. This results in the development of intense anxiety or unexpressed anger and can lead to a resumption of drinking or to the patient's leaving treatment. It is therefore essential to have as complete an understanding as possible of the

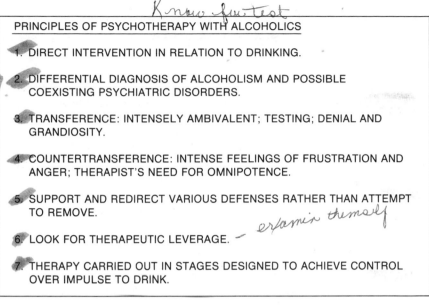

Know for Test

PRINCIPLES OF PSYCHOTHERAPY WITH ALCOHOLICS

1. DIRECT INTERVENTION IN RELATION TO DRINKING.

2. DIFFERENTIAL DIAGNOSIS OF ALCOHOLISM AND POSSIBLE COEXISTING PSYCHIATRIC DISORDERS.

3. TRANSFERENCE: INTENSELY AMBIVALENT; TESTING; DENIAL AND GRANDIOSITY.

4. COUNTERTRANSFERENCE: INTENSE FEELINGS OF FRUSTRATION AND ANGER; THERAPIST'S NEED FOR OMNIPOTENCE.

5. SUPPORT AND REDIRECT VARIOUS DEFENSES RATHER THAN ATTEMPT TO REMOVE. *examine themself*

6. LOOK FOR THERAPEUTIC LEVERAGE.

7. THERAPY CARRIED OUT IN STAGES DESIGNED TO ACHIEVE CONTROL OVER IMPULSE TO DRINK.

Figure 3

patient's developmental history, psychological conflicts, interpersonal relationships, current life situation, and transference and countertransference in order to make the interventions appropriate in terms of *what* defense is being directed, *when* in the course of therapy it is being done, and *how* the intervention is presented to the patient.

Looking for *therapeutic leverage*, as indicated earlier, is an essential part of the early stages of treatment.

Stages of Treatment. The treatment has been observed to progress through several stages (Figure 4). Although the stages can be observed in group therapy and in AA involvement, they are most apparent in individual therapy. The first stage involves the situation in which the alcoholic "cannot drink." This situation exists when there is external pressure on the patient to stop drinking, such as the threat of loss of job, his spouse's leaving, or with the use of disulfiram. In a sense, the alcoholic is forced to stop drinking for at least a short time. His attitudes toward drinking and the denial of his drinking as a serious problem have not changed. The alcoholic has stopped not because he sees it as necessary, but because someone else does. He must be helped by directive counseling to face problems and stress without resorting to alcohol. Involvement of the family in joint sessions with the patient and the referral of the family to Al-Anon are helpful in changing family *know for test*

STAGES OF TREATMENT

STAGES	PATIENT STATUS	TREATMENT
STAGE I	"I CAN'T DRINK" (NEED FOR EXTERNAL CONTROL)	ALCOHOL DETOXIFICATION DIRECTIVE PSYCHOTHERAPY ANTABUSE AA FAMILY THERAPY AL-ANON
STAGE II	"I WON'T DRINK" (INTERNALIZED CONTROL)	DIRECTIVE PSYCHOTHERAPY SUPPORTIVE PSYCHOTHERAPY CONSIDER DISCONTINUING USE OF ANTABUSE AA
STAGE III	"I DON'T HAVE TO DRINK" (CONFLICT RESOLUTION)	PSYCHOANALYTICALLY ORIENTED PSYCHOTHERAPY

I know I have a choice

Figure 4

attitudes about the alcoholic family member and in giving the family greater understanding of the illness of alcoholism. During this stage, patients should be taught to recognize cues that might lead to drinking so that they can develop alternative coping mechanisms. Forgetting to take an disulfiram tablet can be such a cue, and therefore the use of disulfiram can serve as an early-warning system. Often when the patient has stopped drinking early in treatment, he feels extremely confident about his newly acquired sobriety and experiences a feeling of euphoria. This feeling is a reaction formation to his unconscious lack of control over his drinking, which is now experienced as a certainty of control over his not drinking as well as control over other aspects of his life. Patients should be warned to expect such inappropriate feelings. This situation is by its nature very unstable since there has been no significant change in his attitude about drinking nor an ego reduction as described by Tiebout (1961). The situation can easily lead to a return to drinking or, through counseling and/or further Alcoholics Anonymous involvement, to a stage where the alcoholic "won't drink."

This is the stage at which the controls on the compulsion to drink have become internalized and there is no longer a serious conscious conflict about whether or not to drink. At this stage, the individual's

attitude toward the necessity of drinking and the deleterious consequences in resuming drinking are apparent; he has experienced a considerable attitudinal change toward drinking. The conflict about drinking is still present, but at an unconscious level. Evidence of the continued
existence of this conflict is present in fantasies and dreams. This stage
is the level many Alcoholics Anonymous members have achieved. Discontinuation or the intermittent use of disulfiram in stressful situations
can be considered. Further help in developing alternative coping mechanisms for stress and unpleasant feelings should be provided. This stage
represents a reasonably good stage of recovery and is fairly stable, only
occasionally leading to a "slip" after years of sobriety. The reactive grandiosity has now been sublimated (redirected) in the ego-enhancing feelings of control over a previously uncontrollable problem. For active AA
members, their work with other alcoholics serves as an additional outlet
for the need for grandiosity. At least six months to one year of directive
psychotherapy is required to achieve this stage of recovery.

The third stage of recovery involves the situation in which the alcoholic "does not have to drink." This stage can be achieved only
through *insight* into the individual's personality problems and conflicts
and their resolution to a major degree. The alcoholic's habitual use of
alcohol in the past can be understood as a way of dealing with the
individual's conflicts. With the resolution of the conflicts through insight, the individual can achieve more adaptive ways of coping with
internal and external problems. This stage can be achieved effectively
through psychoanalytically oriented psychotherapy and self-under-
standing. It is a stable stage as long as the alcoholic refrains from drinking. Abstinence is relatively easy to maintain at this stage. The duration
of treatment required to achieve this stage of recovery has, in the author's experience, been about one to two years after reaching stage II.

After reaching stage II or III, some patients enter a situation in which
they believe, "I can return to social drinking." Possibly a small percentage of alcoholics can achieve this (Pattison, 1968), but at our present
level of knowledge it is *impossible* to predict which patient this might be.
All alcoholics believe during the initial stages of treatment that they can
return to controlled drinking. Alcoholics who have achieved recovery
(stage II or III) in most cases do not desire to resume social drinking
because of the risk involved. Recent publicity regarding this issue has
raised the question in some recovered alcoholics, but generally they have
been persuaded not to take the chance of resuming social drinking. For
all practical purposes at the present time, abstinence should be a necessary goal in the treatment of *all* alcoholics. Alcohol is not necessary
to life, and it is quite possible to live and even be happy without con-

suming alcohol. This fact should be part of the attitudinal change an alcoholic experiences during the process of recovery.

Termination of Treatment. The termination of treatment with an alcoholic is critical. If the treatment process has been successful, the alcoholic will have established a dependent, trusting relationship with the therapist, and therefore termination will produce anxiety and the possibility of a return to drinking. This termination should be based on mutual agreement between the therapist and patient, a termination date determined, and the final period of therapy involved with the issue of termination.

Termination can occur at stage II or III since both are relatively stable stages regarding control of drinking. A decision has to be made, however, when a patient reaches stage II, as to whether further treatment to achieve insight into the psychological conflict related to his drinking problem and moving to reach stage III in treatment is important to the patient. This option should be left to the patient. Nonpsychiatric physicians can provide the directive counseling and the use of disulfiram, where indicated, to help alcoholics reach stage II. More traditional psychotherapy is required to reach stage III and nonpsychiatric physicians and alcoholism counselors might consider referral of such patients to psychotherapists.

Regardless of whether the patient terminates in stage II or III, the door to return to therapy should be left open. A patient who stops treatment after stage II may determine after a while that not drinking is not enough to help him deal with his feelings and conflicts and might wish to return to treatment to try to achieve insight into his personality conflicts. A patient terminated after stage II may have a slip, and a return to treatment should be available. This slip, however, should not be viewed as a treatment failure, but as part of a rehabilitation process that is not yet complete. Patients who slip in stages II and III generally do not return to continuous uncontrolled drinking because their awareness of their problem and control mechanisms are such that controls can be quickly reinstated. The slip can be looked at as a psychological maladaptation to conflict and anxiety or as a transference reaction, and it is possible to help the patient gain more understanding of his need to drink by analyzing such slips.

This approach to psychotherapy of alcoholics, presented in terms of stages of progression of treatment in relation to varying abilities to control the impulse to drink, provides a framework for a complex and often amorphous treatment process. It provides a goal-directed approach to achievable levels of improvement. Complex therapeutic decisions regarding involvement of the family in treatment, starting or stopping of disulfiram, attendance at AA meetings, use of uncovering techniques, discontinuation of therapy, and others can be considered in relationship to these fairly predictable stages in the recovery process. It is possible to make predictions of outcome of therapeutic intervention or lack of intervention based on knowledge of the stage of recovery the patient has entered. Therefore, such an awareness can make the complex psychotherapeutic process with alcoholics potentially understandable and subject to a certain degree of predictability.

SUMMARY

Alcoholism can be treated psychotherapeutically in individual or group therapy. The underlying psychodynamics consist of conflict with excessive dependent needs leading to the defenses of denial and reactive grandiosity. The use of alcohol serves to reinforce these defenses. Certain principles are necessary for the successful psychotherapeutic treatment of alcoholism: (1) efforts must first be directed at producing abstinence from alcohol; (2) there must be an understanding of the transference and countertransference aspects of the treatment process by the therapist. The treatment process has been observed to progress through fairly distinct stages, consisting of the patient's ability to maintain controls on the compulsion to drink. In treating the alcoholic, one must determine first if the alcoholic has coexisting physical or serious psychiatric disorders that will affect the treatment process. In addition, the social, family, and economic circumstances of the patient must be understood and utilized to provide therapeutic leverage that will enhance the effectiveness of treatment.

REFERENCES

Bacon, M. K., Barry H., and Child, I. L. A cross-cultural study of drinking, II: Relation to other features of culture. *Quarterly Journal of Studies on Alcohol*, 1965, 3, 29–48.

Blane, H. T. *The personality of the alcoholic: Guises of dependency*. New York: Harper and Row, 1968.

Blum, E. M. Psychoanalytic views of alcoholism: A review. *Quarterly Journal of Studies on Alcohol*, 1966, 27, 259–299.

Douglas, D. B. Who is a real alcoholic? Practical help in managing alcoholism. *New York State Journal of Medicine*, 1976, 76, 603–607.

Ewing, J. A., and Rouse, B. A. Failure of an experimental treatment program to inculcate controlled drinking in alcoholics. *British Journal of Addictions*, 1976, 71, 123–134.

Kissin, B., Platz, A., and Su, W. H. Social and psychological factors in the treatment of chronic alcoholism. *Journal of Psychiatric Research*, 1970, 8, 13–27.

Knight, R. P. The psychodynamics of chronic alcoholism. *Journal of Nervous and Mental Disorders*, 1937, 8, 538–543.

22   SHELDON ZIMBERG

Lovibond, S. H., and Caddy, G. Discriminated aversive control of alcoholics' drinking behavior. *Behavior Therapy*, 1970, *1*, 437–444.
McClelland, D. C., Davis, W. N., Kalin, R., and Wanner, E. *The Drinking man*. New York: Free Press, 1972.
McCord, W., and McCord, J. *Origins of alcoholism*. Stanford: Stanford University Press, 1960.
McCord, W., and McCord, J. A longitudinal study of the personality of alcoholics. In D. J. Pittman and C. R. Snyder (Eds.), *Society, culture, and drinking patterns*. New York: Wiley, 1962.
Merry J., Reynolds, C. M., Bailey, J., and Coppen, A. Prophylactic treatment of alcoholism by lithium carbonate. *Lancet*, 1976, *2*, 481–482.
Mindlin, D. F. The characteristics of alcoholics as related to therapeutic outcome. *Quarterly Journal of Studies on Alcohol*, 1959, *20*, 604–619.
Neubeurger, G. W., Miller, S. I., Schmitz, R. E., *et al.* Replicable abstinence rates in an alcoholism treatment program. *Journal of the American Medical Association*, 1982, *248*, 960–963.
Pattison, E. M. Abstinence criteria: A critique of abstinence criteria in the treatment of alcoholism. *International Journal of Social Psychiatry*, 1968, *14*, 268–276.
Pattison, E. M., Coe, R., and Rhodes, R. J. Evaluation of alcoholism treatment: A comparison of three facilities. *Archives of General Psychiatry*, 1969, *20*, 478–488.
Pendery, M. L., Maltzman, I. M., and West, J. L. Controlled drinking by alcoholics? New findings and reevaluation of a major affirmative study. *Science*, 1982, *217*, 169–174.
Sobell, M. B., and Sobell, L. C. Second-year treatment outcome of alcoholics treated by individualized behavior therapy. *Behavior Research and Therapy*. 1976, *14*, 195–215.
Tahlka, V. *The alcoholic personality*. Helsinki: Finnish Foundation for Alcohol Studies, 1966.
Tamerin, J. S., and Mendelson, J. H. The psychodynamics of chronic inebriation: Observations of alcoholics during the process of drinking in an experimental group setting. *American Journal of Psychiatry*, 1969, *125*, 886–899.
Tiebout, H. M. Alcoholics Anonymous—An experiment of nature. *Quarterly Journal of Studies on Alcohol*, 1961, *22*, 52–68.
Vaillant, G. E. *The natural history of alcoholism: Causes, patterns and paths to recovery*. Cambridge: Harvard University Press, 1983.
Wilsnack, S. C. The impact of sex roles and women's alcohol use and abuse. In M. Greenblat and M. Schuckit (Eds.), *Alcoholism problems in women and children*. New York: Grune & Stratton, 1976.
Zimberg, S. Evaluation of alcoholism treatment in Harlem. *Quarterly Journal of Studies on Alcohol*, 1974, *35*, 550–557. (a)
Zimberg, S. The elderly alcoholic. *The Gerontologist*, 1974, *14*, 221–224. (b)
Zimberg, S. New York State Task Force on alcohol problems: Position paper on treatment. *New York State Journal of Medicine*, 1975, *75*, 1794–1798.
Zimberg, S. *The clinical management of alcoholism*. New York: Brunner/Mazel, 1982.
Zimberg, S., Lipscomb, H., and Davis, E. B. Sociopsychiatric treatment of alcoholism in an urban ghetto. *American Journal of Psychiatry*, 1971, *127*, 1670–1674.

2

Working with the Preferred Defense Structure of the Recovering Alcoholic

John Wallace

Introduction

Within the past five years, substantial progress has been made in understanding the origins of alcoholism, the factors that maintain it, and the methods by which it can be treated. Both alcoholism specialists and general mental health professionals have come to construe the disease as biopsychosocial in nature (Ewing, 1983; Tarter, 1983; Wallace, 1978). Most important, alcoholism is now widely recognized as an illness requiring specialized interventions and expertise. Methods useful with other clinical populations may have little direct application in the treatment of alcoholism and may, in fact, result in undesireable outcomes for the alcoholic patient.

In this chapter, I shall attempt to describe a theoretical framework for psychotherapy with alcoholics. This framework constitutes a modal or typical approach to alcoholism therapy, but does not preclude individualized treatments as well. As we have come to appreciate, both the commonality and individuality evident among alcoholics in treatment must be addressed. Accordingly, the general approach to alcoholism psychotherapy presented here, while focusing on commonality, is intended to be consistent with a multimodality approach to treatment.

John Wallace • Director of Treatment, Edgehill Newport, Newport, Rhode Island.

THEORETICAL ORIENTATION

A sophisticated disease concept of alcoholism does not ignore psychological and sociocultural factors. Whereas biological factors are clearly involved in the origin and maintenance of the disease, psychological and sociocultural factors play important roles as well. The naive question "Is alcoholism a disease or a learned problem of behavior?" is now properly construed as inadequate to address the complexity of the illness. More pertinent questions of etiology might very well concern issues involving a triangulation of pharmacogenetics, neurochemistry, and culture, for example, "How do family histories interact with particular brain peptide levels in individuals drawn from cultures varying widely in drinking styles, customs, and practices?"

Biological Factors Are Primary. Recent research clearly implicates biological factors in the etiology and maintenance of alcoholism. Numerous studies in animals on the pharmacogenetics of alcohol preference, consumption, and effects of hypnotic doses reveal that hereditary influence is ubiquitous (McClearn, 1981). Selective breeding in mice and rats has been accomplished and strain differences are well documented.

Human genetic studies (Goodwin, Schulsinger, Moller, Hermansen, Winokur, and Cuze, 1974; Kaij, 1960; Schuckitt, 1981) conducted internationally indicate that the sons of alcoholics have at least a three times greater risk of becoming alcoholics than the sons of non-alcoholics. This increased risk was found in studies where social learning effects were *absent* and was not further increased in studies where both genetic and social-learning effects were jointly present. In addition, the rate of concordance for alcoholism in identical twins is 60% and 30% in fraternal twins. Moreover, young men with alcoholism in first degree family members metabolize alcohol differently than men without such family histories. Higher associated levels of acetaldehyde and less behavioral impairment after three drinks have been noted in young men with alcoholism in first degree family members (Schuckitt, 1981).

A recent study of patients with and without familial histories of alcoholism revealed numerous differences (Frances, Timm, and Bucky, 1980). Patients with familial histories showed more severe symptomatology of alcoholism, more antisocial behavior, worse academic and social performance in school, unstable employment histories, and more severe physical symptoms related to alcohol.

In a recent study by Gabrielli, Mednick, Volavka, Pollock, Schulsinger, and Itil, 1982, young sons of alcoholic fathers showed high frequency EEG activity (above 18 Hz). Hence, fast EEG activity which is an inheritable characteristic and is frequently found in adult alcoholics has been found in EEG records of the 11–13 year-old-sons of alcoholics. Since alcohol is known to slow brain activity, alcoholics may be persons who learn to reduce genetically determined fast brain wave activity by self-medication with alcoholic beverages. Recent work by Bohman, Sigvardsson, and Cloninger (1981), indicates that female alcoholism is also partially genetically determined. In a study of female adoptees in Sweden, a 3-fold increase in subsequent alcoholism was found in adopted females whose biological mothers were alcoholic. For males, a crossfostering analysis revealed a 9-fold increase in male adoptees whose biological fathers were alcoholic (Cloninger, Bohman, and Sigvardsson, 1981).

Numerous studies have centered on the effects of alcohol on brain neurotransmitters and the possible effects of neurotransmitter systems on drinking behavior. Serotonin (5-HT) metabolism is apparently altered by alcohol and lesions of neuron systems containing 5-HT result in increased preference for alcohol in rats (Myers and Melchoir, 1977). On the other hand, alcohol intake in rats can be suppressed by administration of a 5-HT precursor, 5-Hydroxytryptophan (5-HTP).

Alcohol preference may be related to norepinephrine levels (NE). When neuron systems of the rat containing NE are lesioned by a neurotoxin infused directly into the cerebral ventricle, suppression of preference for alcohol is observed (Myers, 1978a).

In short, these studies on neurotransmitter systems suggest that alcoholism may be related to particular biochemical events in the brain.

In the past decade, considerable interest has developed in the possible role of aldehyde-biogenic amine combinations. Acetaldehyde, the first metabolic intermediary of alcohol, along with other adelhydes, in combination with various neurotransmitters yields a family of substances called tetrahydroisoquinolines (TIQs). For example, dopamine plus acetaldehyde yields salsolinol. Dopamine plus dopaldehyde yields tetrahydropapaveroline (THP), an alkaloid that is a morphine precursor.

Administration of TIQs to animals has been shown to increase preferences for ethanol solutions. Myers and his colleagues (Myers, 1978b; Myers, McCaleb, and Ruwe, 1982) for example, have shown that in rats and monkeys when THP is infused into the cerebral ventricles, preferences for astonishingly high concentrations of ethanol (40%) can be established. Moreover, it appears that such preferences are irreversible. These results are remarkable since monkeys do not naturally prefer alcohol to water. Also, the concentrations of ethanol are very high.

Blum, Hamilton, Hirst, and Wallace (1978) have hypothesized that alcohol and opiate addiction may be linked by morphine precursors formed by alcohol-biogenic amine condensation products. In effect, alcoholism may be related to the brain's production of various TIQs. The following findings support an alkaloid isoquinoline role in alcoholism.

1. Elevated THP levels in patients entering alcoholism treatment have been noted.
2. THP and Salsolinol interact with opiate receptor sites, that is, these isoquinolines appear to be similar to opiates.
3. Apparently irreversible preferences for *very high* concentrations of ethanol can be induced in animals by infusions of THP into the cerebral ventricles.

These findings clearly implicate biological factors in the origin of alcoholism. Moreover, research such as this on biological factors has reached a level of sophistication that renders the question of whether or not alcoholism is a disease non-productive, if not absurd.

3 The Psychological Perspective. If biological factors play a primary role in the etiology and maintenance of alcoholism, how may psychological factors be construed? While psychological factors may act to some extent as *antecedent* conditions for the development of alcoholism, it is probable that they act largely as significant *consequences* of the disease. Withdrawal symptoms, for example, are clearly outcomes, rather than causes, of alcoholism. Low self-esteem, denial, poor frustration tolerance, depression, and anxiety may also be outcomes of the disease. Most important, however, is the fact that these physical and psychological outcomes can serve to maintain the disease and complicate recovery.

Psychological interventions with alcoholics can lead to satisfactory results if therapists are able to recognize the typical psychological outcomes of alcoholism and to work with them effectively in early, middle, and late stages of psychotherapy. In effect, the typical psychological outcomes can be viewed as learned coping strategies.

In the following pages, a case is presented for working with these learned coping strategies of alcoholics. This does not imply that these learned coping strategies are the cause of alcoholism. Rather, they are seen as important psychological outcomes of the disease and constitute important factors in the maintenance of active alcoholism. My arguments shall include the following major ideas:

1. Alcoholics can be described in terms of a preferred defense structure. This preferred defense structure (PDS) need not be construed at all in terms of the classical language of defense mechanisms. The alcoholic PDS can be thought of as a collection of skills or abilities—tactics and strategies, if you will—for achieving one's ends.

*Look at
Handout
5*

2. Therapy with alcoholics, as it is currently practiced, too often attempts to remove the alcoholic PDS instead of utilizing it effectively to facilitate the achievement of abstinence. Therapeutic efforts that confront the alcoholic PDS prematurely and too heavily will increase, rather than reduce, the probability of further drinking.

3. Recovery programs successful in producing abstinence, such as Alcoholics Anonymous, partially owe their success to the intuitive recognition of the fact that the alcoholic PDS is to be protected and capitalized on rather than confronted and radically altered.

4. Paradoxically, the very same defenses that the alcoholic used to maintain his drinking can be used effectively to achieve abstinence.

5. Equally paradoxically, the very same defenses that enabled the alcoholic to drink, as well as achieve abstinence, must ultimately be removed if long-term sobriety is to be maintained. However, in many cases such growth must take place over periods of time ranging from two to five years of abstinence.

6. Alcohol therapy must be viewed as a *time-dependent* process. A particular therapeutic intervention for a recently drinking alcoholic may be entirely inappropriate for one who has managed to achieve several years of sobriety and vice-versa.

THE PREFERRED DEFENSE STRUCTURE (PDS) OF THE RECOVERING ALCOHOLIC

For my purposes, I have assumed that an alcoholic PDS exists and that it is the *outcome* of alcoholism, not an antecedent condition. In the following, I do not mean to suggest a single, unvarying profile—one that is characteristic of each and every alcoholic drinker. I am assuming, however, that *some* of these are found in *some* combinatorial pattern in virtually every alcoholic drinker at *some* point in his drinking and recovery from alcoholism.

Denial. Enough has been written about denial as a major defense in alcoholism as to require little in the way of further elaboration here. What has *not* been observed, however, is that aside from the obvious destructive nature of denial in matters concerned with drinking, denial is not without merit. Tactical denial or, if you will, *deliberate* denial of certain life difficulties or problems is a useful and extremely valuable temporary adjustive and coping device. In the case of the alcoholic well-practiced in such behavior, denial as a general tactical mechanism should not be discarded totally. That would be rather like throwing out the baby with the bath water.

But, of course, the recovering alcoholic must stop denying the impact of alcohol upon his major life concerns. That is an obvious truism in alcoholism therapy that need not be altered. Simply because that statement is true, however, it does not follow that the recovering alcoholic must immediately, thoroughly, and completely root out all evidence of denial generally in his personality and behavior. First of all, he can't. Second, he rather likes the tactic of denial—he should, he's leaned heavily upon it for years. Third, at some level or another, he recognizes that tactical denial is a coping strategy he simply cannot do without.

In any case, the important point is as follows: alcoholism may very well be referred to aptly as "the merry-go-round of denial." If my analysis is correct, however, with regard to denial generally, the alcoholic is going to keep going round and round, *long after his drinking stops.* And the very worst thing a therapist could ever possibly do is try to jam the mechanism and block the use of tactical denial entirely.

2 Projection. While much has been written about *disowning* projection (the tendency to attribute unwanted and unacceptable aspects of self to others), there has been very little appreciation of other types of projection in the field of alcoholism. This is most suprising since *assimilative* projection is perhaps the most outstanding characteristic of both drinking and sober alcoholics. Assimilative projection is the tendency to assume that others are very much like oneself and to perceive them as such. Negative or socially unacceptable impulses and traits need not be seen in others. In fact, much of assimilative projection involves many desirable and socially admirable characteristics. As we shall see, the tendency toward assimilative projection has great significance, both for the illusion and substance of identification and also for the understanding of therapeutic communities.

3 All-or-None Thinking. It is often the case that the alcoholic will exhibit a strong preference for certainty. Judgments of people, events, and situations are often extreme. Decision-making does not often seem to take into account the realistically probable. Decision rules are often inflexible, narrow in scope, and simplistic. Perceived alternatives are few, consisting largely of yes-no, go-no go, black-white, dichotomized categories. It is in this sense that the thinking is said to be "all or none" in character. This aspect of the alcoholic PDS has obvious implications for the nature of persuasive communications in therapy as well as for the manner in which information is structured and presented.

In general, it is my experience with alcoholics in a variety of therapeutic contexts that they prefer large amounts of structure. While the drinking alcoholic may certainly appear to prefer uncertainty and unpredictability bordering on chaos, the recovering alcoholic seems to like things to move along in a fairly predictable and structured manner. Meetings of AA, for example, are certainly among the most structured of social encounters.

The qualities of all-or-none thinking, preference for highly certain communications, simple decision-making rules, restricted choices, and highly structured social encounters all have obvious implications for the conduct of therapy and the structuring of therapeutic environments.

Conflict Minimization and Avoidance. Although their behavior while drinking may suggest otherwise, alcoholics do not like interpersonal conflict, nor do they handle it well; nor do they thrive in competitive relationships. As others have suggested, alcoholics do best in relationships characterized by complementarity rather than competition. Complementary relationships are those based upon satisfaction of reciprocally balanced needs. For example, a dominant person and submissive person would constitute a complementary relationship. These attributes concerning conflict minimization and conflict avoidance have obvious implications for both the nature and depth of therapeutic confrontation with the alcoholic. Confrontation tactics should be used by only the most skillful of therapists and only at carefully selected times in the therapeutic process. Angry and hostile confrontation with the alcoholic client is rarely, if ever, appropriate. Moreover, the group therapist working with alcoholics should exercise extreme caution in utilizing the resources of the group to confront a resistant member.

Rationalization. As anybody with only passing acquaintance with alcoholism can testify readily, alcoholics are often masters of rationalization. Many have developed the art and science of wishful thinking to its ultimate form of expression. They have had to. Anybody who can continue to drink in the face of the steadily accumulating disastrous consequences of active alcoholism must surely have learned a trick or two in order to make his drinking appear perfectly reasonable to himself and to others. But, as we have already seen with denial, rationalization can be a useful tactic in dealing with otherwise difficult situations, anxiety-laden happenings, and guilt-provoking personal actions.

After years of making the procuring and drinking of alcohol his number one priority, the alcoholic understands very well how ultimate priorities can be maintained. Paradoxically, it is a relatively straightforward shift from rationalizing drinking to rationalizing other less than desirable behaviors *with sobriety*. That is, in the early stages of abstinence, the recovering alcoholic may quickly discover that while drinking was a crutch, sobriety is an even better one! "Why, I can't do that, I might get drunk!" "I had to choose between her and my sobriety." In essence, the recovering alcoholic may discover that he has a freedom of personal action that few others can enjoy. But such rationalization can be an invaluable tactic in avoiding the reexperiencing of painful emotional cues that previously served as triggers to drinking, for example, guilt, remorse, anxiety, resentment, and anger. Eventually, of course, the recovering alcoholic must face up to his *sober* rationalizations. However, the word to be stressed in that sentence is *eventually*. What the alcoholic very definitely does not need early in his sobriety is a therapist who moves too rapidly.

Self-Centered Selective Attention. Alcoholics, for the most part, tend to look at things from a single perspective—*theirs*. Even in some alcoholics with considerable sobriety, there is often a curious lack of true empathy, a seeming inability to grasp the position of the other. This is not to say that alcoholics are "selfish." The facts are often to the contrary. But an alcoholic can be generous to a fault and still show extreme self-centeredness. As used here the term *self-centered selective attention* refers to the fact that alcoholics tend to be obsessed with self, to perceive the happenings around them largely as they impinge upon self. They attend selectively to information relevant to self, ignore other information not relevant to self, screen out information that is discrepant with their views of themselves, and distort other information that does not fit their preferred self-image.

In a very real sense, alcoholics are often resistant to feedback from others as well as from their own life experiences. This characteristic "blindness" can prove severely distressing and, in fact, maddening to those whose lives are linked to the alcoholic in important ways. It is often the case that drinking alcoholics (as well as recently sober ones) can maintain views of reality in the face of even massively disconfirming feedback. Faced with these obvious contradictions, the therapist may feel that it is his responsibility to apply immediate corrective feedback. Unfortunately, with the alcoholic client that is surely the very worst thing that the therapist could do. One must never forget that the characteristic blindness of the alcoholic is there for reasons, that it is dynamically linked to chronically low self-esteem, feelings of worthlessness, guilt, fear, and what might otherwise prove to be overwhelming anxiety. It is not that the therapist and his client are uninterested in the "truth," whatever that might be. It is really more a matter of *when* "truths" get revealed and also what "truths" need to be invented if the client is to get sober.

Preference for Nonanalytical Modes of Thinking and Perceiving. It often seems to be the case that alcoholics are influenced more by the emotional persuasive appeal than the "rational." Leadership styles that are likely to work with the alcoholic are often charismatic, inspirational, and "spiritual." It is not that alcoholics cannot operate in logical–analytical modes. That would be patently false since alcoholics are as capable as nonalcoholics in approaching matters in a linear, logical, and analytical manner.

Passivity versus Assertion. Although the intoxicated individual may often appear aggressive, assertive, and even frankly hostile, it is often the case that the alcoholic in the initial stages of abstinence prefers passivity over active coping as a general adjustive strategy. Assertion and active coping tend to bring the person into normal conflict with others, and, as we have seen, alcoholics do not thrive in situations characterized by conflict, competition, and win-lose outcomes. In fact, it is precisely in these situations that they tend to pick up a drink.

In actuality, despite the surface picture, the preferences of the alcoholic are for a general life attitude of passivity rather than active assertion.

Obsessional Focusing. Alcoholics are, for the most part, intense people, and, as nearly everyone knows, they are often obsessed people. Intense obsession is no stranger to the alcoholic. In addition to the obsession with alcohol during periods of active drinking, it is not uncommon to find obsessions with work, money, success, sexuality, and so forth. Contrary to popular stereotype, the alcoholic, sober and drinking, is often so obsessed with work as to fully deserve the label "workaholic."

In general, the alcoholic seems to prefer a state characterized by a moderate-to-high activation level. Witness the enormous amounts of stimulating drugs, for example, caffeine and nicotine, consumed by sober alcoholics. Even the so-called states of serenity of many sober alcoholics are intensely focused states of moderate-to-high activation rather than low.

The therapeutic problem in alcoholism therapy is not to alter directly this level of intense obsession, but to *redirect* it. Along these lines, it is interesting to note how the obsession with alcohol, previous drinking, and sobriety continues in the *sober* alcoholic. Recovering alcoholics in AA, for example, often seem obsessed with their programs, with meetings, and with alcoholism generally. Curiously, this same obsession with the problem is what enables them to remain sober when previously it served to maintain drinking.

In essence, the problem in alcoholism therapy is not to reduce obsessional energy, an often impossible task, but to switch the focus of the obsession.

TACTICAL AND STRATEGIC USE OF THE PDS

In the preceding material, I described the alcoholic PDS and hinted at how it might be used effectively to help the alcoholic client achieve abstinence. I do not wish to imply that the above is an exhaustive description of the PDS. However, the major features of that structure have now been considered. We are in a position now to restate the central thesis of this chapter. An alcoholic preferred defense structure exists. It is not only ineffectual but therapeutically disastrous to confront this structure prematurely. The therapist knowledgeable about alcoholics will turn this structure to the advantage of his client and himself by selectively reinforcing and encouraging the defenses of the alcoholic client. The central problem in therapy with the alcoholic is learning how to swing the PDS into the service of abstinence rather than continued drinking.

Eventually, the alcoholic preferred defense structure must be dealt with directly if real changes in personality are to be achieved. When and to what extent such changes should be attempted, however, depends upon characteristics of individual alcoholics as well as upon years of continuous sobriety. In my opinion, in the majority of recovering alcoholics, such changes should not be attempted until several years of sobriety have been achieved.

The therapeutic task in alcoholism therapy at the early stages of abstinence differs radically from that of other psychotherapies. The role of the therapist is not to expose, confront, and modify the defenses of the alcoholic client. Rather, the role of the therapist is to teach the alcoholic client how to use these very defenses to achieve and maintain abstinence. Denial, rationalization, projection, and so forth have for too long been construed in moralistic terms by psychotherapists. In actuality, such mechanisms are perfectly acceptable *tactics* when used deliberately and selectively for particular purposes. In the case of the alcoholic, these tactics have become part of a preferred defense structure throughout years of alcoholic drinking. For a therapist to try to remove these is equivalent to trying to force water to flow uphill.

Little therapeutic imagination is required to see how tactics such as denial and rationalization can be used effectively with the recovering alcoholic. Once the denial and rationalization associated with drinking have been confronted and dealt with, the recovering alcoholic typically is faced with many very real and difficult life problems. A list of these

This is the reason you don't tear down defenses

may serve to remind us of the intolerable internal and external stressors the recovering alcoholic may be required to face. He may have to deal with very serious malfunctions of physical health. His marital situation may remain complicated for many years after his last drink. His finances are often in alarmingly poor condition. He may have alienated everybody who ever meant anything to him. He may be facing nontrivial legal and criminal proceedings, unemployment, disturbed interpersonal relationships, parent-child complexities of unbearable proportions, personal emotional problems of serious dimensions, and so on. What can we do for the person in, not one serious life crisis, but a host of them all at once? It is precisely here that variants of denial and rationalization become important. Through direct tuition, we can help the alcoholic to the position that things will work out if he just will stay sober, that even though his life is complicated at the moment, at least he is sober, that sobriety is his number one priority, and so on and so forth. In other words, we as therapists are appealing to his preferred use of denial and rationalization to give him a toehold on abstinence.

Similarly, by appealing to the alcoholic's preference for assimilative projection, we can get him to identify with other persons whose problems seem to center around something called "alcoholism." If the alcoholic comes to construe himself in these terms, then all of the benefits that can flow from such a self-attribution are his. The label "alcoholic" or "alcoholism" provides the person with a convenient explanatory system for much of his behavior. Moreover, by listening to the experiences of others who make the same self-attribution and who also conveniently explain their behavior by this attribution, the person has a ready source of social reinforcement for his changing belief system. Furthermore, he is now open to considerable positive social influence. And he has been given the key to dealing with otherwise overwhelming anxiety, remorse, guilt, and confusion. In addition, by fixing his lifeline in terms of two clearly demarcated points (i.e., when you were drinking and now that you are sober), we have provided the client with reference points for a belief system that includes the possibility of dealing with the negativity of previous behavior and the possibility of hope for desired future behaviors.

In a very real sense, helping the client to achieve a self-attribution of "alcoholic" and, hence, an explanatory system for his behaviors is a central role of the therapist. It should not be done directly. In fact, the guiding principle of work at this phase of therapy should be, "as little external force as necessary for the attribution to be made." If the therapist literally tries to force the attribution upon the client, one of two things will happen: The client will become defiant and reject the therapist's attribution, or the client will publicly acquiesce but privately disagree.

Psychotherapy with the client at this point is very much the teaching of an "exotic belief." The often heard phrase, "your life was a mess because you were drinking, you weren't drinking because your life was a mess," and the many variants of this phrase are, in actuality, efforts to teach the client the convenient fiction that his problems are entirely attributable to alcoholism. If it enables the client to (1) explain his past behavior in a way that gives him hope for the future, (2) cope with his guilt, anxiety, remorse, and confusion, and (3) provide himself with a specific behavior (staying sober) that will change his life in a desired direction, then the assertion is valuable in early treatment. *The therapist must remember that the recovering alcoholic has a lifetime of sobriety in which to gradually recognize the fact that not all of his personal and social difficulties can be attributed to alcoholism.* In the meantime, the therapist can make very good use of assertions that have their basis in denial and rationalization. In effect, the therapeutic task is one of helping the client to construct a belief system. The fact that this belief system may at the beginning of sobriety contain strong elements of denial and rationalization should not trouble us. One must remember that the recovering alcoholic in initial stages of sobriety is faced with so many serious life problems that he will need a healthy dose of denial and rationalization if he is to survive at all.

MIDDLE AND LATE PHASE TREATMENT

Whereas a supportive psychotherapy that respects the learned coping strategies of the person in early stages of abstention is important, it is equally important that middle and late phase treatment be increasingly more intense. Alcoholics, in order to achieve a comfortable and secure sobriety, must begin to abandon these learned coping strategies in exchange for open, nondefensive, and authentic relationships with self and others. Of course, anxiety is often the price that patients must pay for psychological growth, insight into self, and awareness of feelings. One does not become whole without discomfort.

In middle and later stages of psychotherapy, it is extremely important for both the therapist and the patient to risk manageable degrees of anxiety in order for insight into self and others to increase and for growth to continue. Normally, however, these more intensive therapeutic efforts with alcoholics should not be attempted before one year of sobriety has been achieved. Ideally, they should be begun within two to five years of continuous sobriety.

SUMMARY AND CONCLUSIONS

Throughout this chapter, I have argued for the existence of learned coping strategies (a preferred defense structure) in the alcoholic client. I have further maintained that traditional and even contemporary psychotherapies are largely inappropriate for the recovering alcoholic precisely because they have failed to recognize the value of this alcoholic preferred defense structure. Therapeutic ideologies that consist largely of disguised moralistic stances concerning certain behaviors called "defenses" are likely to do more harm than good in the early stages of treatment.

The central problem in early alcoholism therapy is not one of exposing, uncovering, and modifying the alcoholic PDS. The central problem is one of discovering ways of swinging the PDS into the service of achieving and maintaining sobriety.

Finally, we psychotherapists need to construe alcoholism therapy as a time-dependent process. We must begin to understand that entirely different therapeutic behaviors are called for in various stages of the long recovery period from active alcoholism.

REFERENCES

Blum, K., Hamilton, M., Hirst, M., and Wallace, J. Putative role of Isoquinoline alkaloids in alcoholism: A link to opiates. *Alcoholism: Clinical and Experimental Research*, 1978, *2*, 113–120.

Bohman, M., Sigvardsson, S., and Cloninger, C. R. Maternal inheritance of alcohol abuse: Cross-fostering analysis of adopted women. *Archives of General Psychiatry* 1981, *38*, 965–969.

Cloninger, C. R., Bohman, M., and Sigvardsson, S. Inheritance of alcohol abuse: Cross-fostering analysis of adopted men. *Archives of General Psychiatry*, 1981, *38*, 861–868.

Ewing, J. A. Alcoholism—another biopsychosocial disease. *Psychosomatics*, 1980, *21*, 371–372.

Frances, R., Timm, S., and Bucky, S. Studies of familial and nonfamilial alcoholism. *Archives of General Psychiatry*, 1980, *37*, 564–566.

Gabrielli, W., Mednick, S. A., Volavka, J., Pollock, V. E., Schulsinger, F., and Itil, T. Electroencephalograms in children of alcoholic fathers. *Psychophysiology*, 1982, *19*, 404–407.

Goodwin, D., Schulsinger, F., Moller, N., Hermansen, L., Winokur, G., and Cuze, S. Drinking problems in adopted and nonadopted sons of alcoholics. *Archives of General Psychiatry*, 1974, *31*, 164–169.

Kaij, L. *Alcoholism in twins*. Almqvist & Wiksell: Stockholm, 1960.

McClearn, G. Genetic studies in animals. *Alcoholism: Clinical and Experimental Research*, 1981, *5*, 447–448.

Myers, R. D. and Melchoir, C. L. Alcohol and alcoholism; Role of Serotonin. In W. B. Essman, *Serotonin in Health and Disease*. New York: Spectrum, 1977.

Myers, R. D. Psychopharmacology of Alcohol. *Annual Review of Pharmacology and Toxicology*, 1978, *18*, 125–144. (a)

Myers, R. D. Tetrahydroisoquinolines in the brain: the basis of an animal model of al-
    coholism. *Alcoholism: Clinical and Experimental Research*, 1978, *2*, 145–154. (b)
Myers, R. D., McCaleb, M. L., and Ruwe, W. D. Alcohol drinking induced in the monkey
    by tetrahydroparaveroline (THP) infused into the cerebral ventricle. *Pharmacology, Bio-
    chemistry, and Behavior*, 1982, *16*, 995–1000.
Schuckitt, M. A. The genetics of alcoholism. *Alcoholism: Clinical and Experimental Research*,
    1981, *5*, 439–440.
Tarter, R. E. The causes of alcoholism: A biopsychosocial analysis. In E. Gottheil, K. Druley,
    T. Skoloda, and H. Waxman, (Eds.), *Etiological aspects of alcohol and drug abuse*. Spring-
    field, Ill: Charles C Thomas, 1983.
Wallace, J. *Compulsive drinking: A biopsychosocial model*. Unpublished manuscript, 1978. Ed-
    gehill Newport, Newport, Rhode Island 02840.

3

Critical Issues in Alcoholism Therapy

John Wallace

Introduction

The Ancients recognized that life is often a matter of choosing a safe course between two equally hazardous alternatives. Navigators operating off the coast of Italy were cautioned to find the narrow passage between Scylla, the rock, and Charybdis, the whirlpool, since sailing too close to either meant certain disaster.

This metaphor for danger on the left *and* on the right is still meaningful, especially so for psychotherapy with the alcoholic client. As some psychotherapists are beginning to realize, making choices in psychotherapy is tricky business. Too often, choice results in exchanging one unsatisfactory state of affairs for another.

In the present chapter, I will show that alcoholism psychotherapy consists of a number of strategic choices in the presence of multiple Scyllas and Charybdises—multiple hazardous alternatives.

Denial versus Premature Self-Disclosure

The Scylla of denial is a well-charted hazard in alcoholism therapy. Therapists working with alcoholics are so familiar with their client's unwillingness (or inability) to see the facts of the drinking and its consequences that nothing further need be added here.

John Wallace • Director of Treatment, Edgehill Newport, Newport, Rhode Island.

What is not appreciated, however, is the corresponding Charybdis of premature self-disclosure. In working with alcoholics, we must realize that the denial is there for a purpose. It is the glue that holds an already shattered self-esteem system together. And it is the tactic through which otherwise overwhelming anxiety can be contained.

In psychotherapy generally, anxiety is often the price that is paid for increments in self-awareness and disclosure to others. Unfortunately, in alcoholics, anxiety is also one of the more important inner cues or "triggers" for drinking. It follows then that the most difficult task in alcoholism therapy is to lessen the denial and encourage increased self-awareness and disclosure while simultaneously keeping anxiety at minimal levels. This means that the alcoholism therapist must be content with a gradually deepening self-awareness in his client rather than demanding sudden, dramatic "breakthroughs." Moreover, the therapist must insure a therapeutic context in which high levels of support are available as the client uncovers aspects of self and discloses these to others.

GUILT VERSUS SOCIOPATHY

Among recovering alcoholics, guilt requires careful therapeutic management. Like anxiety, guilt can operate as a powerful inner trigger for continued drinking. Both therapists and recovering alcoholics recognize this fact and, as a consequence, strive to minimize guilt or avoid it entirely. In fact, the excessive moralism surrounding alcoholism historically, and still prevalent in some quarters, leads many persons to take the extreme position that guilt serves no useful psychological or social function.

But while it is undeniably true that many lives have been wrecked by excessive guilt, it is equally true that as many have been lost in the chaos resulting from the absence of a sharply defined set of values and a developed individual conscience.

Normal guilt serves a highly useful function. It acts as an important feedback signal to the person that his actions are no longer in harmony with his central, core beliefs and values. A therapist who attempts to eliminate guilt of this nature is doing his client an ultimate disservice. And the recovering alcoholic who refuses to acknowledge normal guilt may find himself caught in an ever-increasing spiral of rationalization and further self-deception.

Irrational guilt, or "neurotic guilt," is of course another matter. Guilt of this nature serves no useful purpose. Moreover, it often leads to paradoxical effects, serving to maintain the actions that produced it. In the drinking alcoholic, irrational guilt over drinking may trigger further drinking, leading to yet more drinking, and so on. This familiar pattern constitutes a cycle—the *guilt–alcohol abuse vicious cycle*. Once caught in it, the alcoholic can spin from one drunk to another.

But, while irrational guilt can snare the drinking alcoholic, the absence of normal guilt in the recovering alcoholic and a determined refusal to assume responsibility for his actions does not bode well for recovery either.

In alcoholism psychotherapy, neither irrational guilt nor sociopathic values are to be encouraged. Instead, the alcoholic client must come to see that while he need not feel guilty for becoming an alcoholic, nor for previous actions while intoxicated, he is responsible: responsible for doing something now and in the future about his disease, for his present actions, and for meeting the complications stemming from his past in an honest, fair, and just manner.

SELF-BLAME VERSUS BLAMING OTHERS

Blaming is closely associated with excessive guilt in alcoholics. Typically, the alcoholic swings radically from blaming others to blaming self. He may hold his spouse responsible for his drinking, his parents, children, friends, employers, or even "society." Well-meaning but misguided friends and associates of the alcoholic will often help him to make erroneous blame assignments.

But at other times the alcoholic will go to the other extreme— heaping abuse upon himself. When the self-punishment becomes too painful to bear, he will once again attribute his drinking and its associated miseries to external agents.

As with the guilt–alcohol abuse cycle, the alcoholic may find himself caught in a *blame-assignment cycle*. Blaming others will not work since this perception of cause arouses resentment, still another critically important inner trigger for continued drinking. But blaming self leads once again to irrational guilt and further lowering of self-esteem, and these too result in further drinking.

For the alcoholic caught in the blame-assignment cycle, there seems to be no way out. But there is an obvious alternative and the effective alcoholism therapist knows how to make good use of it; *attributions of cause can be made to the disease of alcoholism*. If he must place blame somewhere, the alcoholic can blame the disease of alcoholism. Obviously not all of the client's difficulties are attributable to his alcoholism. But in the early stages of abstinence and treatment, tactical use of this attribution can be very effective.

Despite its recent critics, the disease concept of alcoholism continues to be superior to any available competing theoretical formulation.

Its advantages are as follows:

1. It provides the patient with a simple, easy to grasp explanation of his perplexing and seemingly inexplicable condition.
2. It gives the client the means to reconstruct his past, cope with the present, and plan his future without being overwhelmed by irrational guilt.
3. It enables the patient to reduce the free-floating anxiety associated with a previously unlabeled and, hence, cognitively unstructured, terrifying life situation.
4. It facilitates the client's decision to remain abstinent rather than continue futile attempts to maintain controlled drinking.
5. It reduces the social stigma growing out of the irrationally moral conception of alcoholism.
6. Extensive community and clinical experience have shown that recovering alcoholics who accept the disease concept are more likely to achieve sobriety and, more important, *maintain* it over longer periods of time than alcoholics who do not.
7. Recent scientific findings point directly to significant biological factors in the etiology of alcoholism (Wallace, 1983).

REBELLION VERSUS COMPLIANCE

Therapists working with alcoholics must be prepared to deal with two frequently encountered patterns of client behavior—rebellion and compliance. Neither of these patterns is associated with continued sobriety.

The rebellious client is a formidable challenge to the therapist's skill and patience. Overtly or passively aggressive, this client rejects efforts to help him. He is hypercritical of the therapist, his information, and his therapeutic techniques. Argumentative, negative, and closed-minded, the client is very often preoccupied with finding faults with the treatment center, therapists, and staff rather than with making therapeutic progress.

The dynamics of the rebellious client are quite apparent. If he can force others to adopt a hostile, rejecting, and punitive attitude toward him, then he is "justified" in keeping others at a distance; that is, his own hostility is appropriate. And he is also "justified" in resuming his alcoholic drinking.

An easy-going, matter-of-fact approach is the correct way to proceed with the openly rebellious client. The therapist should monitor his own actions and attitudes, taking care not to allow reciprocal hostility and rejection to develop on his part. The therapist can then avoid giving the rebellious client the "excuse" that he is looking for to drink.

Compliance, although not as overtly challenging to the therapist, is a more insidious pattern than open rebellion. The compliant client is agreeable, pleasant, and seemingly cooperative. In in-house hospital programs, he is usually "model patient" on the ward, quick to agree with virtually anything treatment staff suggests or recommends.

Unfortunately, compliance is not the same thing as the *inner belief and attitude change* necessary for sobriety to be achieved and maintained. The compliant alcoholic client is the patient who, after arousing great expectations in his therapists, will promptly shatter these by getting drunk on the day he leaves the hospital.

In working with either rebellious or compliant clients, the therapist should adhere to the following central principle: *Employ the least amount of external therapeutic force necessary to achieve belief and attitude change.*

I refer to this principle as the *principle of least justification.* It recognizes that the ultimate goal of alcoholism psychotherapy is a self-governing human being with strong inner convictions and controls. If too much external control is applied during treatment, then the source of sobriety is seen as external and the justification for its continuance remains *outside* the client.

Derivations from the principle of least justification make it clear why strong confrontation tactics are questionable in alcoholism psychotherapy. In the case of the rebellious alcoholic, such forceful therapeutic tactics give the client exactly what he is seeking: an external agent as the locus of control and sobriety against whom he can continue to react.

In the case of the compliant alcoholic, strong confrontation tactics will simply yield more compliance. In the presence of the therapist and in the context of the treatment situation, the compliant alcoholic will appear obedient. But once these external constraints are removed, the compliant alcoholic will drink.

Whatever the therapeutic tactics, it is clear that neither rebellion nor mindless compliance is the desired goal of alcoholism psychotherapy. Surrender to the facts of the alcoholism and acceptance of them are the desired alternatives. These are the keys to a long-term, contented sobriety.

ACTING-OUT VERSUS REPRESSION

Impulse control and expression of feelings are particularly troublesome for the alcoholic. When drinking, his behavior is likely to be unpredictable, spontaneous, and impulsive. Moreover, at that time his feelings are close to the surface and easily aroused. Anger, affection, sorrow, self-pity, depression, aggressiveness, sexuality, and so forth are readily evoked in the drinking alcoholic.

But when he stops drinking, this picture of poor impulse control and hyperemotionality changes radically. When abstinent, the "dry" alcoholic swings to the opposite extreme. He shows rigid defenses, tight control over his impulses, flat emotionality, and compulsivity rather than spontaneity. Moreover, he usually resists therapeutic efforts designed to open up areas of feeling.

The fact that the "dry" alcoholic clings to repressive adaptive tactics is not surprising. He has been out of control, not only in his drinking, but usually in his social behavior as well. As a consequence, therapeutic techniques that require the "dry" alcoholic to give up control even temporarily are often difficult to employ. The alcoholic is likely to resist these. In the early stages of abstinence, the recalled images of prior loss of control are too vivid, disgusting, and terrifying for the alcoholic to relax his grip upon himself. Incapable of "letting go," he is likely to keep a tight rein on feelings, actions, and attitudes. Early on in treatment, the therapist should respect these rigid boundaries in his client and not try to breach them prematurely.

Although there are clear advantages in easy-going and moderate therapeutic tactics in the early stages of abstinence, in the long run the recovering alcoholic should be helped to get in touch with his feelings. He must learn to have feelings when *sober*, not only when drinking. The trick, of course, is to help him to realize that simply *because he has feelings and impulses, he need not act them out.*

Neither uncontrolled acting-out nor repression is the desired goal of alcoholism psychotherapy. Rather, the client should be helped to see that awareness and acceptance of feelings and impulses will enrich a sober life, not diminish it.

In dealing with feelings and impulses, however, the therapist is advised to move cautiously, with great care, perceptiveness, and sensitivity. Timing is all-important and the therapist who must have dramatic release of feelings and explosive acting-out of impulses early in the treatment process might better seek these high-intensity experiences with nonalcoholics in group-encounter settings.

OBSESSION WITH THE PAST VERSUS REFUSAL TO CONSIDER IT

If permitted by the therapist, some alcoholics will ruminate endlessly over the past and report its happenings in great detail. In group-therapy settings, this form of alcoholic behavior tends to drive other clients to distraction. In handling this type of client, the therapist must gently but firmly insist that he focus on the present.

On the other hand, therapists will encounter the opposite: clients who refuse to talk about their pasts at all. Refusal to consider the past is as dangerous for the alcoholic as wallowing in it. As the saying goes "the man who dwells in the past will lose one eye, but the man who forgets his past will lose both eyes."

The desired alternative here involves the learning of several important attitudes. First, the alcoholic must come to accept his past *precisely as it happened.* It will not do for him to engage in retrospective rationalization, nor in distortion or minimization of the facts.

Second, the recovering alcoholic must *own* his past. It is his and not anybody else's. Assigning blame to others for all that happened simply will not do.

Third, the alcoholic client must come to see that his past, faced honestly and squarely, is his most valuable tool in helping himself and others. The past is there to be learned from, not shoved aside so that the same disastrous mistakes can be repeated over and over. In helping the alcoholic client come to terms with his past, it is useful to remember Albert Ellis' thought: "It is not so much what has happened to a person that is important, but what a person tells himself about what has happened." Obviously alcoholic clients can tell themselves many different things about their pasts. Some of these accounts can be helpful. Others can be hazardous. Part of the therapist's task is to help the client choose those constructions of the past that hold the greatest promise for a future of sober, contented living.

Fourth, the recovering alcoholic must accept the likelihood that past events may continue to affect his present life situation. In some cases, the effects of prior active alcoholism may be long delayed. Marriages may fail, jobs may be lost, and health problems may develop even years after the drinking has ceased.

The therapist can be an invaluable aid in helping his client see that events once set in motion may have to proceed to their natural conclusions. The recovering alcoholic may not like these delayed costs of his prior drinking. He may rail bitterly against the injustice of it all, especially since he has been sober for several years or more. While the recovering alcoholic has every right not to like such delayed costs, he must nevertheless learn to accept them.

It is clear that neither obsession with the past nor refusal to acknowledge it is the correct attitude or behavior for the recovering alcoholic. An informed therapist will see that his client learns appropriate alternatives. But as with all things in alcoholism therapy, such learnings take time. The therapist should not permit his client to rush headlong into a detailed examination of his past mistakes. Rather, he will encourage a pattern of gradual realization and deepening acceptance.

INDISCRIMINATE DEPENDENCY VERSUS STUBBORN INDEPENDENCE

In discussing interpersonal dependency, we usually pose the question in terms of whether or not one should be "dependent" or "independent." But since human lives are necessarily intertwined in complex ways, it is misleading to cast the issue in these terms. We are all dependent upon one another in varying degrees. The important questions that rarely get asked are as follows:

1. Upon *whom* should I be dependent?
2. For *what*?
3. At what *costs*?

Indiscriminate dependency on others *or* a stubborn, self-defeating pattern of independence is commonly encountered among both drinking and abstinent alcoholics. Neither pattern is appropriate.

In the case of indiscriminate dependency, the alcoholic client is remarkably adept at attracting people who are all wrong for him. Hoping to satisfy love, affectional, sexual, and friendship needs, he very often ends up in destructive relationships with people who are "toxic" for him. The pain and misery of such relationships can take the recovering alcoholic back to drinking more readily than any single, traumatic event.

Not only must the recovering alcoholic develop a discriminating attitude in his basic love relationships, but he must also come to see that a certain degree of selectivity is indispensable in all of his interpersonal and social relationships. Since we must all depend to some degree upon others for *information* about ourselves, others, and events in which we are involved, we must exercise judgment in seeking advice and counsel from others. Too often, drinking and recovering alcoholics seek out others whose perceptions and constructions of reality are even more distorted than their own. Even in therapeutic communities such as Alcoholics Anonymous, a recovering alcoholic can manage to find somebody who will tell him precisely what he needs to hear in order to hold on to attitudes, beliefs, and actions harmful to himself and others.

While indiscriminate dependency is likely to complicate the alcoholic's life further, the answer does not lie in stubborn independence. People need people. And in the case of the alcoholic, the need is even more intense. For too many alcoholics, the belief that they could solve their problem by themselves has led them from one drinking disaster to another. While there surely is some small number of alcoholics who were successful in stopping drinking by themselves, for the majority this has not been possible.

The development of discriminating dependency upon others is the proper therapeutic course with regard to this particular Scylla and Charybdis. The alcoholic client must learn that in social relationships generally, *discriminating trust* is in order. He need not practice general mistrust of others, nor must he avoid relationships of all kinds. The point is that in relationships that really matter to him, he must be clear about the person in whom he places his trust, the things he expects from the relationship, and the costs he may be paying for whatever it is he receives.

COMPULSIVE SOCIALIZING VERSUS ALIENATION

Closely related to the issue of dependency is the issue of compulsive socializing versus alienation. Therapists working with alcoholics must be aware that while alienation is a clearly undesirable alternative, the development of a pattern of compulsive socializing is to be avoided as well. Certainly the recovering alcoholic should attend group-therapy sessions and meetings of Alcoholics Anonymous. But as sobriety lengthens, the therapist should not continue to encourage excessive dependency upon himself, treatment centers, clinics, or other groups. Although the recovering alcoholic will continue to need therapeutic contacts for many years, these should not become the totality of his existence. The goal of rehabilitation should be a normal life—one in which the concerns of family, friendships, work, play, and continuing recovery activities should be in balance.

Just as the alienated alcoholic needs to reach out more to others, the compulsively social alcoholic needs to learn to be *alone* without feeling *lonely*. He needs to learn how to use small amounts of anxiety and discomfort as stimuli for further growth rather than rushing off after immediate relief from these in the warm bath of group support and security. In the early stages of abstinence, it is correct for the therapist to encourage the uncomfortable client to use the telephone or get to an AA meeting. But in later stages, some of this anxiety should be capitalized upon as motivation for deeper self-exploration and further changes in attitudes, beliefs, and actions.

Precisely because it works so well in reducing felt discomfort, group affiliation takes on the properties of a powerful reinforcer. And, as experience has shown, it is a reinforcer that many alcoholics cannot do without if sobriety is to be achieved and maintained. But like many good things in life, group affiliation can become excessive and, in time, detrimental to the total pattern of growth of the person. While a degree of compulsivity in meeting attendance is important in the first one to five years of sobriety, these activities should not preclude a balanced life in later years. *Choice*, not compulsion, should be the ultimate goal of long-term treatment of the recovering alcoholic.

Pain and discomfort are indeed dangerous triggers for drinking early in sobriety, but we must not forget that they are also the necessary motivating conditions for deep inner changes. Therapists who persist in assuming responsibility for their client's feelings of well-being as treatment progresses are making a fundamental error. The recovering alcoholic must learn to "sit still and hurt" when it is necessary to do so. In the long run, he must learn that only he can do something about his inner emotional and spiritual condition.

PERFECTIONISM VERSUS INFERIORITY

Alcoholics are often snared on one of the extremes of perfectionism or inferiority. In some cases, the same individual can fluctuate back and forth between the two. In perfectionism, the client can make himself miserable by trying to do the impossible. Mistakes of any kind are to be avoided at any cost, dress and grooming must be impeccable, performance consistently superior, and behavior beyond reproach. Nobody could possibly sustain such unrealistically high standards, but the perfectionistic alcoholic client will try. Moreover, he is likely to make everybody else miserable by forcing, either explicitly or implicitly, his unreasonable expectations on those around him.

The dynamics of striving after perfection in the recovering alcoholic are readily apparent. This pattern stems directly from the client's low self-esteem, poor self-regard, and self-doubting. A thoroughgoing perfectionism is often the alcoholic's way of coping with these negative self-perceptions and attitudes. Since even one imperfection or mistake is likely to arouse the underlying self-dislike, the alcoholic strives to avoid any at all.

Such all-or-none judgmental attitudes toward self are self-defeating. The perfectionistic alcoholic either grits his teeth and bears up under a tight, nervous, harassed sobriety or returns to drinking. Once drinking, his previous pattern of perfectionism swings back and forth between frank expressions of inferiority, self-doubting, and self-hatred on the one hand and grandiosity on the other.

Grandiosity, a commonly encountered phenomenon among drinking alcoholics, is but a variant of striving after perfection. Its dynamics are also to be understood in terms of low self-esteem. If the alcoholic feels that his inner person is a "small" human being, then the outer person is likely to be portrayed as a "big" one.

If the Scylla of perfectionism and the Charybdis of inferiority are to be avoided, then the therapist must steer a steady course toward a differentiated, realistic self-image in his client. The client's strengths and weaknesses must be explored honestly and realistically. He must be counseled to see that self-acceptance and positive self-regard are not only possible in the presence of self-imperfections, but highly desirable. Moreover, the unrealistic nature of his all-or-none thinking about self and its negative consequences must be made clear.

Perhaps most important, the therapist should facilitate the view that personal shortcomings are either problems capable of solution *or* unchangeable conditions that must be *accepted*. It simply will not do to permit the client to try to maintain the impossible fiction that he is "perfect." Nor will it do to allow him to hate himself.

But neither can the therapist permit his client to "cop out" with the rationalization that whatever he does is acceptable simply because he is a recovering alcoholic! A convenient fiction like that one may be in order in the very early stages of abstinence, but in the long run, if sobriety is to be maintained, such childish personal and social attitudes must yield to more mature and responsible ones. Maturity, whatever else it may mean, is knowing the price of things—not only the prices one must pay for one's own actions, but those that *others* must pay for them as well.

SELF-OBSESSION VERSUS OBSESSION WITH OTHERS

Throughout years of alcoholic drinking, alcoholics tend to become highly self-centered. *Self-centeredness* as used here does not mean *selfishness*. Alcoholics can be very generous people but still be highly self-centered. Self-centeredness in this sense refers to the alcoholic's highly subjective perceptions and his tendency to focus his attention back upon himself.

Self-centeredness can lead quite naturally to obsession with self. When this happens, the alcoholic can make himself miserable by ruminating over his past and present life situations. Minor problems are blown up out of proportion and transformed into seemingly insoluble difficulties. Worry, anxiety, impatience, depression, agitation, and intolerable frustration are the unfortunate outcomes of obsession with self.

Counselors who understand the alcoholic obsession with self will rightly encourage the client to stop being so concerned with self by placing his attention on another person. The alcoholic is often advised to try to help others if only as a form of therapy for himself. But, while the alcoholic should be encouraged to shift his attention from self to others at certain points in the recovery process, therapists should be aware that this practice can lead dangerously close to the Charybdis of obsession with others to the neglect of self.

It is not uncommon to find recovering alcoholics who have become so obsessed with others that they seem to have lost any sense of selfhood and an individuated identity. Recovering alcoholics who work professionally in the field are particularly vulnerable to the dangers of losing self in the demands of helping others, as are active AA sponsors who overextend themselves by agreeing to work with far too many newcomers to their program.

The way out of this particular dilemma is for the therapist and his client to keep in mind that the solution is not an either/or one. Neither obsession with self nor obsession with others is the goal of treatment. While each extreme is tactically useful at various points in recovery, the therapist should help his client to achieve a balance between his own needs and those of others. This requires teaching the client the difficult skill of holding both his own point of view and that of others in mind simultaneously.

It is unfortunate that many have misconstrued the nature of the concept of therapeutic community. Individual uniqueness need not be sacrificed so that community may be achieved. Identification with others does not require one to give up precious aspects of self not shared with others. In fact, a true therapeutic community does not stamp out individuality but encourages and enhances it by providing the necessary social-emotional support for its growth. A stable, clear, and strong self-identity firmly grounded in community is the ideal outcome in alcoholism therapy.

Pessimist versus Pollyanna

Alcoholics will often show extreme expectations. Some tend to focus upon adverse aspects, conditions, and possibilities or to expect the worst possible outcome. Others swing the other way, adopting an irrepressible optimism than can only be shored up with massive denial.

In fact, the "denial high" or "pink cloud" is routinely found among alcoholics in early stages of recovery.

Extreme expectations of either kind—pessimistic or optimistic—should not be encouraged by the therapist. Unrealistically high expectations lead inevitably to the frustration of disconfirmation. And the pain of frustration can lead to drinking. It is even possible that some alcoholics will deliberately choose high levels of expectation so that failure may be insured and a subsequent return to drinking justified.

Recovering alcoholics should be counseled to face life realistically, not in terms of highly improbable outcomes. Neither the Scylla of cynicism and pessimism nor the Charybdis of irrepressible optimism is the long-term desired goal in alcoholism therapy.

SUMMARY

Alcoholism psychotherapy is frequently undertaken and evaluated without a clear sense of the critical issues involved. Treatment programs are developed and launched with only the vaguest notions about "helping the alcoholic," trying some "behavioral therapy," using didactic lectures, transactional analysis, psychodrama, and so on and so forth. This is all rather like putting the cart before the horse.

Theories of treatment should proceed from a clear understanding of the nature of the alcoholic client, his characteristics, the dilemmas he faces, and the choices he has to make.

This chapter has attempted to provide a systematic view of psychotherapy with the alcoholic by exposing the critical issues. It has argued for a theory of psychotherapy that consists of a number of strategic choices. Moreover, it has shown that these choices during the long recovery from alcoholism must be made in the presence of multiple Scyllas and Charybdises—multiple hazardous alternatives. In each case, not only have I identified the hidden dangers at each choice-point, but I have also tried to indicate the most reasonable compromise. I hope this analysis of the critical issues involved in treating alcoholics will be of assistance in the invention of methods and techniques *specific* to the disease of alcoholism.

REFERENCES

Wallace, J. Alcoholism: Is a shift in paradigm necessary? *Journal of Psychiatric Treatment and Evaluation*, December, 1983.

II

TECHNIQUES OF TREATMENT

4

Psychiatric Office Treatment of Alcoholism

SHELDON ZIMBERG

INTRODUCTION

The Need for Office Treatment of Alcoholism. It has been estimated that there are about 10,000,000 alcoholics in the United States. In New York City there are about 400,000 alcoholics. During the past 15 years there has been an increasing number of alcoholism treatment facilities developed in New York City. However, only about 5% of alcoholics in need of treatment are currently receiving it. There is only a handful of psychiatrists, nonpsychiatric physicians, and other professionals who are willing and able to treat alcoholics effectively in their private offices so that only a small number of alcoholics who could afford private treatment receive it. The shortage of trained professionals interested in treating alcoholics in their own offices is even more severe than in institutional settings. This problem is probably of even greater proportion outside large urban areas that do not have large concentrations of health-care resources.

There are about 25,000 psychiatrists in the United States. Very few are interested in treating alcoholics or are knowledgeable about alcoholism. Most psychiatrists believe that alcoholism cannot be treated psychiatrically and therefore refuse to see such patients. When alcoholism is one of several problems of a patient already in treatment, the

SHELDON ZIMBERG • Director of Psychiatry, Joint Diseases, North General Hospital, New York, New York; Associate Professor of Psychiatry, Mount Sinai School of Medicine, New York, New York.

alcoholism is not diagnosed and the drinking is often ignored. These reactions result from the psychiatrists' lack of training in effective alcoholism-treatment approaches and a lack of awareness of a significant degree of success in the treatment of alcoholism. The traditional psychiatric approach to the treatment of alcoholism involves dealing with the defenses resulting from the underlying conflict with dependency and attempting to uncover the roots of this conflict. This approach was discussed in detail in Chapter 1 of this book, "Principles of Alcoholism Psychotherapy." Clearly this traditional psychoanalytically oriented approach has been a failure and must be abandoned. A new way of looking at alcoholism from a psychosocial, physiological, pharmacological, and behavioral perspective is required in addition to understanding the psychodynamics.

Psychiatrists who have retained their medical knowledge and consider themselves physicians first can be the most effective therapists in the area of alcoholism. Their medical knowledge will permit them effectively to detoxify patients from alcohol and use medications such as disulfiram. Psychiatrists should be aware of the limitations of their medical knowledge and should work collaboratively with internists to see that every alcoholic patient has a thorough physical examination and that medical complications of the alcoholism or other coexisting medical disorders are diagnosed and treated. The psychiatrists' knowledge of medicine, in addition to psychodynamics, defense mechanisms, and the transference countertransference aspects of therapist-patient relationships, makes them uniquely qualified to treat alcoholism. However, even if all psychiatrists were to treat alcoholism, still only a small percentage of alcoholics could be in treatment. Therefore, psychiatrists must extend their potential expertise in this area by providing consultation on the treatment of alcoholism to industrial-medicine departments, to other physicians, to other mental health professionals, and to alcoholism counselors.

Types of Office Psychotherapy. It has been considered for many years that the treatment of choice of alcoholism was group therapy. This view was based on the observation that group therapy obviously had greater productivity and was less costly than individual therapy. In addition, the interpersonal relationships established in groups were potent therapeutic aspects in alcoholism. The value and effectiveness of group therapy is discussed in much greater detail in Chapter 5 of this book, "Group Psychotherapy in the Treatment of Alcoholism."

There are, however, several serious limitations in group therapy. The most serious is the fact that attrition of group members requires having to start over again as new members are added to replace dropouts. This situation makes it difficult to get to many complex issues that are affecting members of the group and to determine the relationship of such issues to the drinking problems. Therefore, the author has found that group therapy is often superficial in dealing with conflicts but can be effective in dealing with alcohol abuse. Group therapy is probably the treatment of choice in hospitals or residential programs where groups can be more closely controlled in relation to attrition of group members, but may not be the treatment of choice in ambulatory settings.

Individual psychotherapy permits a therapist to obtain a much greater understanding of the patients' defenses and conflicts and therefore makes the probability of successful interventions or lack of interventions much greater. The beginning stages of group therapy or individual therapy must deal first with the use of alcohol before any effective psychotherapy can take place. The stages of the recovery process were described in Chapter 1, "Principles of Alcoholism Psychotherapy."

Family therapy involves the psychotherapy of the entire family unit and is discussed in Chapter 8 of this book. Family therapy or couples' therapy can be an extremely effective modality in situations in which the interpersonal relationships in the family, particularly between husband and wife, are interfering with the recovery of the alcoholic individual. Group therapy with married couples as an effective treatment is described in Chapter 9.

Alcoholics Anonymous is an extremely effective self-help program. Every alcoholic should have some exposure to AA if for no other reason than to see many recovered alcoholics and thereby gain hope for his own recovery. Those alcoholics who can become deeply involved in AA can have a system of lifetime support for this chronic illness. Therefore, suggestions that patients go to AA meetings should be part of any approach to the treatment of alcoholism. The methods used by AA sponsors as lay therapists are discussed in the Chapter 13, "Folk Psychotherapy of Alcoholics Anonymous."

This chapter will present an analysis of outcomes of patients treated in a psychiatric office setting with individual psychotherapy and at times couples' therapy. The approaches described are based upon the principles of alcoholism psychotherapy contained in Chapter 1 and represent a synthesis of psychosocial, physiological, pharmacological, and behavioral observations applied to the disorder of alcoholism.

METHODOLOGY

This study of psychiatric office treatment of alcoholism was based on an analysis of patients seen in private psychiatric practice during a two-year period. All alcoholic patients who were evaluated and/or treated were included in the study. There was no control group for purposes of comparison, and therefore inferences regarding the treatment of alcoholism in general cannot be made. However, since this group constitutes a sample population of alcoholics who were interested in receiving private psychiatric treatment and who could afford to pay for such services either out of pocket or through insurance coverage, there is value in describing what can be accomplished by a psychiatrist in relation to a disease commonly thought to be untreatable.

From each patient a complete drinking history, psychiatric history, psychosocial and developmental evaluation, and mental status examination was obtained. The patients were referred to an internist for a complete medical history and physical examination. Liver function tests, a complete blood count, and electrocardiogram were obtained, and medical clearance for the use of disulfiram was established.

The patients were told that they were alcoholic and had to achieve abstinence and the ability to live without alcohol as the goal of treatment. They were also told that the therapist would provide them with the tools to assist them in this goal. The initial treatment consisted of detoxification from alcohol, in most cases on an ambulatory basis. Some patients required detoxification on an inpatient basis.

Ambulatory detoxification from alcohol involved telling the patients to discontinue the use of alcohol and take Valium (diazepam) 5 mg three to four times a day with at least one or two doses at bedtime. This dosage regimen was gradually decreased over a one-week period. The patients were given one nonrenewable prescription for 21 5-mg Valium tablets. Patients were never maintained on minor tranquilizing medication beyond detoxification. During this week, patients were seen in the office two or three times to evaluate the severity of withdrawal signs and symptoms and to adjust the medication. The patients were counseled and given support and encouragement during this detoxification process. The patient's spouse or close relative, if one was available, was also seen during this week in order to obtain more information about the patient's problems and interpersonal relationships, as well as to help provide support during the detoxification period.

During detoxification or after it was completed, all patients were encouraged to attend Alcoholics Anonymous meetings. Many patients were initially reluctant to do so because of the denial they manifested in relation to their drinking problem. They were told that AA was the best place to learn about the illness of alcoholism and to see many recovered alcoholics functioning quite well who had even more severe drinking problems than they did. Thus, they could develop hope in relation to their own alcoholism. The decision of whether they would want to become committed members of AA was postponed until they had gone to a number of different meetings and groups and had a good exposure to the AA approach.

This noncoercive and open-ended approach to encouraging attendance at AA meetings enabled many of the patients to go to AA eventually. All spouses and relatives of the patients who were interested in helping the alcoholic individual were encouraged to attend Al-Anon in order to understand the illness of alcoholism better and to assist in the treatment process.

All patients were encouraged to take disulfiram and most complied. The maintenance dose of disulfiram was 250 mg in most cases. They were informed about the things to avoid while taking disulfiram and were given a disulfiram identification card to carry with them. All of the patients who consented to take disulfiram asked how long they would have to take it. They were told that it would be necessary to take disulfiram until they developed internalized controls over the impulse to drink. The stages of recovery from alcoholism were described to them at this point. A period of at least six months to one year was required before disulfiram could be discontinued by mutual agreement. In some cases it was advised that disulfiram might have to be used on an intermittent basis during periods of stress or crisis when drinking might recur.

The patients were treated with individual psychotherapy in most cases on a once-a-week basis. (The techniques and principles of the psychotherapy of alcoholism are discussed in detail in Chapter 1, "Principles of Alcoholism Psychotherapy.") In some cases in which marital problems were a major aspect of the patient's situation, joint husband and wife sessions were held periodically, averaging once a month along with the individual therapy; one of the weekly individual sessions became the joint therapy session. It is probably advisable that this approach of individual and joint therapy be utilized in all cases of married alcoholics in psychotherapy since the family relationships are often crucial in determining the recovery of the alcoholic individual.

The data obtained for this study came from a review of the charts kept on these patients and follow-up telephone calls to patients who were no longer in treatment to determine their current status.

RESULTS

The study was conducted on 23 patients seen during a two-year period. There were 14 males and 9 females. The average age was 44 with a range of 22 to 54. The average duration of their alcoholism was 8 years with a range of 2 to 17 years. The severity of their alcoholism placed 13 of the patients at level 4 of the Alcohol-Abuse Scale (see Figure 2 in Chapter 1) and 10 at level 5.

Additional demographic characteristics of this treatment population indicated that 11 patients were married, 6 divorced or separated, 5 single, and 1 widowed; 5 were Catholic, 11 Protestant, 5 Jewish, 1 Moslem, and 1 with no religious affiliation; all of the patients were middle-class individuals with 19 employed, 1 student, and 3 housewives.

The results of the study can be seen in Table 1. This table indicates that of the 23 patients treated, 14 (61%) were successes. An outcome was considered successful when there was at least one year of abstinence from alcohol with functional improvement in other aspects of life. Of the 14 patients who achieved a successful outcome, 10 patients achieved a stage II level of recovery (internalized controls over the impulse to drink) and 4 achieved a stage III level of recovery (conflict resolution). (See Figure 4 in Chapter 1.)

In the study 5 (22%) patients dropped out of therapy early (6 sessions or less) and 4 (17%) were failures. If we consider the outcome of the 18 patients who remained in therapy, 14 (78%) had successful results.

History of the treatment population indicated that 11 had no previous treatment for their alcoholism, 11 had previous psychiatric treatment which was unsuccessful, and one had previous alcoholism treatment which was unsuccessful.

When first seen for treatment, most of the patients required detoxification from alcohol, with only 2 being sober on initial contact. Of the 21 requiring detoxification, 17 (81%) were successfully detoxified on an ambulatory basis; 4 (19%) required in-hospital detoxification after failure of ambulatory detoxification.

In addition to once or twice weekly individual psychotherapy sessions and joint therapy sessions, all patients were urged to attend Alcoholics Anonymous meetings and to take disulfiram. Of the 23 patients, 13 participated in AA and 10 did not. Among the 14 patients who had successful outcomes, 10 used AA and 4 did not. Among the patients who dropped out and those who failed in therapy, 3 used AA and 6 did not. Although the numbers are too small to determine statistical significance, it is suggested that attendance at AA is associated with a successful outcome.

Disulfiram was used in 19 of the 23 patients and in 13 of the 14 patients who had successful outcomes. There were 2 patients who had complications from the use of disulfiram, which required its discontinuation. One patient developed a toxic hepatitis and another developed an organic brain syndrome. These conditions cleared up after the disulfiram was stopped.

CASE HISTORIES

Case 1. In this case, the patient could not at first comply with the requirements of treatment, was discharged, and finally became engaged in the treatment process.

The patient was a 54-year-old Jewish woman high-school teacher. She was the mother of one married son and had become a widow after the birth of this child. Her husband died of cancer.

She had been in psychiatric treatment on and off for about six years prior to coming for treatment of her alcoholism. She had had one psychiatric hospitalization for depression and had a history of abusing sleeping pills. During the previous four years she had been using alcohol at an increasing frequency and amount. Her drinking consisted of drinking after school and on weekends. Each morning she awoke with withdrawal tremors. She had no episodes of delirium tremens, but had had several blackouts. It was becoming increasingly difficult for her to function in school, and she was absent from school more frequently. She felt she was on the verge of being unable to function any longer as a teacher and might be suspended by her principal.

At the initial evaluation it was noted that she seemed depressed. Her level of alcohol abuse was noted to be level 5. She came to the first session with alcohol on her breath. She was detoxified from alcohol on an ambulatory basis using Valium (diazepam) and remained sober for three weeks. Since there was evidence of overt depression after withdrawal from alcohol, she was started on Elavil (amytriptyline), 25 mg three times a day. She was urged to attend AA meetings and start on disulfiram. She refused to take the disulfiram or attend AA, insisting that she could remain sober just by coming to therapy. She took the Elavil only sporadically.

After three weeks she began drinking again and could not be detoxified on an ambulatory basis. Hospitalization for alcohol detoxification was suggested; however, she refused. During several weeks of trying to convince her to enter a hospital, she continued to drink;

TABLE 1.   CHARACTERISTICS OF TREATED PATIENTS

	Successes[a] 14 (61%)	Early Dropouts[b] 5 (22%)	Failures 4 (17%)
A. Sex			
Male	8	4	2
Female	6	1	2
B. Age			
Average	43	38	41
Range	33–54	22–52	30–51
C. Religion			
Catholic	3	1	1
Protestant	6	2	3
Jewish	4	1	0
Other	1	1	0
D. Marital Status			
Married	7	3	1
Divorced	3	1	1
Single	3	1	1
Separated	0	0	1
Widowed	1	0	0
E. Employment			
Employed	11	5	3
Student	1	0	0
Housewife	2	0	1
F. Social Class			
Lower-Middle	1	2	1
Middle	7	1	1
Upper-Middle	6	2	2
G. Duration of Alcohol Abuse (years)			
Average	7	6	5
Range	3–17	2–12	2–10
H. Level of Alcohol Abuse			
4	8	3	2
5	6	2	2
I. Use of disulfiram			
Yes	13	2	4
No	1	3	0
Complications	2	0	0
J. Type of Detoxification			
Hospital	3	0	1
Ambulatory	9	5	3
None	2	0	0

(continued)

TABLE 1. (continued)

	Successes[a] 14 (61%)	Early Dropouts[b] 5 (22%)	Failures 4 (17%)
K. Use of Alcoholics Anonymous			
Yes	10	2	1
No	4	3	3
L. Previous Treatment			
None	6	3	2
Psychiatric	7	2	2
Alcoholism	1	0	0

[a] One year or more of abstinence with improvement in other aspects of their lives. Stage II level of recovery, 10; stage III, 4.
[b] Six sessions or less.

thereafter she was told that she could not be helped while she continued to drink and to refuse the suggestions that were offered her for the treatment of her alcoholism. She was discharged from treatment and referred to an alcoholism clinic in her area.

She attended the local alcoholism clinic, but her condition continued to deteriorate. She asked the clinic staff to have her hospitalized for detoxification but all their beds were filled. She called the author one evening asking to have herself hospitalized. She was given the AA Intergroup telephone number, and it was suggested that she speak to the hospital desk and request that they find her a bed for detoxification. She called them and was hospitalized. This was the first time that she had made contact with AA.

After detoxification, the hospital staff referred her to a residential treatment program. She spent one month at this program and began to experience a change in attitude. She returned to individual psychotherapy and consented to take disulfiram and attend AA meetings. She has remained sober continually since her hospitalization, a period of about 7 years till the present time (1983).

After six months of disulfiram therapy, she developed hepatitis, possibly secondary to the disulfiram, so it was discontinued. She attended AA regularly at first but could never become completely involved in AA and has subsequently discontinued AA meetings.

After a year of sobriety, we began dealing with some of her underlying conflicts and her relationship to her son, which was overprotective and ambivalent. She gained some insight into her conflicts and into some of the reasons she used alcohol as an escape from unpleasant feelings generated by these conflicts. She reached stage III of recovery and is currently in therapy to develop more insight into her personality conflicts, particularly her passivity, guilt, and self-blame that led to her depression and later the abuse of alcohol.

Case 2. This case presents a patient with a severe drinking problem who was quickly engaged in treatment and made a rapid recovery.

The patient was a 40-year-old single Catholic man who worked making advertisements for a television station. His employer had noted his lack of productivity and encouraged him to seek help for his drinking problem.

The patient presented a history of 20 years of drinking with at least 10 years of problem drinking. He was drinking daily and during working hours. He had tremors, blackouts, and symptoms suggestive of incipient delirium tremens. He had previously stopped drinking for periods of days to two weeks at a time, but currently he was unable to stop. He was coming late to work and having frequent absences. He was experiencing considerable weight loss and appeared to be in poor health.

His past history indicated that he was born in Quebec, Canada, and that his parents were very strict Catholics. He went to religious schools, which he found intolerable because of the discipline. At age 20 he came to the United States and began to support himself. He began drinking at this time. He had no history of previous psychiatric treatment and had not sought help for his drinking problem before this. He was judged to have a level 5 degree of severity of alcoholism, characterized by withdrawal signs and symptoms, blackouts, physical deterioration, and severe problems functioning in his job.

The patient was detoxified on an ambulatory basis and referred to an internist for a medical evaluation. He was noted to have an enlarged liver and abnormal liver chemistries. He was given vitamin supplementation and medical clearance to start on disulfiram. He agreed to be maintained on disulfiram and to attend AA meetings. He found the AA meetings extremely helpful, and he began attending four to five meetings per week.

He maintained his sobriety and experienced a dramatic change in attitude about the need to drink. Antabuse was discontinued by mutual decision after about four months, and he was discharged from treatment after six months. His liver had recovered and he was in good physical condition.

He experienced a rapid improvement in his health, and his attendance and productivity on his job improved dramatically. He felt psychologically extremely good, almost high, and he wanted to give up smoking and rapidly change other aspects of his life that had deteriorated while he was drinking. He was cautioned about this "grandiose" feeling that frequently develops in alcoholics soon after they achieve sobriety, and he was urged to go slowly and gradually deal with his problems. This guidance was necessary to help him avoid overcompensating for the feelings of failure he had while he was drinking.

At discharge he had experienced significant changes in his attitude about drinking, largely through his AA involvement and his identification with a number of recovered alcoholics. He had no insight into his underlying psychological conflicts, but he felt he achieved what he wanted to achieve in relation to drinking. After six months he was discharged. He had reached a level II of recovery and was still actively engaged in AA attendance. He was told he could return to treatment at any time he wished. At a one-year follow-up telephone call he was sober, functioning well at his job, and attending AA.

Case 3. This case presents a patient who failed in the treatment process.

The patient was a 51-year-old Protestant man who was separated from his second wife. He was an artist who had a number of paintings hanging in museums. He had not had any shows in several years and was not able to make a living from the sale of his paintings. He worked as a professor of art at a college.

He had at least a 30-year history of drinking and ten years of a severe problem drinking. During this time of heavy drinking, his creativity and productivity in painting had declined and a promising career as a painter was at a stalemate. He had separated from his wife about a year prior to treatment and was living with a younger woman in his loft. He saw his wife and two daughters frequently and his wife would nurse him when he became ill from a drinking episode. She was always ready to help him no matter what. The woman he was living with was also an artist. She did not approve of his drinking and frequently berated him.

His first wife had left him for another man about 15 years before. He went to another state in another part of the country and married his second wife soon after. She was completely devoted to him.

His drinking pattern was that of a binge drinker with weeks to months of not drinking or drinking socially and not becoming intoxicated. When he did drink heavily, he drank to a stupor and became physically ill with gastritis and withdrawal manifestations.

He had been in group therapy with a psychologist for about two years prior to coming to treatment for his alcoholism. His drinking episodes were becoming more frequent and severe, and he decided to seek help for his drinking since the group therapy was apparently not helping him in this area.

At initial evaluation he had been drinking and was noted to be at a level 5 of severity of alcohol abuse. He had a physical examination, which revealed an enlarged liver and abnormal liver chemistries. He was willing to take disulfiram, and medical clearance was obtained. He was referred to AA but went to only three meetings. He said that he was not really like the people he met at the meetings and that his problem was not nearly as bad as theirs.

On disulfiram and weekly psychotherapy sessions he achieved about six months of sobriety. He could not resolve the conflict of whether to give up his second wife and marry the woman with whom he was living. His wife was seen on several occasions and encouraged to go to Al-Anon. She agreed to go, but never actually went to a meeting. His girl friend was also seen in order to try to understand this relationship. She did not approve of his drinking and encouraged him to continue in treatment and go to AA. She was applying increasing pressure on him to marry her, threatening to leave him. The patient found this conflict almost intolerable.

After six months of sobriety, he stopped the disulfiram and began drinking heavily again. He could not be detoxified on an ambulatory basis and was hospitalized for detoxification. He was sent with his wife's help to an alcoholism residential treatment program. He stayed six weeks, but did not experience any change in attitude. His wife reported that he had been drinking while out on pass from the program.

When he returned he had short periods of sobriety on disulfiram but stopped the drug and began drinking again. He refused to attend AA.

It was noted that he had some evidence of recurrent depression and brief periods of being somewhat elated. The use of antidepressants in the past had not been successful. The possibility that he was suffering from manic-depressive illness was considered, and he was started on lithium carbonate at a maintenance serum level of about 1.0 meq/liter. After three months there was no change in his mood or drinking behavior. It was suggested that he be admitted to another alcoholism residential treatment facility, but he refused because he said he could not afford to be away from his teaching duties any longer.

After another six months of treatment he was still drinking, and he was told he could no longer be treated at this time. He was referred to an alcoholism clinic for continued treatment and told he could return any time he was willing to engage in a more intensive effort to achieve sobriety.

At follow-up he had not gone to the alcoholism clinic but was seeing a local physician who was treating him with vitamins and minor tranquilizers. He was continuing to drink, but he said at a lesser intensity.

Case 4. This case presents a patient who dropped out of treatment early.

The patient was a 52-year-old married Catholic man who was the vice-president of a large banking company. This was his second marriage. His wife was considerably younger than he and they had recently had a baby girl.

The patient had been the owner of a financial company that had gone bankrupt. He subsequently obtained a high executive position in a banking firm. He had been drinking heavily for about 12 years, but did not have any overt physical consequences of his drinking. He had had a myocardial infarction about one year previously and his doctor advised him to discontinue drinking. He tried but was unable to do so. He drank at lunchtime and in the evenings. He had a level 4 of alcohol abuse. There was no psychiatric history or any previous attempt to seek help for his drinking problem. His wife strongly urged him to go for help for his drinking because of her concern for his health.

The patient was seen in consultation and detoxified on an ambulatory basis. Discussion with his cardiologist indicated that disulfiram at .125 mg (half the usual dose) would be medically acceptable for maintenance. The patient and his wife were seen in joint sessions and the treatment program outlined. He was to be maintained on disulfiram, attend AA meetings, and have weekly psychotherapy sessions. His wife was urged to attend Al-Anon.

The patient was reluctant to start on disulfiram or attend AA. He discontinued therapy after three sessions.

Follow-up indicated that this patient has continued to drink but to a lesser degree.

Case 5. This case presents a patient with a long history of alcoholism who had been unresponsive to previous alcoholism treatment.

The patient was a 44-year-old married, Jewish lawyer. He had a 17-year history of alcoholism that included several hospitalizations, an episode of delirium tremens that occurred about 10 years ago, and several attempts at alcoholism treatment. These attempts included AA attendance, disulfiram, group therapy with a psychiatrist who specialized in alcoholism treatment, and most recently an internist who specialized in alcoholism treatment.

In recent years his drinking pattern had changed from daily to a period of abstinence for 1 to 2 months' duration, which would then be followed by binges of several days to a week's duration. He came into treatment at a point when he appeared to be losing control of his periods of abstinence and his binges were becoming more frequent. He always planned his drinking to occur at times when it would least interfere with his work, but his more frequent binges were beginning to affect his work performance and create marital problems.

The patient was started in individual psychotherapy and disulfiram, but refused to go to AA.

During the beginning stages of treatment, he would stop taking disulfiram, wait a few days, and start a binge. This continued for several months until he was told he could not continue in treatment if he continued to drink. He came to one session drunk, at which time he was extremely depressed and full of anger at his father who had died about four years previously.

Prior to this session, the patient had denied any feelings about his father or, in fact, any disturbing feelings or thoughts of any kind. A joint session with his wife confirmed the presence of depression when he was drunk and his angry feelings at his father. He began to realize for the first time that he drank not only because he wanted to do so, but also as a way of coping with a great deal of emotional conflict.

The author's acceptance of him when he was drunk and his beginning awareness of having repressed a great many feelings that were liberated by intoxication enabled him to accept the need for sobriety. He took the disulfiram on a regular basis and began attending AA meetings. He was able to identify with some of the members for the first time and went on to achieve continuous sobriety.

The profound, dependent relationship he had established with the author in the transference was threatened by the possibility of discontinuing therapy and was enhanced by his being accepted when he came to a session drunk. This represented a breakthrough in the treatment. The transference was not interpreted. He achieved a stage II recovery level because, as his drinking ceased, his defenses in relation to his underlying conflicts were strongly reinstituted. He was able to achieve more than three years of continuous sobriety with only two slips of binge drinking lasting two to three days during the four years after these first three years of sobriety.

Case 6. This case presents a patient who was not seen during the study period but was treated more recently by the same methods. The case is useful because it demonstrates a successful outcome of a patient referred from a company employee assistance program and medical department.

The patient was a 54-year-old Catholic man, single, living with his mother. He was an officer of a large insurance company and was referred by the company for alcoholism treatment because it was noted he was taking increasingly long lunch hours, was no longer as productive as he had been, and was observed to have alcohol on his breath frequently when he returned from lunch. This company had an effective alcoholism screening program, but generally sent all their alcoholic patients for inpatient treatment of 4 to 6 weeks duration. Such a referral was not possible in this case, because the patient could not leave his elderly mother alone.

The patient had a six-year history of excessive drinking. He would drink heavily during lunch hours and after work. He would never drink at home because of his mother's disapproval. He would also drink heavily at bars or friends' apartments on weekends and sometimes not come home until the next day which caused his mother serious concern. In the past year or two his drinking had begun to interfere with his capacity to work effectively. He was referred to the medical department by his supervisor where he was noted to have an enlarged liver and abnormal liver chemistries and was referred to outpatient treatment because he refused referral to an inpatient program. He had a level 4 severity of alcoholism.

His history revealed that his father left when he was an infant and that he had had virtually no contact with him all of his life. He believed, however, that his father was an alcoholic and his alcoholism was the cause of the divorce. He was brought up solely by his mother who had to work to support them. She worked very hard over the years and the patient had become totally dependent on her. Her health had been failing recently and the patient was quite concerned about this.

When the patient came to treatment, he denied rigorously that drinking was a problem. When confronted with the medical findings and the poor work report, he grudgingly accepted that he may have been drinking too much during lunch time. He was started on disulfiram and referred to AA. He took the disulfiram, but only went to two or three AA meetings. He was very concerned about losing his job and was willing to try to stop drinking, not because he thought it was necessary, but because he knew the implications of his continuing to drink on his position in the company. He had worked for this insurance company for more than 30 years and could not think of losing his job. He continued to stay sober for three months after treatment and then went on a weeks' vacation. He stopped the disulfiram and began drinking excessively.

When he returned from vacation, he told the author of his serious slip but pleaded that the medical director of the company not be told. This information was, however, conveyed to the medical director in accord with the signed release obtained from the patient at the beginning of treatment. The medical director made it clear to the patient that he would be suspended if he continued to drink. The patient got the message and remained abstinent for another two months, but without AA involvement.

After an additional two months of abstinence he got drunk during a Thanksgiving Day party at a friend's apartment. He had a blackout, did not return home for two days, and did not contact his mother. His mother called the author and was terribly upset. When the patient returned home, he was full of guilt and remorse. In therapy the patient finally acknowledged that he could not control his drinking and would attend AA more frequently.

The author advised the company's medical director to provide the patient with daily, supervised administration of disulfiram. The shame associated with going to the industrial nurse to obtain the disulfiram further convinced the patient of his need to come to grips with the alcoholism.

He found an AA group near the job that he could attend during lunch time and became a committed AA member. He had hit bottom and surrendered. Further, he felt considerable relief at his acceptance and the support he received at AA, yet he was reluctant to engage in any uncovering therapy. His use of disulfiram returned to self-administration and eventually he was taken off disulfiram. He has experienced two years of continuous sobriety and has weathered a crisis during which his mother was severely ill and hospitalized without drinking.

Case 7. This patient presents a women alcoholic who had a serious drinking problem complicated by the presence of depression. This patient was also not in the original study but was a patient treated in recent years.

The patient was a 53-year-old Catholic, single woman living alone. She had a five-year history of severe alcoholism. She had had three detoxifications and one inpatient rehabilitation treatment experience. She had lost an excellent job as an executive secretary with an oil company and was presently working as a secretary for an insurance company. It was a job of much less responsibility than her previous job.

Her drinking problem was characterized by continuous drinking for short periods of time, abstinence of 3 to 4 months duration, and a severe drinking episode that generally required hospital detoxification to stop. When seen by the author she was an inpatient at a private psychiatric hospital where she was being treated for the alcoholism and the presence of a severe depression.

The patient gave a history of recurrent episodes of depression and feelings of severe inadequacy at her job and inferiority in relation to her boss. These episodes occurred at 2 to 3 month intervals, at which time she would go on a drinking binge. She attended many AA meetings and was desperately trying to control the impulse to drink since she knew her company would no longer tolerate her continued drinking and resulting hospitalizations.

When discharged from the psychiatric hospital, the patient was involved in therapy once a week and started on disulfiram (125 mg a day because 250 was making her too sleepy). Within two months after beginning therapy she developed a severe depression and was started on anti-depressant medication. Even on low doses of several anti-depressants she developed side effects of irritability and agitation and could not tolerate them. Finally she was started on Surmontil (trimipramine) in doses up to 100 mg a day and this relieved the depression. She did not drink when she became depressed because she had been on Antabuse. She maintained sobriety for about a year and during a holiday stopped the disulfiram and began drinking heavily again. She was eventually sent to a four-week inpatient treatment program.

Upon returning from the program, she was determined to deal with the alcoholism and became more involved in AA and began to qualify as a speaker after six months of abstinence. She has gone on to have two years of continuous sobriety and is maintained on disulfiram and Surmontil. She is seen on a once a month basis and has been promoted in her job. Although she still has insecurities, her self-esteem is much improved and the depressive episodes are less severe and of shorter duration. Lithium therapy was considered but her adverse reaction to medication and her reluctance to try lithium prevented its use.

DISCUSSION

This chapter has presented the experience of a psychiatrist treating alcoholics in a private psychiatric office setting. The treatment methods employed were primarily individual psychotherapy along with the intermittent use of joint couples' therapy. In addition, disulfiram was used with most patients. All patients were encouraged to attend Alcoholics Anonymous meetings and spouses to attend Al-Anon meetings. The principles and techniques utilized in the psychotherapy of alcoholism and the observable stages of recovery are described in detail in Chapter 1 of this book.

The results obtained suggest two important issues for consideration.

The first issue to consider is that private psychiatric office treatment can be effective in a majority of alcoholic patients, even those with severe alcoholism (level 5 of alcohol abuse), if carried out with appropriate treatment techniques. In fact, the results obtained by the author with alcoholic patients is comparable to results he has obtained with depressed patients. Therefore, alcoholism is an eminently treatable condition and the attitudes of avoidance, rejection, and hopelessness felt by most psychiatrists in relation to the treatment of alcoholism are not justified.

Residents in psychiatry should be offered experience in the diagnosis and treatment of alcoholism, and practicing psychiatrists should be offered such courses in continuing medical-education programs. In fact, the experience of such a course on Psychotherapy of Alcoholism offered by the author and his colleagues at the Mount Sinai Post-Graduate Medical School in New York City indicates that there are many individuals interested in obtaining knowledge of the specialized approaches required to treat alcoholics.

It is apparent that, with the enormous magnitude of the alcoholism problem in this country, even if all psychiatrists were to treat a substantial number of alcoholics in their practices, they would reach only a small fraction of those in need. However, the knowledge and experience of the psychotherapeutic approaches to the treatment of alcoholism can be broadly extended by psychiatrists acting as consultants to various health programs, community agencies, and industrial medical departments, as well as training and supervising other physicians, professionals, and alcoholism counselors in these methods.

The second issue to consider is the validity of the belief that group therapy is the treatment of choice in the treatment of alcoholism. There are certain advantages to group therapy and these are discussed in detail in Chapter 5 of this book. However, the author noted that many of the patients he treated were "turned off" by previous group therapy experiences and others without such prior experience were not willing to go to a group. If group therapy had been the only treatment choice available to such patients, they would have dropped out of treatment. An outcome evaluation study of the treatment of socioeconomically deprived alcoholics in an alcoholism clinic setting (Zimberg, 1974) indicated that abstinence was significantly associated with patients who "had more intensive individual psychotherapy and family therapy."

In addition, the basic principle underlying this approach to psychotherapy is intervention, as described by Tiebout (1962) and supported by the experience of Curlee (1971) and Moore (1972). First intervention is directed at the drinking and subsequently to the many crises and problems that exist after the alcoholic stops drinking. For these interventions to be effective, on target, and at the right time, the patient's underlying conflicts and personality structure must be well understood. The activist aspects of direct intervention in psychotherapy has a greater risk of causing patients to drop out of treatment than the passive noninterventionist approach of psychoanalytic psychotherapy. This greater knowledge of the patient and his individual needs and vulnerabilities is difficult to achieve in group psychotherapy settings, which almost always deal with issues relating to interpersonal relationships and more superficial problems. Therefore, individual psychotherapy is a more effective treatment modality for those alcoholics who have serious underlying psychological conflict and for those who wish eventually to obtain some insight into the psychological conflict that contributed to their drinking behavior.

SUMMARY

The results of individual psychotherapy with alcoholics conducted in a private psychiatrist's office have been presented. There were 23 patients treated, with a 61% recovery rate, 22% who dropped out of treatment early, and 17% who failed to recover. In most cases, patients were detoxified on an ambulatory basis and maintained on disulfiram. The primary treatment was individual psychotherapy with intermittent couples' therapy for married patients. All patients were encouraged to attend AA meetings and spouses were encouraged to attend Al-Anon meetings. This study demonstrates that alcoholism can be effectively treated in a psychiatrist's office. In addition, individual therapy may be the treatment of choice for many alcoholics.

REFERENCES

Curlee, J. Combined use of Alcoholics Anonymous and outpatient psychotherapy. *Bulletin of the Menninger Clinic,* 1971, *35,* 368–371.

Moore, R. A. Psychotherapeutics of alcoholism. *Proceedings of the Second Annual Alcoholism Conference of the National Institute on Alcohol Abuse and Alcoholism,* June, 1972.

Tiebout, H. M. Intervention in psychotherapy. *The American Journal of Psychoanalysis,* 1962, *22,* 1–6.

Zimberg, S. Evaluation of alcoholism treatment in Harlem. *Quarterly Journal of Studies on Alcohol,* 1974, *35,* 550–557.

5

Group Psychotherapy in the Treatment of Alcoholism

Sheila B. Blume

Introduction

This chapter will discuss group psychotherapy as it is widely applied in the treatment of alcoholism today. For our purposes, a therapy group may be defined as a group of clients or patients, usually six to ten in number, who meet regularly with a professional leader or leaders for the purpose of overcoming identified personal problems. The leader of the group is responsible for screening and selection of the members and for the formulation of specific goals and a plan of treatment for each. This distinguishes group therapy from Alcoholics Anonymous, a treatment method which is covered elsewhere in this book (Chapter 10). Specific group variations, such as family therapy and psychodrama, are also covered elsewhere (Chapters 6 and 8), although techniques borrowed from these treatment methods are very helpful in the psychodynamic-eclectic group therapy discussed here. Recommendations on format, structure, and technique are based chiefly on the author's fifteen years' experience treating alcoholic patients at the Charles K. Post Alcoholism Rehabilitation Unit at Central Islip Psychiatric Center, New York.

Sheila B. Blume • Medical Director, Alcoholism and Compulsive Gambling Programs, South Oaks Hospital, Amityville, New York.

WHY GROUP THERAPY?

The most frequently given reason for employing group psychotherapy in alcoholism treatment is economy. A single therapist, it is argued, can see six to eight patients in a one-and-a-half- to two-hour period, whereas treating the same number in individual sessions would consume six to eight hours of therapist time. This argument is only partially correct, since the group therapist must be prepared to spend time with individual group members before or after group sessions, and will also spend time in screening new members, in family conferences with group members, and in arranging other needed services for group participants. Record keeping will also consume more therapist time in group treatment. Group therapy does, however, offer the distinct advantage that the absence of one or two group members does not result in blocks of lost therapist time, as does the "no show" client in individual treatment.

More important reasons for the popularity of group psychotherapy in alcoholism have to do with the nature of alcoholism itself and of the alcoholic patient entering treatment. Regardless of the premorbid personality of the alcoholic person, as a result of his or her extreme dependence on alcohol as a problem-solver, the alcoholic becomes emotionally isolated from other people and often has only superficial and manipulative relationships with those around him. The therapy group breaks through this isolation, encouraging the development of emotional interrelatedness and interdependence with peers. In general, the more an alcoholic person can be induced to talk about his problems and feelings to others, the less likely he will be to drink about them.

A second characteristic of the alcoholic person entering therapy is his tendency, in struggling for a new means of adjustment to the traumata of life, to become overly dependent on his therapist. This tendency is a far greater problem in individual therapy than in group therapy, where interdependence on peers replaces the single intense relationship with the individual therapist. The statement from alcoholic patient to therapist, "You are the only person in the world who understands me," although meant as a compliment, should be taken as a warning sign. The recovering alcoholic should feel that many people—family, friends, fellow alcoholics, AA members, and helping professionals—are capable of understanding his needs and feelings if he chooses to communicate them. Thus, a variety of people may serve as resources in times of stress to help him avoid a return to drinking.

Many alcoholic patients are initially resistant to the suggestion that they join Alcoholics Anonymous. Fears and preconceptions about the nature of AA lead the new patient to rationalize: "I'm not a joiner," "Listening to the stories of other people would only depress me," or "I couldn't possibly tell other people about myself." The experience of group psychotherapy, by overcoming such objections, prepares the alcoholic person to understand and profit from the AA program.

Group therapy is also of value in assisting the newcomer to therapy to accept the new positive identity "recovering alcoholic." Before treatment, the label "alcoholic" is applied to him by others in his life in a negative, stigmatizing way. Within the group, the successfully recovering alcoholic is a hero or heroine, afforded high status. Outsiders tend to be labeled "civilians." Formation of this positive identity is an important advantage of both residential programs and Alcoholics Anonymous. It is shared in an outpatient clinic or private practice setting only by group treatment methods.

Group therapy presents an advantage to the therapist, who is able to observe directly the interpersonal behavior of each group member. The opportunity to compare actual behavior with self-perceived and self-reported behavior is another advantage of group psychotherapy. Group techniques also lend themselves easily to experiential training by allowing the trainee to function as cotherapist within the group. In addition, group therapy offers considerable personal benefits to the therapist, who learns from the group members. It is also great fun.

TYPES OF GROUPS IN ALCOHOLISM TREATMENT

Educational Groups

The orientation or alcohol education group in lecture-discussion format is a valuable tool in alcoholism treatment. Many inpatient and outpatient programs offer such groups to beginning patients and their families while the initial intake evaluation is in progress. They serve as an excellent introduction to the group experience. In educational groups, members are free to speak up but may also remain silent without experiencing group pressure to reveal themselves. Shy members have the opportunity to observe that those who do make self-revelations are well received by others in the group. At the same time, a solid foundation of shared information about alcohol and alcoholism is built. This saves the later, personal-problem oriented groups from having to educate each new member in the basics of alcoholism, and thus allows more intense concentration on individual feelings and behavior.

Closed versus Open Groups

Closed therapy groups are those in which all participants begin group treatment at the same time and remain together. Such groups are usually time-limited. Open groups are ongoing, with new members added as others complete treatment or drop out. The meeting room and therapist usually remain constant, but occasionally the leadership will also change without dissolution of the group. The choice of closed or open format is more often dictated by the setting in which treatment takes place than the preferences of the group members or therapist.

The closed group tends to build more intense relationships, since all members share in the entire history of the group. On the other hand, prospective members must wait for a new group to organize, and a large number of dropouts for any reason may make the group too small to be effective. Members who have completed the full course of therapy sessions but remain in obvious need of further help must begin again in a new group.

Open groups allow more flexibility in that the length of treatment may be tailored to individual need. Vacancies may be filled as they arise, and a member who has dropped out may reenter the same group at a later time. However, in the open group the leader must take a more active role since he or she serves as the connecting thread and group historian. The newcomer in an open group often feels at a disadvantage compared to the "old-timers." It is up to the therapist to see that "in" jokes and references to sessions past are explained. If a life experience related previously by one of the older members of the group would be of value to a newer member, it is the responsibility of the leader to encourage that member to retell the story. The repetition itself can be of some value in that it allows the therapist to observe the way in which the group member reevaluates the experiences of his life as therapy progresses.

Homogeneous versus Mixed Groups

For the reasons mentioned under Why Group Therapy? above, there is considerable advantage to be gained by treating alcoholics together in all-alcoholic groups. An exception to this is the couples' group in which a number of alcoholics and their marital or sexual partners, some of whom may not suffer from alcoholism, attend together.

Other characteristics such as age, sex, education, religion, race, sexual preference, ethnic group, and social class have been mixed successfully in therapy groups for alcoholism. Some authors have advocated separate groups for alcoholic women; such groups have the advantage of focusing more effectively on specific women's issues. The same argument has been given for special groups for homosexual alcoholics and for adolescent alcohol abusers. The major disadvantage of all-male or all-female groups is their tendency to stereotype the opposite sex, for example, "All men are after the same thing," "Women are always out for your money," "You can't trust a man," "Nobody can understand a woman." It is the job of the therapist to challenge such easy rationalization if such a group is to be effective.

Setting Up the Group

Confidentiality

Crucial to the success of any therapy group is the feeling of trust on the part of its members, allowing them to share painful experiences and hidden parts of their lives. This trust cannot be achieved without strict adherence to the principle of confidentiality on the part of all group members. Clear rules on the subject should be made explicit before therapy begins, and any exceptions to be expected (e.g., on the part of the group leader to other staff members, or as required by law, etc.) should be made clear. Penalties for breaking the rule should also be spelled out in advance. The therapist should screen out any prospective group member who he has reason to believe may be a potential blackmailer, since this possibility is the most serious danger of group treatment.

Ground Rules

Additional ground rules should be spelled out clearly for all members. These include rules concerning lateness, absences, attending meetings under the influence of alcohol or drugs, treatment termination and reentry, and the responsibilities of the leader and of the other members. A signed agreement or therapeutic contract will give added weight to the individual member's commitment. Some groups make concomitant attendance at AA or the taking of Antabuse a requirement for membership.

Selection and screening of members is basically the responsibility of the group leader, who should have available a full case history including evidence of any coexisting organic, neurotic, psychotic, or character disorder.

A preliminary interview to explore the patient's feelings about group treatment and to discuss the group-therapy process is also desirable. In some therapy groups, the prospective member is interviewed in a final step by the group itself, which must unanimously approve his or her inclusion.

Room Arrangement

The major requirements for a therapy-group setting are quiet and privacy. If all seats in the room are not equal, the leader should avoid sitting in the most comfortable chair or the focal point of the room. Although some groups meet sitting at a table, it is of considerable advantage in observing body posture and nonverbal communication if the members of the group sit in a circle without any obstruction between them.

GOALS AND TECHNIQUES OF GROUP PSYCHOTHERAPY IN ALCOHOLISM TREATMENT

General Goals

Sobriety. In the treatment of alcoholic people, the therapist must take a positive stand in favor of sobriety. Real therapeutic work in changing attitudes and behavior patterns will be impossible if the patient continues his alcoholic drinking. An attitude on the part of the therapist that tells the patient, "Do what you want; it's your life; I don't care," has not produced therapeutic success. Although responsibility for sobriety rests squarely with the patient, the group leader indicates his position by repeated introduction of the theme of the value of sobriety into the group discussion. This is accomplished by interjecting appropriate comments or questions after the discussion of some past or future event in the life of a group member. Examples are: "What would be the worst possible way you could handle that situation?" "What measures can you take to avoid drinking in that situation?" "How could you have played that one sober?" "You made it through that difficult time without a drink. How did you manage it?"

Overcoming Denial. There are at least two levels of denial in the alcoholic patient. The first is the denial of the presence or magnitude of the drinking problem. This denial is the problem that commonly blocks entrance into treatment and may recur after treatment has begun. Once the initial denial has been overcome, a second level is sometimes encountered: the denial that there are any problems other than the drinking itself. Both of these denials may be handled in the therapy group as they arise.

Two general approaches to denial are direct confrontation and the more indirect method of attacking the reason for denial. Confrontation is successful only in the patient who is well integrated into the therapy group and has made a strong emotional investment in the group process. Even with such a member, confrontation by the leader is best accomplished in terms such as, "Just a minute, didn't you tell us a couple of weeks ago that. . .," or, "I seem to remember your saying. . .," rather than, "You're a liar," or worse yet, "You're denying." Fellow group members may confront more directly.

The indirect approach takes into account that denial is predominantly an unconscious mechanism of defense against perceived threat and includes attempts to find out or even guess the reason for the use of this defense. The reason will vary and the approach will be tailored to the perceived threat. For example, if the denial is one of sexual problems, the reason may be that the patient perceives admitting to impotence as an intolerable blow to self-esteem. This can be approached by having others in the group who are ready to face this problem discuss their own sexual histories and in particular their previous fears of putting such a history into words. Identification with other group members provides the most effective help in working through denial in a group setting.

Motivation. In the process of psychotherapy with alcoholic patients, motivation must be a continuing concern. The motivations for entering treatment initially are varied and often based on pressures generated by others in the environment in the form of "either-or" choices. From this beginning, the therapist works toward an ideal self-motivation for recovery, based on the desire to live life free of alcohol. Just as "recovering alcoholic" becomes a highly valued identity during the therapy process, sobriety becomes an important component of self-esteem. Motivation may wax and wane in response to the emotional state of the individual, and thus provides a clue to early detection of the onset of depression or other distress. In successful therapy, motivation should build progressively toward the ideal. It is therefore of value for the group leader to ask each member periodically, "Do you want to stop drinking?" and "Why?" The answer will help monitor each member's progress.

Recognition and Identification of Feelings. Alcoholic people drink for a wide variety of reasons, but there are two that present the greatest hazard to alcoholics striving for sobriety. The first of these is drinking to relieve painful feeling states. When drinking, the alcoholic may even consume alcohol in anticipation of such feelings. Thus, various emotional states come to be perceived as the state of needing a drink and are poorly recognized or sorted out one from another. In the process of living without this drug, it becomes important for the alcoholic to identify and label his emotional states in order to make an adequate response to his distress. Positive feelings may also be poorly identified by the drinking alcoholic, who perceives them as the urge for a drink to celebrate or confuses them with his drug-induced euphoria. These positive feelings are the building blocks of self-esteem during recovery. Recognition and identification of feeling states thus becomes a major component of therapy. This is accomplished by asking such questions as, "How do you feel right now?" "How did you feel then?" A response such as "lousy," "not good," or "great" should be refined by such questions as, "Can you name the feeling more exactly?" A patient who can tell when he is frightened, angry, or lonely, for example, is in a position to choose an appropriate response to this predicament.

Recognition and Identification of Behavior Patterns. The second troublesome reason alcoholic people drink is to manipulate the environment and others around them. For example, they may drink to avoid responsibility for words or acts, to make others angry, or to "get even." Such behavior patterns are sometimes referred to as games, as in the literature of transactional analysis (Steiner, 1971). Identification and recognition of such recurring patterns is also crucial to the process of developing more adequate behavior. The questions "Have you ever behaved like that before?" and "How far back can you trace that pattern?" are useful in accomplishing this goal. At times, the patient's destructive behavior pattern will have been present long before his alcohol abuse.

New Ways to Handle Old Problems. Successful adjustment to life without alcohol requires new responses to situations that would have prompted drinking in the past. These responses must become habitual through successful repetition. AA members often use slogans such as "First things first" and "Easy does it" to help them handle states of distress. In a similar vein, group members may develop slogans or mottoes tailored to their own personal problems. These slogans will then be used at times of stress as reminders of their new responses. Such statements as "not guilty" or "I don't have to please my father" can be very effective in individual cases. Other examples will be given below. Group members will help one another develop and practice these new responses.

Development of an Emergency Plan. Each recovering alcoholic should have a well-thought-out plan to respond to unforeseen events that create emotional turmoil. This plan may be written on a card and carried and should include the names and telephone numbers of people who may be called in an emergency. Members of the group may serve as special resources for one another in such emergencies in addition to AA members, clergymen, clinics, hot lines, etc.

Enjoying Life without Alcohol. Finally, a general goal in alcoholism treatment is helping the patient to develop sources of pleasure in his sober life. Identification with other group members and their suggestions will be of value. It is often helpful to point out such pleasures as they come up in group discussion. The question, "Would a drink have made that (happy feeling) better?" helps the group appreciate the development of such pleasure sources.

Specific Goals

In addition to the goals above, which apply to the treatment of all alcoholic people, specific goals must be developed related to the personality, interpersonal relationships, and life situation of each individual. Examples of such goals and related techniques follow.

Problems with Responsibility. Some alcoholic persons take upon themselves too much responsibility for the feelings and behavior of others in the environment. They feel called upon to make and keep others comfortable and happy at all times. They cannot draw a firm boundary to their own responsibility. A helpful slogan for such patients is "That's his (her, their, your) problem." Members of the group will help draw the boundary line until it is internalized.

Overly selfish people who have felt little concern for others in their lives can be helped through the group process to develop a better sense of responsibility. This can be done by pointing up situations and comments in the group in which they are helpful to others and rewarding these liberally. Such patients can sometimes be maneuvered into positions where they help a fellow patient, are given charge of the group in the leader's temporary absence, or are given other responsibility in the group. Such patterns are then transferred to outside situations.

Guilt. Related to problems of responsibility are special guilt problems in alcoholic people. A therapy group, acting like the chorus in a Greek play, will speak for the general values of society. In this capacity, the group does an excellent job of differentiating between realistic and unrealistic guilt. The group has little tolerance for unrealistic guilt, to which it assigns the negative label "self-pity." Such labeling helps the guilt-ridden member differentiate between the two. The guilt feelings felt to be realistic by the group because of the actual deeds of the member are assuaged through the process of identification with others in the group. A confession of a past deed for which the member feels realistically guilty is followed by similar stories from others of actions they also truly regret. The therapist may then ask how any of the group attempted to apologize or make amends, and a realistic discussion of the process follows. This usually produces significant relief of realistic guilt.

Anger. Many recovering alcoholics have individual problems surrounding anger and frustration. Some patients have difficulty expressing anger in any way at all. They have been trained in childhood that any such expression will be met with punishment. This problem is handled by waiting until such a patient has good cause to be angry within the group and then challenging him. The challenge will add to the inner anger until nonverbal expression will make his anger clearly visible to all. Role-playing or doubling (see Chapter 6) will enhance this confrontation. When the patient finally expresses his anger, he is cheered and rewarded by the group. The original anger-provoking situation is quickly resolved (for example, by apology) and the experience is perceived positively. After practice within the group, such patients may go through a brief period of getting angry at everyone around them, but this situation corrects itself rapidly. Role-playing and assertiveness training are also useful in giving such patients experience in expressing anger appropriately and in facing angry responses from others.

Passive–aggressive patterns of behavior may be handled in a similar manner, with the group reinforcing direct appropriate expressions of anger. The mottoes, "I have a right to be angry" and "Since I don't like absolutely everybody, why should absolutely everybody have to like me?" are appropriate to some patients in this group.

Trouble controlling anger is also a frequent problem among alcoholics. Such patients have often grown up angry, feeling cheated by life and those around them. They should not be treated with the same "let it all hang out" strategy as patients with the first two categories of anger problems.

Tracing the anger to its original sources in group psychotherapy is helpful to the patient with anger problems. Allowing the patient to discharge his anger directly toward this source in role-playing or to an empty chair can also be useful. Specific techniques of controlling anger can be taught by group members who have better control. "Unloading" angry feelings by talking to other, sympathetic people is practiced in group, as is modulated expression of anger as opposed to unfocused rage. Mottoes helpful to such patients have included, "Consider the source," "Why am I overreacting?" "She's not my mother," and "I won't let you get under my skin."

Depression. People who are depressed usually show it in a group session by remaining quiet. The therapist should make an effort to draw the depressed person out slowly and patiently until he has expressed his feelings, including crying or mourning if appropriate. This allows the group to comfort the depressed person and sympathize with him. The therapist can then use the group setting to help the patient win a series of small victories to regain a feeling of some mastery over self and enviornment. A helpful question, once the depression begins to lift, is "Do you deserve to be happy?" Once the patient admits he has that right, the leader can ask him to go to each member, make eye contact, and repeat, "I deserve to be happy," until he says it with some conviction. The group is quite supportive in such an exercise. "Not guilty" is an excellent motto for some depressed people.

Fear. Many people suffering from alcoholism have learned to drink when fearful or anxious and may look for other sedative drugs for this purpose during recovery. Group therapy can help such a person learn to overcome his fear without chemical help. The best remedy for fear may be learned by watching a parent introduce his young child to the ocean at a beach. Exposure to the feared object or situation in small but progressive doses, from a secure base, is the method used, similar to the principle in systematic desensitization. Within a therapy group, the fear is first discussed and explored so that fear based on misunderstanding or misperception can be eliminated. Next, the fear is faced in small doses, in either role-playing within the group or homework assignments or both. In the case of an imminent fearful situation which must be faced (e.g., a court appearance), another group member, preferably one who needs practice in helping others, can accompany the patient. In preparing for a confrontation of which a group member is afraid, a useful technique is to role-play the siutation and have the patient reverse roles, becoming the adversary. Then have him act out the worst thing that this adversary could possibly do (his deepest fear), reverse to his own role, and finally discuss the real probabilities of the situation with the group. Assertiveness training and relaxation training are other techniques of value to patients with fear problems.

Four generalized fears often encountered in treating alcoholism are fear of closeness, fear of rejection, fear of failure, and fear of success.

All may be present in the same individual. These fears will be reflected within the group as well as in past and present experience outside the group. The leader should encourage members openly to overcome such fears within the group, as a useful first step toward tackling them in other life situations.

PROBLEMS IN GROUP TREATMENT OF ALCOHOLISM

The problems that occur in all psychotherapy groups also appear in alcoholism treatment. The therapist must guard against scapegoating of one member by the group, allowing one member to dominate the group sessions, or allowing superficial conversation or prolonged storytelling to replace focusing on relevant feelings, interactions, and behavior patterns. In addition to these general problems, others peculiar to alcoholism treatment also arise.

Closure

Because extreme negative emotions may precipitate drinking in alcoholic patients, it is important to avoid ending the group session leaving individual members in a state of unresolved conflict. This is particularly important in an outpatient setting. A member showing great distress toward the end of a session can be helped by a review of his emergency plan and an expression of group support. A look backward at progress since beginning treatment may also be of value. Since conflict within the group is necessary for change to occur, closure becomes an important extra problem in alcoholism groups.

Intoxication

As mentioned earlier, the group should have ground rules concerning attending meetings under the influence of alcohol. The intoxicated member may be allowed to attend and listen, or to participate, but should not be allowed to monopolize the session. The group must avoid offering positive reinforcement to the drinking behavior. On the other hand, both group and leader should make clear their positive expectation that the member will be present and sober at the next meeting. Drug abuse may be handled in a similar way.

Wish for Special Attention

Although this problem arises in all therapy groups, it may manifest itself in an alcoholic group by repeated drinking or "near-drinking" episodes calling for extra individual attention from the leader or other members. Such a pattern should be pointed out to the patient and recognition given when he is able to curb this tendency and to depend on inner as well as outer resources. Although the group leader may see group members individually for matters that would otherwise take up group time inappropriately, such as referrals for other services, prolonged parallel individual consultation is seldom advisable. The goal for a group member wishing to discuss a problem privately with the therapist is usually exploration of the reasons for the consultation and reassurance that the matter is quite appropriate to discuss in the group.

SUMMARY

Group psychotherapy is a widespread and popular approach to the treatment of alcoholism. It can be employed successfully along with AA, Antabuse therapy, vocational rehabilitation, and other methods. Alcoholism groups provide both special advantages and special problems. The brief bibliography will provide additional material on the subject.

REFERENCE

Steiner, C. Games alcoholics play. New York: Grove Press, 1971.

SUGGESTED READINGS

Brown, S., and Yalom, I. D. Interactional group therapy with alcoholics. Journal of Studies on Alcohol, 1977, 38, 426-456.

Doroff, D. R. Group psychotherapy in alcoholism. In B. Kissin and H. Begleiter (Eds.), The biology of alcoholism. Vol. 5. New York: Plenum, 1977.

Feeny, D. J., and Dranger, P. Alcoholics view group therapy. Journal of Studies on Alcohol, 1976, 37, 611-618.

Fox, R. Group psychotherapy with alcoholics. International Journal of Group Psychotherapy, 1962, 12, 56-63.

Fox, R. Modifications of group psychotherapy for alcoholics. American Journal of Orthopsychiatry, 1965, 35, 258-259.

Killins, C. G., and Wells, C. L. Group therapy of alcoholics. In J. H. Masserman (Ed.), Current psychiatric therapies. Vol. 7. New York: Grune and Stratton, 1967.

Macphail, D. Personal experience of group-therapy for alcoholism: A critical examination. Lancet, 1965, 2, 75-77.

Mandic, M. The structure of therapeutic group of alcoholics. Alcoholism, 1978, 14, 158-163.

Mullan, H., and Sangiuliano, I. Alcoholism: Group psychotherapy and rehabilitation. Springfield, Ill.: Charles C. Thomas, 1966.

Sands, P. M., and Hanson, P. G. Psychotherapeutic groups for alcoholics and relatives in an outpatient setting. *International Journal of Group Psychotherapy,* 1971, *21,* 23–33.

Sands, P. M., Hanson, P. G., and Sheldon, R. B. Recurring themes in group psychotherapy with alcoholics. *The Psychiatric Quarterly,* 1967, *41,* 474–482.

Scott, E. M. A special type of group therapy and its application to alcoholics. *Quarterly Journal of Studies on Alcohol,* 1956, *17,* 288–290.

Strayer, R. Social integration of alcoholics through prolonged group therapy. *Quarterly Journal of Studies on Alcohol,* 1961, *22,* 471–480.

Tomsovic, M. Group therapy and changes in the self-concept of alcoholics. *Journal of Studies on Alcohol,* 1976, *37,* 53–57.

Vannicelli, M. Group psychotherapy with alcoholics, special techniques. *Journal of Studies on Alcohol,* 1982, *43,* 17–37.

Vogel, S. Some aspects of group psychotherapy with alcoholics. *International Journal of Group Psychotherapy,* 1957, *7,* 302–309.

Westfield, D. R. Two years' experience of group methods in the therapy of male alcoholics in a Scottish mental hospital. *British Journal of Addiction,* 1972, *67,* 267–276.

6

Psychodrama and the Treatment of Alcoholism

Sheila B. Blume

Introduction

Just as the terms *psychoanalysis* and *psychoanalytic* are used in three broad senses—first, to describe a method of treatment and research; second, to describe a body of theory based on data obtained using this method; and third, to describe a set of techniques derived from the formal method but applicable to other settings—the terms *psychodrama* and *psychodramatic* are used in the same three senses.

Psychodrama as a Formal Method of Treatment. The formal psychodrama is a type of group psychotherapy that differs from traditional group methods in its stress on action rather than description. The insights reached in psychodrama are action-insights derived from the actual experience of living the past, present, or future in dramatic form. Action takes place in the "here-and-now," on a stage, and with the help of a trained director and other members of the group. The scenes enacted may move freely in space and time in the real world and also into dreams or fantasies, in order to explore aspects of the subjective reality of an individual. The emotional overtones and meanings associated with an event or relationship, called by Moreno (1959) its "surplus reality," are explored through a variety of specialized techniques. Catharsis of emotion is achieved through the here-and-now experience of this subjective reality.

SHEILA B. BLUME • Former Director, New York State Division, of Alcoholism and Alcohol Abuse.

Psychodrama also serves as a laboratory for human behavior in which new experimental ways of dealing with life problems may be tried, new roles may be assumed, and one's own behavior may be seen through the eyes of others. There are three segments in the formal psychodrama: warm-up, enactment, and sharing. These will be described in detail under The Formal Psychodrama, below. Psychodrama as a group method has been incorporated into programs for the treatment of alcoholism over the last 15 to 20 years (Cabrera, 1961; Fox, 1962; Weiner, 1965; Blume, Robins, and Branston, 1968; Von Meulenbrouck, 1972; Blume, 1974, 1977; Wood, Del Nuovo, Michalik, Schein, and Bucky, 1978).

Psychodrama as a Body of Theory. Psychodrama was invented and developed by Jacob L. Moreno (1889–1974), a pioneer in both the theory and practice of group treatment methods. Much of the theory of psychodrama will be found in Moreno's writings, along with the theories of sociometry and of the dynamics of group interaction.

Moreno considered the "encounter" to be the basic tool of psychotherapy, defining it as a complete interpersonal experience between two people. The encounter differs radically from the psychoanalyst-analysand relationship, as well as from the traditional doctor–patient or teacher–student relationships. The goal of all therapy, and of psychodrama in particular, is to liberate the spontaneity of the patient, his ability to vary feeling and behavior. This spontaneity allows him to develop new and more adequate responses to the problems of his life. Creativity is defined as the ability to produce an adequate response to a new situation or a new and more successful response to a familiar one. Creativity is seen by Moreno as a major criterion of emotional health.

Moreno speaks of the "social atom" as the sum of all meaningful human relationships in the life of an individual and of "surplus reality" as the many complex emotional associations which provide added dimensions to any human interaction. It is the exploration of the surplus reality of the individual's experience that differentiates psychodrama from simple role-playing or acting from a written script.

In psychodrama, it is consistently observed that one individual is able to play the role of another, whom he has neither seen nor met, sufficiently well to provide a genuine encounter with the person in whose psychodrama scene he plays a part. Participants are constantly amazed at the genuine nature of the interaction in a psychodrama session and will often remark, "That's exactly what *she* said!" or "That's *him* all right!" Moreno developed the concept of "tele," derived from the Greek word meaning "far," to explain the understanding that develops between members of a cohesive group. This telic relationship accounts for the congruence of choices made by members of such a group beyond that possible by chance alone. Part of the formal psychodrama session is devoted to the development of a cohesive group feeling among the participants. Choices made by the protagonist (the subject of a psychodrama session) will reflect his telic relationships with others in the group. Moreno was very much interested in the structure of human groups. He developed the science of sociometry as a way to measure and describe this structure by asking group members to make a number of specific choices. The theory of sociometry has proven useful in a great variety of group settings, but particularly in the psychodrama group.

Sociodrama is the term applied to the use of psychodramatic methods to explore intergroup and intragroup rather than interpersonal and intrapsychic problems. A shared problem of the group is selected to be worked out on the stage rather than an individual personal problem. Sociometry is of considerable value in structuring such sessions. An exposition of these and other concepts may be found in the works of Moreno (1959, 1964, 1969, 1972, 1975).

Psychodrama as a Set of Techniques. The techniques developed by Moreno derived originally from his knowledge of the theater and his studies of the play of children. He experimented early in his career with spontaneous dramas such as the "talking newspaper" and established his Theater of Spontaneity in Vienna in 1922. Only gradually did this experimental theater become a method of psychotherapy. Techniques developed in psychodrama have been widely applied to other forms of treatment, and to child-rearing, education, training, and human-engineering settings.

The comments below concerning the use of psychodrama in alcoholism treatment are based on the author's 12 years of experience with psychodrama as part of the treatment program at the Charles K. Post Alcoholism Rehabilitation Unit at Central Islip Psychiatric Center in New York.

WHY PSYCHODRAMA IN ALCOHOLISM TREATMENT?

Studies of persons entering treatment for alcoholism show that as a group they are isolated, anxious, depressed, low in self-esteem, and often cut off from their feelings. They have become dependent on alcohol as a means of relief from painful emotional states and characteristically utilize the defenses of denial and rationalization to maintain their drinking behavior. Although longitudinal studies suggest that these alcoholic people may not have started out with these traits (McCord and McCord, 1962; Jones, 1968, 1971; Loper, Kammeier, and Hoffman, 1973), the alcoholic patient in treatment presents this complex clinical picture plus a full range of associated psychological, social, and sexual problems. Treatment strives to break through the human isolation and to relieve the alcoholic's anxiety and depression through insight and corrective emotional experience. The psychodramatist sees the therapeutic encounter as the ideal tool for this purpose. He sees each patient surrounded by his own social atom, which can be explored and enlarged through treatment. He sees each human interaction as an opportunity to examine the surplus reality that constitutes the subjective experience of each individual, leading to both insight and corrective experience.

Psychodramatic methods also facilitate the exploration of those sources of frustration, depression, anxiety, anger, loneliness, and despair which led the individual to rely on drinking for relief in the past. They allow the patient to try out new creative solutions to these life problems as they are identified. A patient can experiment, on the psychodrama stage, with expressing his feelings instead of hiding them or, on the other hand, controlling his emotional expression instead of flying into a rage. He can try staying in a situation instead of running away, or he can beat a timely retreat instead of remaining and accepting abuse. He can try giving in or holding out, expressing love or expressing anger, saying "yes" or saying "no."

Because of the emphasis on action in the here-and-now, the patient can be brought in touch with feelings from which he is otherwise cut off, freeing his spontaneity. Playing roles in the psychodramas of his fellow patients also develops spontaneity, since there is no way he can rehearse or prepare in advance what he will say. Shy or repressed patients may start off playing simple roles as characters peripheral to a scene, such as a bartender, waitress, or bus driver, or even an animal, to help them overcome their self-consciousness about participating.

The development of tele, the emotional cement of the group, can be helpful in overcoming individual isolation. Interrelatedness and identification developed in the psychodrama group can then be transferred to other therapy groups or to Alcoholics Anonymous.

Psychodrama can also prepare the alcoholic patient for difficult future situations. Behaviorist views of alcoholism stress environmental cues and stimuli that trigger drinking behavior. Such situational cues can be recreated in psychodramatic terms and alternative behaviors practiced. Psychodrama facilitates active rehearsal for situations of great stress such as job interviews, social affairs, being speaker at an AA meeting, or facing former drinking friends.

A frequently encountered problem in the treatment of alcoholic patients is their tendency to develop strong dependency ties to the therapist. This is less so in group psychotherapy than in individual therapy, but even less so in psychodrama. The director is never thrust into the role of giving advice, interpreting the patient's behavior, or doing favors for the patient. On the other hand, the protagonist usually forms an affectionate bond with the director in a psychodrama session, as he does as well with his double (see Techniques to Intensify Emotional Involvement and Expression and to Reach Action-Insight, below), certain auxiliaries, and members of the group who share feelings with him.

The formal psychodrama is seldom used alone as a treatment method. It is usually part of an organized alcoholism program, in either an inpatient, day care, or outpatient setting. It is combined with alcoholism education, individual and group psychotherapy, family treatment, AA, and other approaches. In such a multimodality treatment setting there is a spillover of material and techniques. Difficult problems arising in the therapy group will be chosen as subjects for psychodrama. Members of the audience particularly moved by a psychodrama session will find new areas to explore in individual or group therapy. Members of therapy groups will break spontaneously into role-playing, doubling, or role-reversal. Problems arising between groups of patients or patients and staff will be worked out sociodramatically.

A recent study by Wood and his colleagues at the U.S. Navy Alcoholism Rehabilitation Center at San Diego compared two groups of alcoholic patients (Wood et al., 1978). One group of 36 patients was treated with four psychodrama sessions weekly, while the second group of 65 patients participated in small-group therapy. Their treatment was otherwise identical. The patients in the psychodrama group had been selected for this therapy modality by their counselors. Although the two groups did not differ demographically, the psychodrama group showed significantly lower scores on five Comrey Personality Scales before treatment. In spite of these indications of greater initial pathology, this group did not differ from the controls at posttreatment testing. Both groups made significant gains in many areas, with the psychodrama group showing significantly greater gains in the area of activity. This interesting study, demonstrating the value of psychodrama in alcoholism treatment, should be followed up by a comparison of outcomes for these groups.

THE FORMAL PSYCHODRAMA

Setting. The formal psychodrama is held if possible in a room with a raised platform or stage. This stage helps to demarcate the action area and separate it from the audience. A stage with several levels allows the symbolic use of these steps to represent levels of reality or levels of involvement in the action. A small balcony easily reached from the stage lends added possibilities in dramatizing relationships and enacting scenes. Variable lighting and the availability of spotlights also provide added dimensions to the psychodrama enactments. Although helpful to work with, none of this special equipment is absolutely necessary. A large room may have one area set aside as a stage simply by grouping the chairs in a semicircle. Height and distance can be obtained in the absence of a balcony by having a participant stand on a table or chair. Props required are very simple. A few chairs, a small table, a pillow, a cup, or a newspaper are usually easily obtainable and sufficient for most sessions. The room used for psychodrama should allow privacy. Casual visitors walking in and out will interfere with group cohesion and may break the continuity of the session.

Size of the Group and Time Required. Formal psychodramas are often conducted in quite large group settings as demonstrations or open public sessions. In the ongoing treatment of the alcoholic patient, however, smaller groups of between 10 and 30 are preferable. The larger size allows for the inclusion of small numbers of students or visitors without overwhelming the patient group.

The time allotted for a session will vary with the treatment setting. A minimum of one and a half hours is usually required to allow sufficient time for warm-up, enactment, and sharing. Time must also be available for a certain amount of postpsychodrama interaction with group members who seem unusually moved by the session, particularly in outpatient settings. If possible, it is desirable to schedule some other therapeutic activity following the psychodrama.

Roles in the Formal Psychodrama. The director is the primary therapist and bears overall responsibility for the psychodrama. The director should be appropriately trained and experienced in the method. He may have a background in psychiatry, psychology, social work, counseling, or any of the psychotherapies. No single field of study in mental health is prerequisite for training in psychodrama. Training may be obtained through the Moreno Institute in Beacon, New York, or at other training institutes in the United States and abroad.

Participants in ongoing psychodrama groups should be screened by the director, who should be acquainted with the patient's history, diagnosis, and present situation. It is important that any medical conditions that would limit the patient's physical ability to participate, such as heart disease, epilepsy, or low-back problems be known to the director so that he may proceed accordingly.

The director conducts the warm-up, chooses the protagonist (the subject of the psychodramatic enactment), directs the enactment in cooperation with the protagonist, and leads the sharing. A feeling of trust must exist between director and protagonist. The director encourages this by working with the protagonist within his own subjective reality and accepting that reality. The director does not order the protagonist around or force him to go into any material the protagonist does not feel ready to handle. He may urge the protagonist on or ask him to try alternatives, but never forces the issue. The protagonist agrees to confide in the director and group and to follow the suggestions made to him with as much spontaneity as possible. He trusts that the director will see to it that he is not injured in the process, but rather gains valuable insight and experience.

Roles other than that of the protagonist are played by group members called "auxiliaries" or "auxiliary egos." These may be staff members, trainees, or patients who are members of the group. The director usually allows the protagonist to choose his own auxiliaries ("Is there anyone in the room who could play your mother? Choose someone that reminds you in some way of her or could be her.") so that the tele developed between group members can be given maximum play. On the other hand, he may ask a trained auxiliary to step in for a special purpose or choose a shy group member for a small role in order to help him overcome his reluctance to get up on stage. Auxiliaries may play roles of the opposite sex and of ages different from their own. The auxiliary attempts as far as possible to abandon his own identity and adopt that of the person whose part he has assumed. There are a number of techniques available to help the auxiliary assume his role.

The remainder of the group constitutes the audience. The audience takes active part in both the warm-up and sharing. During the enactment, the individuals in the group react to the scenes on stage and identify with the participants. At times, the audience may cheer or applaud. At other times the audience may play a group role as called for in the action, such as an AA group, a baseball team, or the children in a summer camp.

Possible Dangers of Psychodrama.   Like any other psychotherapeutic method, psychodrama is a potent tool that can harm as well as heal. For this reason the role of director should not be assumed by an untrained person. In the heat of an enacted scene a protagonist will often express long-buried feelings such as sexual desire, hatred, or the urge to kill. The director must be trained and prepared to handle such situations in a way that will allow the protagonist to integrate these feelings with others in his life without experiencing undue horror or guilt. The director must be able to reach closure in each enactment, bringing the final scene to an end in a positive, supportive way. The protagonist must not be left hanging in an unresolved conflict or in a posture of utter hopelessness as the enactment ends. For a description of closure, refer to Techniques to Effect Closure, below.

The director must also see that the psychodrama group does not scapegoat one of its number and must keep in touch with the feelings, mood, and responses of the audience as well as those of the participants on stage. If he feels that the audience is losing interest or reacting negatively, he may stop and ask for feedback. This is often helpful, since the audience may have noticed something important that he has overlooked. At minimum, it keeps the audience involved and prevents their abandoning the protagonist.

If the group has trouble sharing with the protagonist at the conclusion of the psychodrama, the director must stimulate interaction. He and the auxiliaries may share their own feelings and experiences. This will prevent the protagonist from feeling isolated and will help him reenter the group.

The author's experience with psychodrama has been confined to the treatment of the alcoholic patient who is free of psychosis. Although psychodrama has been employed in the treatment of psychotic patients in other settings, its use with psychotic alcoholics has not been reported.

The Warm-Up.   As the group assembles for a psychodrama session, each member carries into the room, not only an individual life history and set of problems, but also a current mood, attitude, and set of expectations. Time of day, weather, season, preceding activities and events, and physical factors will influence the mood of the individual. Group members' interactions before the session begins will influence each other's feelings as well. The director may be present as the group assembles or enter later. He observes the seating arrangements chosen by the members of the audience, their levels of activity, their postures, and other nonverbal cues. From these and his own casual interactions with members of the group, he gets a sense of mood and level of group cohesion. The director also enters the room with his own set of feelings and expectations. It is the function of the warm-up period to develop sufficient interrelatedness among the group members and between the group and director to allow the therapeutic enactment to begin.

The warm-up may involve anything from a brief verbal interaction in a group that is accustomed to working together, to a prolonged introduction and formal group exercise in a large group new to one another. In general the director tends to move around the stage and encourage members to do so as well, so that they prepare for action. Members of the group are called up on stage and asked to choose others to join them. As the director interacts with these members, he trusts his own empathic or telic sense to choose a protagonist with whom he feels he can work.

As the warm-up concludes, the director asks the other participants to resume their seats in the audience and begins to focus on the protagonist whose particular subjective reality will be enacted. A general or specific problem is chosen by mutual agreement. The director conducts a very brief interview on stage, sufficient only to choose the scene in which to begin the action. At the conclusion of the warm-up, the director may alter the lighting in the room to dim the audience area and brighten the stage.

The Enactment. To move from warm-up to enactment, the director helps the protagonist set the scene. If the problem is a patient's relationship with her mother, for example, the director may ask where she usually sees her mother or where she last saw her. She may be asked to create that setting on the stage by physically placing chairs to represent furniture, indicating the placement of windows, doors, and pictures, and describing her feelings about the room as she walks through it in the here-and-now. If she seems insufficiently warmed up, she may be asked to play the role of an object in the room and comment on the room's history and the people it has seen.

The protagonist is asked to choose auxiliaries to play the roles of others in the scene. Each auxiliary is warmed up to his role by the protagonist with the director's help. The protagonist always addresses the auxiliary as the person in his life in the here-and-now. For example, a protagonist has chosen a fellow patient to play the role of his wife. She will be encouraged to ask, "What do you call me?" "What am I like?" He may reply, "I usually call you Honey, although your real name is Harriet. You call me Honey too unless you're angry, and then it's Richard. You are in your late 50s but can pass for 35 and you're proud of it." The director may ask the protagonist to reverse roles with the auxiliary and become his wife. The director may then interview him in that role ("Your husband tells us that you're 58. You certainly don't look it! Tell us how you feel about that." "How do you feel about your marriage?") or ask for a self-presentation ("Mrs.———, please tell us about yourself.") When the auxiliaries feel sufficiently warmed to their roles, the action can begin.

Scenes generally move from the less emotionally charged to the more emotional. A protagonist trying to handle his relationship with a dying parent may start with a childhood memory and work through an adult encounter before enacting a deathbed scene. A current problem situation may lead backward to a childhood experience or forward to a future event. An enactment that begins as the recreation of a protagonist's dream may lead to an important interpersonal encounter. The director strives to help the protagonist approach his problems with new insight and spontaneity. Special techniques used to intensify involvement and emotional expression, such as the double or alter ego, are described under Techniques to Intensify Emotional Involvement and Expression and to Reach Action-Insight, below.

The enactment ends with some kind of conclusion or closure to the problem presented. This may involve a successful replay of an originally unsuccessful life experience, a reconciliation with an important person, or a break with some aspect of the past. The director asks the protagonist and sometimes the auxiliaries to sit with him on the stage to begin the sharing. Lights are turned up if they have been dimmed, and the audience again becomes part of the action.

Sharing. The formal psychodrama ends with a period of sharing of feelings and experience. The members of the group have the opportunity to share with the protagonist and one another the reactions and feelings that developed during the session. They are asked to confine their comments to personal expressions of their own experience and refrain from analyzing the protagonist's actions, asking questions, or giving advice. The statement, "I feel you were really jealous of your brother" is not accepted as a shared feeling. "I had a brother too, and I was so jealous of him that I guess I never really got to know him as a person," or "I can identify with your brother in that scene, because I have an older sister who acted a lot like you did. I'm still not close to her" would be accepted. Members of the group who feel particularly close to the protagonist may share a handshake or an embrace as well as a comment. Sharing helps the protagonist and the group to reenter the real world. Group members often express new insights into their own problems gained during the session and thank the protagonist for his help. Some typical examples are: "I used to drink the way you did. I really saw myself up there as you went through that scene. I always used to say I was only hurting myself with my drinking, but now I can see that wasn't true. I'm going to have to work out a way to let my kids know that."

"This session really helped me understand why I'm always uncomfortable around my in-laws, and always looking for an excuse to get out of the house. Maybe they're not such terrible people, but the problem is really between my wife and me." "I can see that I make myself lonely by driving people away with my drinking. There are plenty of people in my life too who are willing to help if I let them." "I really admire the way you spoke up to your boss. I've always been scared to death of authority."

A statement made in the sharing will sometimes lead to an invitation to be protagonist at the next session or a suggestion to bring the problem up in group or individual therapy.

TECHNIQUES USED IN PSYCHODRAMA

Subjectivity. The subjective reality of the protagonist is always respected. He is not expected to present a total picture of his life or a balanced view of each member of his social atom. He presents only the aspects important to the scene enacted. He is instructed to correct the auxiliaries or his double if what they do or say is not appropriate. The director will often have him reverse roles with the auxiliary to correct him and regain the flow of the scene. If the director is unsure, he will stop and ask the protagonist, "Is this right? Is this the way it was?" Auxiliaries try to take their lead from the protagonist rather than inventing directions of their own. The director, however, may suggest a line of action to an auxiliary, such as, "See if you can get her to tell you whether she's been drinking" or "Don't give in so easily this time," if he is interested in developing an insight or obtaining deeper emotional involvement of the protagonist.

Time and Space. One of the greatest advantages of psychodramatic technique is its ability to move in time and space. A relationship may be explored forward and backward in time and in both reality and fantasy. This time flexibility allows the same scene to be replayed over and over, each time exploring a new dimension, and finally experimenting with new problem-solving approaches.

The stage may be divided into areas representing time periods such as past, present, and future, childhood and adulthood, or active alcoholism and sobriety. When the protagonist is in the designated area of the stage, he is in that period of time. Auxiliaries may be asked to play the role of the protagonist past, present, or future, drunk or sober, so that he may interact with those aspects of himself.

Space may be used to symbolize emotional relationships. A father who is perceived as powerful and critical may stand on a table while talking to the protagonist. A mother who is seen as distant and unconcerned may turn her back or be placed at the edge of the stage. A protagonist pleading or humbling himself may be placed on one knee. An auxiliary may be instructed to move closer to the protagonist when he feels warmth and love communicated and to move away when he feels rejection.

The "family portrait" is an interesting application of this principle. A subject is asked to place auxiliaries representing the various members of his family in postures and spatial relations to one another which symbolize emotional relationships. He then may place himself or an auxiliary representing himself in the grouping. Such an exercise may serve as an effective warm-up. The subject is asked to step out of the picture and address the family members, expressing his feelings about them, thus beginning the enactment. The same technique may be used during an enactment to clarify the interrelationships in a group being studied on stage. The protagonist may be asked to construct the grouping and then alter it to represent his ideal conception of how it should be. This helps develop insight into ways to improve the disturbed relationships in his life.

The stage area may represent the protagonist's life space, so that he may symbolically throw a person out of his life by pushing an auxiliary (or a chair, which may be thrown or kicked) off the stage. Some protagonists have gently escorted such an auxiliary out of the psychodrama theater, down the hall, and out the front door of the building in a fine exercise of spontaneity. In alcoholism treatment it is often useful to have an auxiliary play the role of alcohol or drinking. This helps the alcoholic protagonist and audience understand the role of drinking in their lives. Alcohol as a character may insert itself in a current family portrait. It sometimes ends up ejected from the stage but calling out, "I'll always be waiting out here if you want me."

Adjustable lighting helps create shifts in time and space on the stage. However, in its absence, the protagonist can be asked to look through an imaginary window and describe the scene, and the director can help by taking off a jacket if the scene shifts to summer or by remarking on the cold and darkness, etc.

Techniques to Help Set the Scene. It is helpful in beginning an enactment with a frightened or repressed protagonist to warm him to the scene as thoroughly as possible. Physical action in moving the chairs around on the stage is helpful in releasing spontaneity. Walking around the scene while describing it also helps. As noted under The Enactment, above, the protagonist may be asked to play the role of a picture on the wall or some other object in a room. If the scene is outdoors, the entire psychodrama theater and the space around it may be used to represent the scene, and the protagonist may be asked to walk around the theater observing, commenting, and thinking aloud. If the scene is a beach and the audience is the sea, he may "swim" through the theater.

Auxiliaries may help set the scene through doubling (see below) or playing appropriate roles. Adjustments of lighting as well as appropriate sound effects provided by the audience also help.

Techniques to Warm Up to a New Role.   The auxiliary asked to play a role in a psychodrama has a difficult task. He is asked to become someone he knows little or nothing about, sometimes literally a character in someone else's dream. In an ongoing alcoholism treatment situation, the auxiliaries are either staff members or fellow patients who usually know the protagonist and already identify with him in a number of ways. They do not usually know the role they are to play from the protagonist's point of view, however. In order to warm up the auxiliary, the director may ask the protagonist and auxiliary to reverse roles. The protagonist then makes a self-presentation, is interviewed, or strikes up a dialogue in his reversed role. The director checks with the auxiliary before starting the action to make sure he knows what he is expected to do. The director may help an auxiliary with suggestions during the action.

The major technique used for turning the auxiliary into the character being played is role-reversal during the enactment itself. For example, a protagonist recreates a scene in which he comes home late from work. The auxiliary playing his wife angrily accuses him of drinking. They argue and he blurts out, "Why the hell did you marry me instead of Jack anyhow?" The auxiliary may do one of several things: reflect the question, "Why do you think I married you?"; ignore the question, "Damn it, you're drunk again"; or respond, "I've often wondered that myself." On the other hand, the director will often stop and reverse roles, asking the auxiliary, now in the role of the husband, to repeat his last line, and giving the protagonist, now playing his wife, a chance to answer the question himself. At times a protagonist virtually plays both roles himself, with the auxiliary simply repeating comments he has already made.

The director may provide an auxiliary with a double. If an auxiliary is stiff or self-conscious in a role, the director may ask the double (see below) to trade roles with the auxiliary, or allow someone else to play the role. Such choices are made as the action develops according to the needs of the situation.

Techniques to Intensify Emotional Involvement and Expression and to Reach Action-Insight. Since recognition and expression of emotion are goals of psychodrama in alcoholism treatment, the director strives to involve the protagonist as much as possible in the emotional reality of the scene. Catharsis of negative feeling sometimes uncovers buried feelings of love and warmth toward an important person and allows forgiveness or reconciliation. Feelings of fear or resentment may be buried under surface feelings of respect or gratitude and may also be uncovered. Protagonists present very different levels of ability to express their feelings on stage.

To intensify recognition and expression of emotion, the technique of the "double" or "alter ego" is employed. The double stands next to and slightly behind the protagonist so that he sees and hears the same communications from the others in the scene. He adopts the same general posture as the protagonist and follows him in moving about the stage. Through this posture, communication, and his telic relationship with the protagonist, he gets a sense of the protagonist's feelings, which he then verbalizes. "I feel uncomfortable up here," "This guy is really getting me angry," or "God, I need a drink" are typical examples. If the statement of the double is accurate, it helps the protagonist get in touch with his feelings. If it is not, he will reject the statement, correct the double, or just ignore him. Often the protagonist calls out "Right!" or "You said it" when the double is on target. The double may sometimes, representing conscience or inner thought, ask a question or make a comment such as, "What's wrong with me? Why can't I tell him what I really feel?" or "If I pick up that drink now, it won't end there."

When the protagonist is in conflict with himself, multiple doubles may be chosen to represent his conflicting desires or values. In treating alcoholic patients, the *to drink or not to drink* conflict is often explored in this way.

Role-reversal is another technique for intensifying emotion, as is the use of "mirroring." In the mirroring technique, action is stopped and the audience is asked if one or more members would like to act out in pantomime some aspect of the human relationship being enacted on stage. Observing his action in such a "mirror" helps the protagonist understand his behavior and see aspects of himself otherwise hidden. Such understanding is referred to as action-insight because it derives from active involvement rather than contemplation or intellectual analysis.

Techniques to Develop Insight into the Feelings and Behavior of Others.   The reversal of roles between the protagonist and others affords a unique opportunity for the protagonist to understand the points of view of the important people in his life. Dr. and Mrs. Moreno have recommended role-reversal as a useful technique in normal child-rearing. Often such an experience represents the first time an individual has ever tried to understand others. The protagonist may protest that he cannot possibly guess what the other person may think. This is usually a form of resistance, which may be overcome with gentle urging or role-modeling by the director.

The protagonist can also learn a lot by being pulled out of a scene and observing a replay of the same situation with someone else playing his part. This is similar to the technique of mirroring. If the protagonist is stuck in a rut and cannot think of an adequate solution to a problem on stage,the director may invite others in the group to try the protagonist's role in the same scene, utilizing their own spontaneity to search for a solution as the protagonist observes and comments.

Techniques to Effect Closure.   Once the life problem presented by the protagonist has been explored in the psychodrama session, the director moves to conclude the enactment and begin the sharing. In order to do so, the director must reach a natural stopping point, or closure, which does not leave the protagonist in a state of unresolved conflict or utter defeat. Since the time allotted to the session is limited, the director must keep an eye on the clock and choose an objective for the session that can be accomplished in the time available. Some scenes will reach closure naturally as a result of their enactment alone—for example, with a reconciliation or a breaking off of a relationship. In other cases, the director will suggest a means to close.

Closure may sometimes be reached by asking the protagonist to confront each of the other characters in the enactment in turn and tell them exactly how he feels about them. The director may ask the protagonist to replay the problem scene trying a new approach. Members of the audience may help if the protagonist is stumped.

The director may switch scenes from one of past defeat to a future scene of success. For example, a man bitter about his wife's desertion may choose an ideal second wife from the audience and enact a scene ten years in the future, when, sober and happily remarried, he looks back upon his old experience. A patient reliving a scene of parental rejection he cannot otherwise handle can be given an ideal parent who loves him in a final scene. If a protagonist seems overwhelmed by many current problems, the director may ask a number of auxiliaries to link arms around him in a tight circle, representing his present problems. The protagonist must physically break out of the circle through his own efforts, cheered on and applauded by the group. A protagonist who has been settling old business with a long-dead person in his life may finally bury that person, conduct a funeral, and mourn him.

Types of Warm-Ups. The type of warm-up used in a given session will depend on the emotional state of the group and director. A small ongoing group may be ready to work before the session begins, with a protagonist and problem already chosen. A larger, less cohesive group in which many members are afraid of participating presents a very different problem.

In such a group the director may invite a group member on stage with him "just for a minute" to study the seating arrangement and postures of members of the audience. He is then asked to rearrange the group to his taste, usually asking those hiding in the rear to come down front. When this is done with good humor, and the backing of the director, it is usually much enjoyed by shy, inhibited people.

Getting the audience to stand up and move around is also useful in developing interrelationships and freeing spontaneity. Many warm-up exercises involve dividing the audience in pairs or small groups and giving them a simple task such as "Choose one of your group to be drunk and the others try to help him" or "One of you wants to drink and the others try to stop him." As the groups report back on their experiences in the exercise, a protagonist is chosen for the deeper exploration of a problem.

Another warm-up frequently used is asking a group member to come up on the stage and say a few words about himself, then bring another member on stage to do the same, and resume his seat. As the "human chain" continues, the director is able to make contact with a sufficient number of group members to choose a protagonist.

The group may be warmed up by means of a guided fantasy. The group members are asked to relax and close their eyes. The director suggests the beginning of the fantasy, for example, "You receive a package as a gift. It is beautifully wrapped. You wonder what's inside and who sent it. Open it," or "You've just won a raffle; a trip to anywhere in the world with anyone you like." The participants complete the fantasies, then come on stage one by one to describe them, until an appropriate protagonist is selected.

An empty chair may be placed on stage and the members of the

PSYCHODRAMA AND THE TREATMENT OF ALCOHOLISM

group asked to imagine anyone they choose in the chair. Selected participants then have the opportunity to converse with this person psychodramatically. A similar warm-up involves composing a letter to someone with whom the group members have unfinished business.

Group members may be asked to remember something personal, such as their first drink, their last drink, a scene from childhood, a time when they felt content in the past, a vivid dream, or a moment of intense pleasure. Any of these memories will lead to a psychodramatic enactment. Many other warm-ups are improvised on the spot in response to the needs of the moment.

APPLICATION OF PSYCHODRAMA TECHNIQUES IN ALCOHOLISM EDUCATION AND TREATMENT SETTINGS

In addition to their use in the formal psychodrama session, described under The Formal Psychodrama, above, psychodramatic techniques find wide application in other methods of alcoholism treatment. An excellent example is the technique of role-reversal, which can be used in program administration, interviewing, individual psychotherapy, couples' therapy, family therapy, and group psychotherapy, and as a teaching device. A patient who is asking to leave treatment prematurely may be given psychodramatic insight into his behavior, through role-reversal (Blume et al., 1968). A patient at a staff conference may reverse roles with the interviewer, and in effect interview himself. A patient begging for advice in an individual therapy session may be asked to change seats with the therapist and reply to the request himself. Role-reversal is tremendously helpful in marital and family therapy in developing insights into others' points of view. In a therapy group the technique may be used in the same way to analyze group dynamics. On the other hand, for example, a group member who has delivered a long complaint about someone in his life outside the group can be asked to sit in another chair and answer the complaint in the role of the other person. The use of a double will intensify the impact of the role-reversal in the staff-interview or group-therapy setting.

Group role-reversal is a useful technique for teaching groups who visit an alcoholism treatment unit (Blume, 1971). Instead of the usual lecture and tour of the building, the group is given a brief introduction to alcoholism treatment and is seated in a circle in alternate seats with an equal number of patient volunteers. After introducing themselves to one another, the group is instructed that they are to reverse roles. The visitors become patients in treatment for alcoholism and the patients become visitors (social workers, medical students, or whatever).

In these roles a group discussion is begun. The patients in their new roles delight in asking the newly designated "patients" about their drinking, their motivation, their insight, and their treatment. The visitors cast suddenly in this role must search themselves for an understanding of the alcoholic person and the patient role. Soon they also warm to the task of questioning the "visitors" about their views on alcoholism and how they as professionals feel qualified to help. The leader tries to keep the discussion moving and give all participants a chance to contribute. The roles are then reversed again for feedback and further discussion. The session ends with each participant in turn sharing his or her reaction to the session.

Psychodrama techniques lend themselves very well to the training of alcoholism therapists. One such training group begins with a guided fantasy dealing with an alcoholic person. "Picture an alcoholic standing before you. Try to see the person as clearly as possible. Notice the posture, the clothing, the facial expression, the hair. The alcoholic person now begins to come slowly toward you. Finish the fantasy in any way you like." Each therapist in this fantasy will summon up the image of an alcoholic person important in his life. Often it is a difficult patient with whom the therapist is failing or has failed. Sometimes it is a relative or close friend. At times, when the therapist is a recovering alcoholic, he sees his former self. In each case there is an encounter relating to the treatment of alcoholism, the surplus reality of which can be both explored psychodramatically and analyzed from a didactic point of view. Since the participants always choose important people, the enactments are always interesting and emotionally significant. Similar training groups can be run using alternate warm-ups designed to bring out the attitudes, frustrations, and personal feelings of therapists about their work.

Sociodrama applies psychodramatic techniques to the exploration and solution of intra- and intergroup problems. Sociodramatic methods can be used to approach problems that arise between groups of patients or between patients and staff in a residential treatment setting. The warm-up delineates the problem in general terms. The director may ask the group to measure its own attitudes by having the two ends of the room represent the extremes of opinion on the subject and having each person place himself in the room according to his opinion, a proportionate distance from each end of the room. A spokesman or small group is chosen to represent each point of view and the group reassembles. After each side presents its views, the director asks the spokesmen to reverse roles. This process continues, developing mutual understanding so that some solution can be reached.

Case Histories

M.L., a 51-year-old self-employed businessman had just entered the unit for alcoholism rehabilitation when he found that his business was in peril and could be saved only by an immediate trip to Europe. He was full of anxiety and had virtually no confidence in his ability to remain sober during the trip, but he also felt that if he drank his mission would be unsuccessful. He was unable to take disulfiram for physical reasons. He was invited to be protagonist in psychodrama on the morning of his leaving the unit. He told the group of his predicament and his fears, shaking visibly and in great distress. The director began the enactment with a scene two weeks in the future, in which the protagonist, having returned successfully from Europe and reentered the program, was invited on stage to tell the group how he had managed the trip sober. It was made clear that the trip was successfully behind him. He relaxed visibly, smiled at the group and told of his trip. The director then had him enact the scenes of his greatest temptation: the airplane, the business meeting, and alone in the hotel room. With the aid of a double, he demonstrated how he used memories of his treatment and the AA philosophy to resist the urge to drink. Since the outcome was predetermined by the director, the protagonist handled these scenes well. The group was very supportive. He was able to manage the trip successfully in real life, and he reported back that the psychodrama enactment had helped greatly. Some of the scenes on the stage had actually occurred, and having handled them on stage gave him confidence. He felt almost amused to see "life mimic art."

H.F., a 41-year-old divorced alcoholic woman, the only child of a borderline psychotic mother, was severely abused during her childhood. She had broken off contact with her mother in adult life in spite of severe guilt feelings about the break. As her life began to change for the better as a result of her treatment, she began to have the irrational fear that her mother would reappear in her life and take away her newly found happiness. She was protagonist in a psychodrama in which this fear was explored. Her mother (played by an auxiliary) phoned her and first begged to resume their relationship, then threatened. The protagonist, with the help of a double, was able to express first her guilt, then her deeply felt anger toward her mother. She realized by the end of the scene that her mother could hurt her only if she herself allowed it. She was much relieved and went on to a stable recovery from her alcoholism. Some years later, her mother did contact her and they met a few times. She stated that the psychodrama and the insight she gained from it were very much on her mind during these encounters and helped her to resist without guilt her mother's attempts to reestablish a destructive relationship.

Summary

The formal psychodrama as a method of group psychotherapy, the insights derived from psychodrama into spontaneity and creativity, and the techniques derived from psychodrama used in related settings have all been successfully applied to the treatment of the alcoholic patient. Psychodrama is usually part of an organized multimodal rehabilitation program. As such it adds the important dimension of here-and-now action to the treatment process. It is also useful in the administration of such a program and in the training of treatment personnel.

References

Blume, S. B. Group role reversal as a teaching technique in an alcoholism rehabilitation unit. *Group Psychotherapy and Psychodrama*, 1971, 24, 135–137.

Blume, S. B. Psychodrama and alcoholism. *Annals of the New York Academy of Sciences*, 1974, 233, 123–127.

Blume, S. B. Psychodrama in the treatment of alcoholism. In N. Estes and E. Heinemann (Eds.), *Alcoholism, development, consequences and interventions*. (2nd ed.) St. Louis: C. V. Mosby, 1982.

Blume, S. B., Robins, J., and Branston, A. Psychodrama techniques in the treatment of alcoholism. *Group Psychotherapy and Psychodrama*, 1968, 21, 241–246.

Cabrera, F. J. Group psychotherapy and psychodrama for alcoholic patients in a state rehabilitation program. *Group Psychotherapy*, 1961, 14, 154–159.

Fairchild, D. M. The use of psychodrama in treating the alcoholic patient. *Alcoholism Review*, 1973, 12, 7–12.

Fox, R. Group psychotherapy with alcoholics. *International Journal of Group Psychotherapy*, 1961, 12, 56–63.

Jones, M. C. Personality correlates and antecedents of drinking patterns in adult males. *Journal of Consulting and Clinical Psychiatry*, 1968, 32, 2–12.

Jones, M. C. Personality antecedents and correlates of drinking patterns in women. *Journal of Consulting and Clinical Psychology*, 1971, 36, 61–69.

Loper, R. G., Kammeier, M. L., and Hoffman, H. M.M.P.I characteristics of college freshmen males who later became alcoholics. *Journal of Abnormal Psychology*, 1973, 82, 159–162.

McCord, W., and McCord, J. A longitudinal study of the personality of alcoholics. In D. J. Pittman and C. R. Snyder (Eds.), *Society, culture, and drinking patterns*. New York: Wiley, 1962.

Moreno, J. L. Psychodrama. In S. Arieti (Ed.), *American handbook of psychiatry*. Vol. 2. New York: Basic Books, 1959.

Moreno, J. L. *Psychodrama*. Vol. 2. New York: Beacon House, 1959.

Moreno, J. L. *Psychodrama*. Vol. 1. New York: Beacon House, 1964.

Moreno, J. L. *Psychodrama*. Vol. 3. New York: Beacon House, 1969.

Moreno, J. L. Psychodrama. In H. Kaplan and B. J. Sadock (Eds.), *Comprehensive group psychotherapy*. Baltimore: Williams and Wilkins, 1972.

Moreno, J. L. Psychodrama. In A. M. Freedman, H. I. Kaplan, and B. J. Sadock (Eds.), *Comprehensive textbook of psychiatry—II*. Baltimore: Williams and Wilkins, 1975.

Paley, M. G. Human drama in the treatment of hospitalized alcoholics. *Alcohol Health and Research World*, 1979, *4*, 43–47.

Van Gee, S. J. Alcoholism and the family: A psychodrama approach. *JPN and Mental Health Services*, 1979, *17*, 9–12.

Von Meulenbrouck, M. A serial psychodrama with alcoholics. *Group Psychotherapy and Psychodrama*, 1972, *25*, 151–154.

Weiner, H. Treating the alcoholic with psychodrama. *Group Psychotherapy*, 1965, *18*, 27–49.

Wood, D., Del Nuovo, A., Michalik, M., Schein, S., and Bucky, S. Psychodrama with an alcohol abuse population. *Group Psychotherapy and Psychodrama*, 1978.

7

Behavioral Modification Methods as Adjuncts to Psychotherapy

atached top (handwritten)

John Wallace

Introduction

Behavioral modification methods are a collection of techniques useful in attempting to change behavior directly without reference to assumed underlying motivational factors. For the most part, these methods have their roots in modern theories of learning. However, they can be used effectively despite one's theoretical or ideological persuasion. They are not tied exclusively to a simplistic, learned behavior model of alcoholism that excludes biological factors, nor are their uses restricted to efforts to teach alcoholics how to control their drinking. Behavioral methods can be used in helping alcoholics to achieve initial abstention from alcohol and an eventual self-fulfilling sobriety.

In this chapter I will discuss the relevance of the behavioral modification tradition for psychotherapy of alcoholism. Along with accepted methods, I will discuss techniques of my own invention that have evolved directly from the practical business of alcoholism treatment.* Total behavioral treatment approaches, such as aversion therapy, are not considered.

---

* I am indebted to Muriel Zink for certain ideas concerning behavioral modification methods with alcoholics.

John Wallace • Director of Treatment, Edgehill Newport, Newport, Rhode Island.

109

Correct me, I don't understand Counselor task Help me understand (handwritten)

GENERALIZED HABIT-PATTERN-DISRUPTION TECHNIQUES

For many alcoholics, drinking is a greatly overlearned behavior. It is associated with many physical and social cues or stimuli. As a consequence, the *initiation* of drinking is under widespread external stimulus control. Drinking can begin in numerous situations in which the alcoholic has no conscious intention of drinking and, on occasion, cannot even remember when he actually started. Generalized habit-pattern-disruption techniques are designed to increase the alcoholic's awareness of situational determinants of his drinking and other behaviors.

Practicing the Opposite. In this method the alcoholic patient is directed to reverse the order and nature of his typical activities. He is asked to shave first in the morning if he had previously showered first and then shaved. He is instructed to leave and enter his bed from the right side if his typical pattern was to do so from the left. He is encouraged to perform simple activities like teeth brushing with his left hand rather than his right.

In general, the focus in this method is to concentrate upon simple, usual activities rather than more complex ones. Its purpose is to stimulate awareness of habitual ways of approaching and responding to typical situations. It is designed to promote the general outlook that the patient is actively and purposively engaged in changing his life. It also serves as an aid to emerging discriminations in the patient with regard to old ways of doing things and new ways.

Substitute Activities. The patient is encouraged to seek out alternative activities that do not involve drinking or drinking environments. If there was an identifiable temporal pattern to the patient's drinking, substitute activities are devised for these time periods. For example, a female patient sober for several months could not understand why she continued to feel agitated, anxious, and depressed. A careful analysis of her prior drinking revealed that her drinking usually began on Friday afternoons and continued on into the weekend. A further analysis revealed that her negative feelings in sobriety usually centered around Fridays and weekends. She was counseled to develop a schedule of enjoyable activities that did not involve drinking starting at Friday afternoon and carrying on through the weekend. After following this temporal rearrangement of her typical activities, she reported positive changes in mood, tension level, and general outlook.

Disruption of Typical Social Activities and Relationships. Because of the potency of previous social situations and relationships to perpetuate drinking, efforts are made to restructure the patient's social behaviors. He is counseled to stay away from old drinking situations and old drinking "buddies." Bars, poolrooms, night clubs, taverns, homes of friends who continue to drink heavily or alcoholically, and other such situations are to be avoided. For the alcoholic who drank "on the street," activities that place him in support systems that do not involve heavy drinking are located. Alcoholics will often resist such suggestions. They will try to remain sober while continuing to associate with actively alcoholic or heavily drinking friends. In some cases they will try to hang out in old drinking haunts, drinking soft drinks rather than beer, wine, or liquor. In most instances these continued associations with persons and places from the alcoholic past eventuate in a return to dangerous drinking.

Following the Drunk Through. Alcoholics rarely consider the likely negative consequences when initiating a given drinking episode. When I question patients as to what they had been thinking about when they decided to drink, various answers are forthcoming. Many patients say, "Nothing, I just wanted to drink." Others answer that they "wanted to get comfortable." "I wanted to get a glow on," is a common response along with "I wanted to get a little high."

Following the drunk through is a technique in which the delayed negative consequences of drinking are imagined along with the initial positive ones. Typically, I ask the patient to imagine himself in his own movie. I ask him to imagine vividly the entire drinking episode in terms of its serial progression from initial drinking to the finish. At each stage of the exercise, the patient is asked to pay close attention to his feelings.

This technique is similar but not identical to the formal behavioral modification procedure known as *covert sensitization* (Cautela, 1966). Covert sensitization is an attempt to condition imagined aversive stimuli to an imagined situation in which drinking might commence. Following the drunk through is not a conditioning procedure; it is an attempt to give the alcoholic a conceptual tool through which he can simulate the likely temporal arrangement of events and consequences of drinking. It is, in effect, an attentional-shifting device, one that forces the alcoholic beyond the initial positive expectations to awareness of delayed negative consequences. In this sense, the exercise is an attempt to disrupt the temporal sequencing of cognitive and behavioral events.

Attendance at Meetings of Alcoholics Anonymous. Efforts should be made to have the patient at least try out AA on an experimental basis. Patients should never be forced directly into such meetings, but the therapist should be willing and able to counter usual misconceptions, prejudices, and distortions of fact about AA. Attendance at AA meetings is, in effect, a behavioral change in the life of the alcoholic of significant proportions. Going to such meetings alters his typical schedule of activities, enables him to make new friendships, exposes him to a host of social supports and reinforcements, and permits him to gather information about other alcoholics and the disease of alcoholism very directly. In many respects AA itself is a behavioral change program in that it advocates practical methods of achieving and maintaining sobriety in the context of a community social-support network. *Positive reinforcement* (social recognition and status for staying sober), *social modeling* (the accessibility of role models and their behaviors for learning how to stay sober), *desensitization* (anxiety and guilt reduction through sharing of common experience, laughter and general merriment over past alcoholic behaviors, and a general atmosphere of social acceptance), and *cognitive behavioral change* (cognitive restructuring of self, behavior, and alcoholism) are aspects of AA that are most congruent with modern versions of behavior therapy.

DISCRIMINATING SOBER VERSUS ALCOHOLIC BEHAVIORS

Research has not generally supported the notion that an "alcoholic personality" exists and predates the onset of active alcoholism. Whether such a personality exists in isolation from the alcoholic experience itself is probably unknowable. It is more fruitful to think of the many commonalities apparent among alcoholics as *common outcomes* of alcoholism rather than as antecedent conditions. Along with sharing commonalities with other alcoholics in terms of outcomes, each alcoholic may also be seen as possessing unique responses to the disease and the particular form it has taken in his own life. It is useful in psychotherapy with the alcoholic to focus on both common and unique outcomes of alcoholism in terms of a collection of attitudes, feelings, beliefs, and behaviors that must be discriminated and contrasted with some alternative collection. In this sense, then, it is useful to talk about a drinking personality and a sober one. Techniques for sharpening this discrimination are important tools in the psychotherapist's repertoire of change methods.

Writing a Behavioral Inventory of Drinking. The simple act of helping the patient to write a behavioral inventory of his drinking is an effective means of sharpening the discrimination between alcoholic behaviors and sober ones. The patient is instructed to begin with his first remembered drinking episode, to write down exactly the circumstances and his actions, and to list the overt consequences. In this inventory no attempt is made to establish motivations for drinking or to gain insights into reasons for drinking. The writing is purely behavioral in the sense that it focuses entirely on situations, actions, and consequences. It is usual to proceed forward in time either in single years or blocks of years covering significant drinking episodes and periods from the beginning of the drinking up until the present. In the group context the therapist can use the patient as informant and write down the more significant details of the drinking history on a chalkboard so that these may be shared with all group members. In the group setting the behavioral inventory of drinking can be a dramatic technique, one loaded with sudden awarenesses and feelings. In a sense it is similar to the behavioral technique known as *flooding*, in which the patient is confronted with a rather massive stimulus configuration concerning a feared object, a lost loved one, or an anxiety-provoking situation. Many alcoholics have never viewed their drinking histories as a whole, but rather as fragmented and partial recollections. When confronted with the massive facts of their past behaviors, they are often visibly startled and provoked to new levels of awareness. And in the group setting this reaction is intensified. Of course the decision to utilize this technique in the group setting is dependent upon a number of factors—the patient's ego strength, trust in other group members, levels of guilt and anxiety, and so forth.

In addition to aiding discrimination between the alcoholic person and the sober one, this technique fosters an important temporal distinction. The patient is invited to consider his *past* and to differentiate it from his *present.* In a sense the behavioral inventory of drinking is one way for the patient to "punctuate" his life—to place a period or marker at a given point and to separate this from the present and the possibility of an alternative future. The idealized self-image or sober personality is seen as an open-ended and permeable self-construct capable of growth and change over time.

Cognitive Behavioral Sharpening. In this technique the patient is invited to have a conversation with himself. It is particularly effective in the group setting and is in fact a method I have derived from Gestalt group therapy (Perls, 1969).

The patient is given his choice of which of two chairs to sit in to begin the exercise. After choosing he is asked to announce which of his persons—the sober one or the alcoholic one—is seated in that particular chair. He is then asked to consider the other chair as containing his other person and then told to begin a conversation with the hypothetical other. In my experience patients rarely refuse the exercise and enter into it willingly. I am careful to keep reminding the patient of the distinction that is represented by the spatial separation of the chairs. I say such things as "O.K., the sober you is sitting in this chair, the other you is over there."

The patient is asked for a description of the sober person. After he has given this, he is asked to move across the space and to seat himself in the other chair. Once he is there, I ask, "Who is in this chair?" I then ask the patient to describe the drinking person. I then instruct the patient to return to the original chair, and again I remind him of who is in the first chair. Often the reminder is in the form of a question: "Now who is in this chair?" I ask the patient to talk to the other person, the hypothetical drinking person, with regard to such things as intentions, plans, wants, wishes, and aspirations. The situation is then reversed and the patient talks from the perspective of the drinking person to the hypothetical sober one. The patient is encouraged to continue his conversation, moving back and forth between the chairs throughout the exercise.

The purpose of this exercise is to sharpen and clarify the inner conflict commonly encountered in patients early in their recovery. The patient quickly realizes that he wants both to drink and to stay sober and, moreover, he is a mass of other contradictory impulses, attitudes, feelings, goals, intentions, and beliefs. The exercise provides the structure in which the patient can freely verbalize these contradictory response tendencies.

This exercise also reveals the clarity and strength of the patient's discrimination between his alcoholic person and his sober one. While the patient is encouraged to *own* both collections of behaviors, he is also encouraged to maintain a sharp, clear distinction between two different response repertoires, life styles, and modes of being in the world. In my experience a patient capable of doing this is taking a necessary though not sufficient first step toward continued sobriety. Patients who show great confusion and are unable to maintain the simple cognitive–spatial distinctions demanded have not yet achieved the identity separation necessary.

Naming the Alcoholic Person. A simple but often effective technique is to invite group members to name their alcoholic person. Patients by and large take to this activity with enthusiasm and quite a bit of fun. The names that they give their drinking personalities are informative. A proper, elderly female alcoholic who drank mostly at home labeled her alcoholic person "Honey West." "Big Slick," "Tarzan," "Don Juan," "F. Scott Fitzgerald," "Crazy Horse," "Pug Nacious," and "Lonely Sam" are some of the names I have collected from alcoholics to describe their drinking personas. These of course reflect the self-perceptions of drinking alcoholics. Aside from diagnostic interest, this naming process can be used effectively as a further technique to sharpen sober–drinking distinctions.

In a group context, once all members have named their drinking personas and shared these with the group, I divide them into pairs. Each member of the pair interviews the other's drinking persona and explores the meanings behind the name. Finally, each member of the pair reports back to the group the things he has discovered about the other's drinking persona. This leads to a general sharing of present feelings and perceptions of various members by the entire group and the manner in which these present perceptions contrast with the material from the interviews.

RESOLVING THE ALCOHOLIC IDENTITY CRISIS

Very often alcoholic people enter therapy with a serious crisis of identity. This identity confusion is the result of the repeated assault of intoxicated thoughts, feelings, and actions upon the primary or sober personality. The alcoholic is often in a painful state of cognitive dissonance, a predictable outcome of repeated circumstances wherein private, cherished *beliefs* about self are contradicted by public intoxicated *actions*. Techniques to resolve such problems of identity are available.

Fixed-Role Therapy. A technique that I have found useful is one that I have derived from George Kelley's invention (1955), fixed-role therapy. I have found it particularly useful in broadening the patient's behavioral repertoire, inventing sets of complex role performances, and salvaging valuable and positive aspects of the drinking personality that might otherwise be suppressed, devalued, or discarded completely. It is particularly valuable in cases in which the patient construes the drinking personality in totally negative terms and the sober one in impossibly perfect and positive terms. One alcoholic female with whom I worked, for example, persisted in construing her drinking personality as a "whore" and her sober one as a "nun." The tensions generated by this obviously unworkable self-construction contributed to relapse after relapse. A description of this case may illustrate fixed-role therapy.

In the group context I asked the patient to describe her dichotomized self-construction. Her drinking person was described as promiscuous, lively, selfish, exciting, sexy, witty, fun-loving, happy-go-lucky, and devil-may-care. Her sober self was described as dull, boring, plodding, serious, responsible, frigid, thoughtful, caring, religious, and guilt-ridden. With the help of feedback from group members, the patient came to see that her drinking personality contained many positive qualities, while her sober personality as she had constructed the role showed many negative ones.

She was asked to consider a *third* complex set of role constructs and behaviors for herself that combined the best of both possible identities. With the help of group members, the patient constructed a new role identity for herself. During the next week, she consciously tried to act out the role in her social interactions. This *behavioral enactment* led to *feedback* in the real world, which was then considered in group therapy again. The patient, other group members, and the therapist discussed *role fit*—the extent to which the patient felt capable of enactment of the original prescribed role. The results of this scrutiny of role fit led to *role modification* in which the possible behaviors from the original role were retained and the impossible or difficult modified. Armed with a new set of behaviors and supporting self-cognitions, the patient again tried a period of behavioral enactment in the real world with resulting feedback. Once again role fit and role modification were discussed in group and further modifications were developed.

Fixed-role therapy, then, can be seen as a process in which ideal role constructs and behaviors are discovered and then tested in continuous cycles of behavioral enactment, feedback, appraisal of role fit, and role modification.

Positive Reinforcement of Sober Actions, Attitudes, and Values. From a behavioral perspective, it is entirely legitimate for the therapist to reinforce patterns of behavior, attitudes, and values consistent with sobriety. Care must of course be exercised here since such therapist behaviors could be construed by the patient as manipulative, patronizing, controlling, and possibly even demeaning. Social reinforcements, however, are not only a matter of specific utterances, phrases, or other tangible behaviors and material goods; they are also defined by the manner in which they are administered in the larger context of symbolic meanings that grow out of the interaction. I usually genuinely share in the patient's amazement and delight in his newfound ability to stay sober. When he reports specific decisions reached or situations handled sober, I ask him to consider how he might have handled these while drinking. I then ask him to consider what these sober experiences tell him about who he really is, what he is really like, and what he seems to want out of life after all. All of these occasions are used to support the patient's growing self-identity as a competent, responsible, and *sober* person.

In the beginning of therapy, I support *any* self-categorizations by the patient that realistically appraise his problems with alcohol. "Problem-drinker," "in trouble with alcohol," "potential alcoholic," and "possible alcoholic" are typical labels that patients apply to self. I invite the patient to explore more deeply these self-categorizations and the implications of each. In the majority of successful therapies, the patient does eventually arrive at a self-categorization of "alcoholic." Some authorities regard this labeling process as relatively unimportant, while others think it possibly destructive to the patient's progress. Although at the tactical level I do not make an issue of how the patient labels himself, I do not regard the process or the substance of labeling of self an "alcoholic" as unimportant or countertherapeutic. Construing self as "alcoholic" is an important new identity for the patient, one that will enable him to reconstruct his past along different conceptual lines, reexamine his present, and plan his future actions accordingly. In some patients the role identity of "sober alcoholic" is all that they have to cling to in lives beset by unbelievable complexity, devoid of opportunity, and surrounded on all sides by the wreckage of the past. It is, in fact, the only thing that gives meaning to the past, makes the present bearable, and promises hope for the future.

When self-categorizations as "alcoholic" begin to appear in the patient, I support, encourage, and elaborate these in terms of what they represent—an emergent, new, and in some cases exciting self-identity with terribly important implications for the immediate and future well-being of the person.

In some treatment centers and AA groups, material reinforcers are formally distributed at various stages of sobriety. Certificates, tokens of various colors coded to indicate months of sobriety achieved, pins, rings, and other such items are awarded. While I have no idea of the effectiveness of such devices, I have observed them to be meaningful to some patients, who seem to require tangible and fairly immediate indications of progress. Other patients, however, regard such things as trivial in their recovery programs. Still other patients appear to avoid them altogether.

Reinforcement procedures have been used successfully by Hunt and Azrin (1973) and Pickens (1979).

METHODS FOR ACHIEVING RELAXATION

Patients often complain of difficulty in achieving a relaxed state in sobriety. Tension, anxiety, and insomnia are commonly encountered. Methods for dealing with these are available.

Progressive Relaxation. Techniques for deep muscle relaxation derived from work by Jacobson (1974) are of some use for certain alcoholics. In this approach, relaxation is viewed as a response and the skills associated with it trainable. Basic to this approach is the learning of a discrimination between a state of muscle tension and a state of relaxation. For example, the patient is first instructed to clench his fist, hold it, and feel the tension that results. He is then instructed to suddenly release the tension and note the bodily cues and sensations associated with relaxation. Various muscle groups of the body are progressively tensed and relaxed and the associated cues discriminated. The patient's breathing is also manipulated through a series of commands to inhale, hold the breath, and then exhale slowly. The breathing exercises are also an aid to the learning of the discrimination between states of tension and relaxation. Through a systematic application of these procedures, the patient learns to bring the relaxation response under self-control. A complete description of progressive relaxation therapy is beyond the scope of this chapter. Fortunately, however, a variety of taped programs suitable for both clinic and home practice are available from commercial sources (Procter, 1975).

In my experience with systematic relaxation programs with alcoholic patients, I have had mixed results. Progressive relaxation requires discipline, determination, and home practice in between clinical sessions. While these methods are often greeted with an initial burst of enthusiasm, many patients quickly find them boring and uninteresting. More seriously, a large number will not sustain practice outside the clinical setting.

Biofeedback Techniques. A variety of biofeedback devices is now available for use with alcoholic patients. As with many novel treatments, fairly extraordinary claims accompanied the early introduction of these techniques (Birk, 1973). Mushrooming enthusiasm for these devices seemed at times to suggest a popular fad rather than considered scientific judgment. Despite the application of biofeedback techniques to a wide variety of disorders and clinical evidence for their effectiveness, controlled, large-sample research is lacking. What evidence we do have suggests some optimism and some pessimism. Sterman's (1973) research on *sensory-motor rhythm* (a 12–15 Hz rhythm recorded from sensory-motor cortical areas) is a model of rigorous research. His findings indicate that biofeedback control of rhythm can dramatically reduce seizures in patients previously uncontrolled by even extreme medication regimens.

Schwartz and Shapiro's (1973) studies of biofeedback control of essential hypertension indicate caution but some promise as well. Paradoxical results have been reported in the long-term application of finger temperature control of the treatment of migraine. Excellent results have been reported with regard to EMG (electromyograph) feedback for generalized muscle relaxation and control of tension headaches.

With regard to alcoholism *per se*, the research literature on biofeedback techniques is suggestive of promise but not definitive. Studies have been largely anecdotal, very-small-sample experimental research, or methodologically problematic. In one study by Steffen (1975), a small number of alcoholic subjects did show reduced muscle action potentials following EMG therapy, but did not differ in number of drinks ordered after treatments. Studies on alpha rhythm (8–12 Hz rhythm recorded from dominant occipital area) by Passini, Watson, Dehnel, Herder, and Watkins (1977) suggest that biofeedback control of alpha production may reduce certain kinds of anxiety while leaving others unaffected.

In my experience with selected alcoholic patients, I have found EMG feedback to be an effective procedure for training muscle relaxation. My clinical work with the EMG was confined to an inpatient 21-day treatment-program context. Under these conditions, regular sessions could be scheduled and carried out. Training always began with electrode placement on the frontalis muscle and was then generalized to other locations. In some instances I used the technique simply as a dramatic illustration to a patient that he could, in fact, relax without resorting to alcohol or other chemicals. In others I used the procedure as a part of a therapeutic interview in which biofeedback data were introduced to counter the patient's continued denial of affect-laden material. In still other cases I systematically taught the patient the skills of relaxation. On one occasion, with a patient who complained that he could not fall asleep under any circumstances, I employed the following procedure:

I put the patient to bed in his room, covered him with a blanket, and hooked him up to the EMG with electrode placement on the frontalis. I explained the nature of the feedback signals and what they meant, set the feedback signal volume control low, and left the room. I returned 20 minutes later to find the patient asleep! I promptly woke him up and asked him to explain the meaning of his behavior. He was clearly astonished that he had fallen asleep so easily and that he had done so without alcohol or sleeping medications. This incident not only changed the way in which he construed his insomnia problem but also led to a high level of motivation to pursue a systematic training program of EMG therapy. Moreover, this experience increased the patient's motivation in other treatment modalities as well.

While my experiences with EMG biofeedback training were generally positive, I found alpha training of limited value. In the context of a 21-day, multimodal inpatient treatment program, alpha training proved too complex a procedure. Moreover, despite early enthusiasm, patients seemed to tire quickly of the disciplined attention required. Finally, a number of my patients seemed to show appreciable baseline alpha production *prior* to treatment. In these cases *magnitude* rather than frequency seemed to be the problem since low-magnitude 8–12 Hz waves were noted in the records. The research literature is inconsistent on this point, with some investigators reporting a preponderance of beta activity (fast waves) in alcoholics while others report no differences between alcoholics and nonalcoholics in baseline alpha production. Still others report slight differences but very large overlap between distributions for alcoholics versus nonalcoholics.

Despite inconsistent findings, biofeedback devices are clearly worthy of continued investigation in alcoholism therapy. Control of sensory-motor rhythm might prove of value in dealing with seizures during withdrawal as well as chronic seizure disorders in recovered alcoholics. As is well documented, the incidence of hypertension is higher among alcoholics than among nonalcoholics (Klatsky, Friedman, Abraham, Siegelaub, and Gerard, 1977). This chronic hypertension must of course be differentiated from the transient elevation of blood pressure routinely noted in many alcoholics in the early stages of withdrawal and treatment. Biofeedback procedures involving blood-pressure control are certainly worthy of further investigation in alcoholism therapy. Finger temperature devices (thermistors) may have application in the treatment of migraine in particular alcoholics, while EMG feedback therapy may prove of worth in the treatment of tension headaches in selected alcoholic patients in addition to achieving reduced muscle tension generally in such patients.

Breathing, Meditation, and Self-Commands.   In helping alcoholics to achieve relaxed states, it is sometimes useful to consider a variety of techniques that involve breathing, meditation, and self-commands.

Alcoholic patients sometimes show difficulty with irregular breathing patterns and particularly hyperventilation. I have found it useful to teach patients to consciously slow their breathing and to moderate it in terms of rhythmic patterns. Breathing in to a count, holding to a count, and then exhaling gradually is one way to accomplish this. On occasion, I have asked agitated and excited patients to bring their breathing into "sync" with my own. Concentration on breathing helps to achieve relaxation in two ways. First, it acts as an attentional-focusing device that distracts the patient from ruminating over anxiety-provoking material. Second, a deliberate change of the breathing to slow, rhythmical patterns reduces the effects of lowered carbon dioxide levels in the blood that sometimes occurs with fast, irregular breathing patterns. In cases of frank hyperventilation, I not only teach the patient

AMA   against medical
            advice

AD S   Alcohol Drug
            Syndrome

---

three months elapse and you don't
the parent, you will close the case,
days after the end of the first
will send few or no CA/SP's to the
er as you will probably have few or

t quarter) and the case was closed in
be sent to the Coalition by April
in the third quarter.

more than one service plan in the
nt to the Coalition because the case
r services, begin another CA/SP.
, 2nd CA/SP, etc. on the form by
he additional CA/SP to the Coalition
the end of the fiscal year,
e to complete #5 "Date of Plan").

contact person responsible for
o children and for indicating the

— don't initial

breathing techniques, I instruct him on how to breathe into a paper bag fitted over his nose and mouth. This procedure increases the percent carbon dioxide in the inhaled air.

Various meditation techniques have shown some value for inducing relaxed states in selected alcoholic patients (Benson and Wallace, 1972). Transcendental meditation is the more popular of these with some evidence available for judging its effectiveness. And, of course, meditation has long been a recommendation of one of the steps to recovery in Alcoholics Anonymous.

Self-commands are useful devices for reinstating relaxed states. During relaxation, the patient is taught to associate certain self-produced cues with the relaxed state. In tense situations he can attempt to partially reinstate the relaxed condition by evoking these cues or self-commands. Typical self-commands are as follows: *calm; easy does it; slow down; relax.* In some cases, entire phrases can be used. The serenity prayer popular in Alcoholics Anonymous is a useful self-command. I have observed alcoholics using the following to good advantage: *This too shall pass. Don't make a big deal of this. Keep it simple. What difference does any of this make anyway? Let go and let God!*

FEAR-REDUCTION PROCEDURES

Recovering alcoholics often show numerous fears. These can involve such simple things as driving a car to more complex matters of "rejection" and "failure."

Systematic Desensitization Procedures. Introduced by Mary Cover Jones (1924) in the earlier part of this century and further elaborated by Joseph Wolpe (1958), Arnold Lazarus (1971), Marvin Goldfried and Gerald Davison (1976), and many others, systematic desensitization is a technique presumably based upon learning theory. The idea behind systematic desensitization therapy is quite simple: a person cannot be anxious and relaxed at the same time. As a consequence, if the person can be made to make a relaxation response in the presence of a feared object or situation, the usual fear response will be inhibited or blocked. The trick, of course, is in getting the patient to make the relaxation response in a situation that normally arouses fear. This is accomplished in two ways. First, the patient is taught deep relaxation techniques. Second, the feared object is analyzed in terms of what is called a *hierarchy.* The hierarchy is formed from the many components of a complex physical or social stimulus configuration. Each component is scaled from low to high according to its anxiety- or fear-eliciting properties.

Elements low in the hierarchy are dealt with first. In a deeply relaxed state, the patient is asked to imagine vividly the element lowest in associated fear. For example, a person fearful of dogs might be asked to first image a piece of fur. When the patient is able to relax in the presence of this real or imagined element low in the hierarchy, a second element higher in the hierarchy is introduced. Gradually, the patient is exposed to all of the elements in the hierarchy until he is able to maintain relaxation in the presence of the feared object. By systematically pairing the relaxation response with elements of increasing potency, the fear is thought to undergo extinction.

Apparently logical, the model is not without its theoretical problems. Recent research has indicated that fear desensitization can occur without explicit instruction in relaxation. Moreover, fear reduction has been reported through methods that proceed from an entirely opposite position: a sudden and rather massive bombardment of the patient with all aspects of the feared situation (flooding).

Bearing in mind these issues of underlying theoretical principles, it is still possible to recommend systematic desensitization for particular patients. After all, subsequent research has not shown that the technique does not work; it has shown that the technique does work, but probably not for the reasons its proponents have claimed.

Behavioral Rehearsals and Enactments. People in general devote an enormous amount of time to fear rehearsal. Alcoholics are no exception. Fear rehearsal is indicated by phrases of the "what if" variety: What if this should happen? What if that should happen? What would I do if she should decide to leave me, if my boss should fire me, if my kid should get sick? and so on. Moreover, it is intriguing to note that many people spend most of their imaginative energies rehearsing failure rather than success.

A variety of methods can be brought to bear upon these related matters of fear rehearsal and failure preparation. Perhaps one of the simplest and most ingenious techniques is Albert Ellis' cognitive behavioral elaboration of the feared situation (1962). Ellis invites the patient to consider the "worst possible thing that could happen." Then he asks realistic questions such as, "What would you do then?" or "What do you imagine would happen then?" In many cases either the patient discovers that he has the resources to cope with even the most disastrous of circumstances he can imagine or he realizes that the situation has been blown out of proportion.

Direct efforts to alter typical fear and failure rehearsals are also in order. The patient is asked to imagine himself as capable, confident, and successful rather than incapable, filled with self-doubts, and a failure. With regard to specific situations facing him, the patient is asked to imagine himself vividly in the forthcoming situations. Various response alternatives are discovered and these are rehearsed mentally. Throughout, emphasis is placed upon positive thinking, and any indications of this type of thinking are reinforced by the therapist. Negative thinking is either ignored by the therapist or actively confronted and discouraged. The patient is encouraged to visualize himself in specific situations, but instead of concentrating upon the possibility of failure, he is instructed to see himself performing competently and successfully.

Behavioral enactments are role-playing devices that simulate the conditions under which the patient is required to perform. These simulations may range from simple two-party interactions to more complex arrangements such as psychodrama and group role-playing. Group role-playing enables the therapist to use *social modeling* procedures. In these, the patient observes competent role models performing alternative responses to difficult social situations. These enactments of real-life situations can be conducted in such a way as to increase the probability of successful role performances by the patient in forthcoming events.

In a sense, fear and failure rehearsals can take place only in a person tyrannized by the future. Just as some persons allow themselves to become victims of their biographies, others permit themselves to become victims of biographies yet to be written. In the alcoholic patient, future focusing or dwelling in the psychological future can be dangerous business. The emphasis in AA upon taking life 24 hours at a time is intelligent, realistic to a point, and effective. *Time binding* is an important idea that the alcoholism therapist can use to advantage. By continuously reinforcing cognitive activity centered on the psychological present and discouraging excessive future focusing, the therapist may be able to disrupt self-defeating patterns of fear and failure rehearsal.

ALTERING ATTITUDES TOWARD SELF

Problems of low self-esteem are a common outcome of active alcoholism. Feelings of inferiority, disliking of self, and the extremes of self-hatred and loathing are common in alcoholism. These are among the most difficult characteristics to change. In certain cases these may continue to plague the recovering alcoholic even years after sobriety has been achieved.

Assertive-Behavior Training. According to Miller (1978), the less assertive the alcoholic, the more alcohol he or she is likely to consume.

Training in being more assertive may not only give the patient appropriate behaviors to use in his self-interest but may produce generalized effects upon self-esteem and other cognitions about self (Materi, 1977).

In my clinical experience with alcoholic patients, I have found them to possess very limited repertoires of assertive and aggressive responses. Quite typically the patient's repertoire consists of extremely mild aggressive responses and intense hostility, the latter erupting only when the patient is intoxicated. There are, of course, exceptions. Some patients, drunk or sober, respond habitually with high-level aggressive responses and intense hostility. In these cases, assertive behavior training must be approached with caution, since the problem is one of reducing aggression, not increasing it. In still other cases, highly aggressive behaviors simply do not occur—drunk or sober.

But for the majority of alcoholics with whom I have worked, the problem has been one of developing mild to moderate levels of aggressive responding. The emphasis is upon developing a series of such responses of varying levels of intensity, reducing the necessity for either open hostility or complete suppression of anger.

Training in assertion can take place in groups specifically organized for this purpose. In general group-therapy contexts, the therapist can capitalize upon spontaneous events to conduct a brief assertive-behavior training session. Such training can also be accomplished in individual psychotherapy sessions.

Assertive responses can constitute specific actions or verbalizations. Actions may include such things as breaking off a destructive relationship, confronting an unfair or unrealistic supervisor, refusing to do something one really does not want to do, asking for a salary increase, pursuing a love affair, or confronting a neighbor over objectionable behaviors. Verbalizations may include such things as leveling about one's feelings, stating what one will and will not permit, making demands, and giving warnings.

Self-Rewards. In dealing with low self-esteem it is sometimes helpful to encourage the patient to set up a schedule of self-rewards. Self-rewards not only increase the probability that desirable patterns of behavior will be maintained but are symbolic gestures to the patient that he regards himself as fully deserving of such things and worthy of receiving them.

Behavioral Actions in the Real World. Self-esteem can scarcely be considered in isolation from the real-life behaviors of the patient. While some of the patient's negative self-regard is grist for the analytic mill, some of it is clearly a function of his actual behaviors outside the clinical setting. As a therapist, I do not take the position that everything my patient does is simply more material for analysis. I sharply confront destructive behaviors that are not in the patient's interests. With patients who persist in acting out reprehensible behaviors in their real-life situations, I very often say something like the following: "Of course you feel negative about yourself. How could you feel otherwise given the facts of your present behavior?" Such statements are clear indications to the patient that psychotherapy is not a procedure to make him feel good and to assuage his realistic guilt as he continues to make messes of his own and other people's lives. Psychotherapy is about *change*—change in attitudes, cognitions, feelings, and *behavior*.

In helping recovering alcoholics feel good about themselves, I frequently ask them to begin doing things that will support positive self-regard. I generally suggest that each day the patient make it a point to do one small thing for somebody else. As a general rule, I try to encourage the patient to bring his private behavior into line with his public behavior. In my experience, alcoholics do not feel good about themselves nor do they maintain their sobriety when their private lives are characterized by dishonesty, deception, and deceit.

Finally, with regard to increasing self-esteem in alcoholics, I find the ideas of AA concerning the making of amends helpful. For certain patients who cannot comfortably accept their past behaviors, I encourage them to become willing to make amends for these and, when realistic, to do so. Of course, one must first appraise the potential sadism of the recipients of such amends as well as the masochistic potential of the patient! Nothing is to be gained from a situation that further damages the self-esteem of the patient or invites him to engage in further intropunitive behavior.

Self-Management Methods. Miller (1979) and Meichenbaum (1977) have discussed self-management training as a means of changing maladaptive coping skills. In self-management training, a number of components are used. A patient is first provided with a cognitive framework for engaging in a self-management activity. He is taught self-monitoring as a means of arriving at an accurate and useful self-evaluation. Consistent with the cognitive and self-monitoring frameworks, change procedures are introduced. These change procedures are: (1) Learning relaxation techniques; (2) exposing of maladaptive elements in the patient's belief system; (3) changing inappropriate cognitive styles; (4) altering the relationships between cues and behavioral consequences; (5) generalizing newly learned self-management skills to the real world (Neuman, 1983).

TREATMENT GOALS

It is unfortunate that behavioral methods have come to be associated with controlled drinking (e.g., Sobell and Sobell, 1978; Pattison, Sobell, and Sobell, 1977). As shown throughout this chapter, behavioral methods can be employed for a variety of purposes in helping alcoholics get sober. Methods such as desensitization, reinforcement, covert conditioning, self-management, biofeedback, relaxation training, and assertion training can be extremely useful tools for the clinician treating patients in the early phases of sobriety. Azrin (1976), for example, has shown how reinforcement theory can be applied in a community setting. Studies in blood alcohol discrimination by Nathan (1983) and his colleagues, although largely of theoretical interest, may eventually lead to practical application. Neuman (1983) suggests possibilities for behavioral therapy in conjunction with "physiological aids" and Christian psychological approaches.

Miller (1979, 1983) has discussed behavioral methods that may help certain problem drinkers moderate their consumption of alcoholic beverages and avoid negative consequences of consumption. Whether Miller's methods would work with alcoholics is not evident from the data he presents nor the literature he reviews.

The scientific literature on controlled, attenuated, moderate, or social drinking among alcoholics has not been characterized by the rigor, objectivity, methodological sophistication, and soundness one normally expects of treatment interventions that involve high risk to patients (Wallace, 1983,a,b). Whereas some proponents of controlled drinking persist in casting the debate in a "science versus ideology" dichotomy, the available scientific evidence indicates that caution rather than advocacy is in order. Further studies on controlled or nonproblem drinking goals has raised doubts about the feasibility of these goals for alcoholics. Pendery, Maltzman, and West's (1983) failure to confirm Sobell and Sobell's (1973) earlier work on controlled drinking has raised serious questions concerning the scientific adequacy of much of the data in this area. Although the work by Armor, Polich, and Stambul is still cited by some as scientific evidence for controlled drinking by large numbers of alcoholics following treatment, subsequent research by these same authors (Polich, Armor, and Braiker, 1980) reported a long-term, sustained nonproblem drinking rate of only 7%. Corrected for several sources of error, this rate is more likely 4% and agrees closely with a long-term nonproblem drinking rate of 3% recently reported by Pettinati and her colleagues (1982).

A long-term nonproblem drinking rate of 3% is of no practical importance in alcoholism treatment at this time. With treatment centers now reporting long-term abstention rates of better than 50% (e.g., Patton, 1979), the ethical and scientific choice is quite clear: *Until convincingly demonstrated otherwise, abstention remains the only practical course for alcoholics wishing to avoid the awesome personal, social, psychological, medical, and spiritual costs of this disease.*

Summary

In this chapter, I have tried to show the relevance of behavioral modification procedures to alcoholism psychotherapy. Variants of the following have been presented: Habit pattern disruption techniques; cognitive behavioral change methods; relaxation, assertion, and biofeedback training; reinforcement, desensitization, and self-management approaches.

With regard to the continuing debate involving abstention versus controlled drinking, it was pointed out that behavioral methods and indeed behavioral psychology, need not be restricted to controlled drinking treatment goals. Behavioral methods can serve as very useful adjuncts to psychotherapy in the service of helping alcoholics achieve abstention and maintain sobriety.

References

Armor, D. J., Polich, J. M., and Stambul, H. B. *Alcoholism and treatment*. Santa Monica: Rand Corporation, 1976.

Azrin, N. H. Improvement in the community reinforcement approach to alcoholism. *Behavior Research and Therapy*, 1976, 14, 339–348.

Benson, H., and Wallace, K. R. Decreased drug abuse with transcendental meditation: A study of 1,862 subjects. In C. Zarafonetls (Ed.), *Drug abuse proceedings of the international conference*. Philadelphia: Lea and Febiger, 1972.

Birk, L. *Biofeedback: Behavioral medicine*. New York: Grune and Stratton, 1973.

Cautela, J. R. Treatment of compulsive behavior by covert sensitization. *Psychological Record*, 1966, 16, 33–41.

Davies, D. L. Normal drinking in recovered alcohol addicts. *Quarterly Journal of Studies on Alcohol*, 1962, 23, 94–104.

Ellis, A. *Reason and emotion in psychotherapy*. New York: Lyle Stuart, 1962.

Goldfried, M. R., and Davidson, G. C. *Clinical behavior therapy*. New York: Holt, Rinehart, & Winston, 1976.

Hunt, G. H., and Azrin, N. H., A community reinforcement approach to alcoholism. *Behavior Research and Therapy*, 1973, 11, 91–104.

Jacobson, E. *Progressive relaxation*, Chicago: University of Chicago Press (Midway Reprint), 1974.

Kelly, G. *The psychology of personal constructs* (Vol. 2). New York: W. W. Norton, 1955.

Klatsky, A. L., Friedman, G. D., Abraham, B., Siegelaub, A. B., and Gerard, M. J. Alcohol consumption and blood pressure. *Annals of the New York Academy of Sciences*, 1977, *296*, 1194–2000.

Lazarus, A. A. *Behavior therapy and beyond*. New York: McGraw-Hill, 1971.

Materi, M. Assertiveness training: A catalyst for behavior change. *Alcohol Health and Research World*, 1977, *1*, 23–26.

Meichenbaum, D. *Cognitive-behavioral modification: An integrative approach*. New York: Plenum Press, 1977.

Miller, P. M. Behavior therapy in the treatment of alcoholism. In G. A. Marlatt, and P. E. Nathan (Eds.), *Behavioral approaches to alcoholism*. New Brunswick, N.J.: Center for Studies on Alcohol, 1978.

Miller, W. R. Problem drinking and substance abuse: Behavioral perspectives. In N. A. Kraseneger (Ed.) *Behavioral analysis and treatment of substance abuse*. Research Monograph Series, No. 25, Washington, D.C.: National Institute on Drug Abuse, 1979.

Nathan, P. E., and Bridell, D. W., Behavior assessment and treatment of alcoholism. In B. Kissin and H. Begleiter (Eds.), *The biology of alcoholism, Vol. 5, Treatment and rehabilitation of the chronic alcoholic*. New York: Plenum Press, 1977.

Neuman, J. K., Behavior therapy of substance abuse: An overview and discussion of future directions. In E. Gottheil and K. Druley (Eds.), *The etiologic aspects of alcohol and drug abuse*. Springfield, Ill.: Charles C Thomas, 1982.

Passini, F. T., Watson, C. G., Dehnel, L., Herder, J., and Watkins, B. Alpha wave biofeedback training in alcoholics. *Journal of Clinical Psychology*, 1977, *33*, 292–299.

Pattison, E. M., Sobell, M. B., and Sobell, L. C. *Emerging concepts of alcohol dependence*. New York: Springer, 1977.

Patton, M. *Validity and reliability of Hazelden treatment follow-up data*. Center City, Minnesota: Hazelden Educational Services, 1979.

Pendery, M., Maltzman, I., and West, L. J., Controlled drinking by alcoholics? New findings and a reevaluation of a major affirmative study. *Science*, 1982, *217*, 169–175.

Perls, F. S., *Gestalt therapy verbatim*. Lafayette, La.: Real People Press, 1969.

Pettinati, H., Sugerman, A., DiDonato, N., and Maurer, H., The natural history of alcoholism over four years after treatment. *Journal of Studies on Alcohol*, 1982, *43*, 201–215.

Pickens, R. A behavioral program for treatment of drug dependence. In N. A. Kraseneger (Ed.), *Behavioral analysis and treatment of substance abuse*. Research Monograph Series No. 25, Washington, D.C.: National Institute on Drug Abuse, 1979.

Polich, M. J., Armor, D. J., and Braiker, H. B. *The course of alcoholism: Four years after treatment*. ADM 281-76-0006 Santa Monica, California: Rand Corporation, 1980.

Proctor, J. *Relaxation procedures*. New York: Biomonitoring Applications, 1975. (Cassette recording.)

Schwartz, G. E., and Shapiro, D. Biofeedback and essential hypertension. In L. Birk (Ed.), *Biofeedback: Behavioral medicine*. New York: Grune and Stratton, 1973.

Sobell, L. C., and Sobell, M. B. Individualized behavior therapy for alcoholics. *Behavior Research and Therapy*, 1973, *4*, 49–72.

Sobell, L. C., and Sobell, M. B. *Behavioral treatment of alcohol problems: Individualized therapy and controlled drinking*. New York: Plenum Press, 1978.

Sterman, M. B. Neurophysiological and clinical studies of sensorimotor EEG biofeedback training. In L. Birk (Ed.), *Biofeedback: Behavioral medicine*. New York: Grune and Stratton, 1973.

Steffen, J. J. Electromyographically induced relaxation in the treatment of chronic alcohol abuse. *Journal of Consulting and Clinical Psychology*, 1975, *43*, 275.

Wallace, J. Ideology, belief, and behavior: Alcoholics anonymous as a social movement. In E. Gottheil and K. Druley (Eds.), *The etiologic aspects of alcohol and drug abuse*. Springfield, Ill.: Charles C Thomas, 1982.

Wallace, J. Alcoholism: Is a shift in paradigm necessary? *Journal of Psychiatric Treatment and Evaluation*, December, 1983.

Wolpe, J. *Psychotherapy by reciprocal inhibition*. Stanford: Stanford University Press, 1958.

8

Family Therapy of Alcoholism

CELIA DULFANO

INTRODUCTION

Since her father's death, Francie had stopped writing about birds and trees and My Impressions. Because she missed him so, she had taken to writing little stories about him. She tried to show that, in spite of his shortcomings, he had been a good father and a kindly man. She had written three such stories which were marked "C" instead of the usual "A." The fourth came back with a line telling her to remain after school.

"What's happened to your writing, Frances?" asked Miss Garnder.

"I don't know."

"You were one of my best pupils. You write so prettily. I enjoyed your compositions. But these last ones . . ." she flicked them contemptuously.

"I looked up the spelling and took pains with my penmanship and . . ."

"I'm referring to your subject matter."

"You said we could choose our own subjects."

"But poverty, starvation, and drunkenness are ugly subjects to choose. We all admit these things exist. But one doesn't write about them."

"What does one write about?" Unconsciously, Francie picked up the teacher's phraseology.

"One delves into the imagination and finds beauty there. The writer, like the artist, must strive for beauty always."

"What is beauty?" asked the child.

"I can think of no better definition than Keats': 'Beauty is truth, truth beauty.'"

Francie took her courage into her two hands and said, "Those stories are the truth."

CELIA DULFANO • Private Consultant, Family Therapy and Alcoholism, Newton, Massachusetts.

"Nonsense!" exploded Miss Garnder. "Drunkenness is neither truth
nor beauty. It's a vice. Drunkards belong in jail, not in stories . . . ."
(Smith, 1943)

Miss Garnder's attitude toward alcoholism was typical 30 years
ago. The first step in our struggle against alcoholism was winning
acceptance of the idea that alcoholism is not a sin, but a disease, and
that the alcoholic is not an unsalvageable bum, but a human being,
with human needs to be satisfied.

While this understanding was being established, we made advances in developing specific services for the alcoholic. Detoxification
units were opened, outpatient departments were broadened, and halfway houses were offered to the homeless alcoholic. These were significant achievements.

But *A Tree Grows in Brooklyn* (Smith, 1943) also shows what we
professionals neglected to look at until recently: that alcoholism affects
the whole family, not just the problem drinker. For years treatment
was focused on the alcoholic alone. If we talked about other members
of the family at all, they were seen only as individuals affected by the
alcoholic. But in many cases the alcoholic is part of a whole network
of people. The alcoholic affects these people, and they affect the alcoholic. This network can be a powerful influence in the alcoholic's life.

On the one hand, the motivation for stopping drinking and maintaining sobriety may come from the alcoholic's ties with the world.
The threat of loss of job or spouse may impel a reluctant alcoholic to
seek treatment (Finlay, 1966).

On the other hand, the alcoholic's environment may maintain his
drinking behavior. As the alcoholic begins to build up a tolerance to
alcohol, his functioning becomes impaired and his behavior changes,
making him or her give up role tasks and concomitant responsibilities.
The system around the alcoholic changes to accommodate the disability. By the time we reach the alcoholic for treatment, an environment
that resists the removal of the alcoholism may have been created (Jackson, 1954).

For these reasons, consideration of the alcoholic's environment is
mandatory in treatment. When there is a family, the treatment of that
part of the environment becomes essential.

In the past "the alcoholic" was usually presumed to be a man. We
talked of "the wife of the alcoholic" and "the children of the alcoholic."
When AA first approached alcoholism as a family illness, the husband
was seen as the alcoholic, and Al-Anon was offered mainly to the

alcoholic's wife. Even today, very little has been written about the husband of the alcoholic (Edwards, Harvey, and Whitehead, 1973).

There were a few early thinkers who saw that alcoholism is a problem that extends beyond the individual alcoholic. Bacon (1945) analyzed the problem of excessive drinking patterns in the family from a sociological point of view. Bailey (1968; Bailey, Haberman, and Shein-berg, 1965), Price (1960), Cork (1969), and others talked about the other members of the family. But everyone saw family members only as individuals who needed individual care.

As alcoholism became recognized as a treatable disease rather than a sin, and as social attitudes toward women changed, we were able to consider the alcoholic woman. We also became aware of alcoholism in the very young and the very old.

Now we are beginning to consider men and women, the young and the old, in terms of their family relationships instead of as isolated alcoholic individuals. Instead of talking about "the alcoholic's family," we are beginning to consider "the family afflicted with alcoholism." In fact, the entire family is becoming the focus of therapy.

Up to now, family therapy and alcoholism treatment have generally been kept separate. Professionals in both fields have been reluctant to work in the other. But the combination of the two fields can create an effective, far-reaching approach to alcoholism and its related problems. The impact of alcoholism on the family can be dealt with directly, and in some cases valuable preventive work can be done. Furthermore, the interactions that feed back from the family into the alcoholic syndrome can be dealt with directly in therapy.

Family therapy does not ignore the individual alcoholic. Individual needs and dynamics are a vital part of the therapeutic focus. But changes in the individual and satisfying his needs will be brought about by changing the family system. The goal of therapy is a changed system: a family structure that can support the alcoholic and the other family members as competent human beings.

FAMILY THERAPY

Most therapy in the past was aimed at the individual as a separate organism. "Primary change was effected by providing 'the patient' with insight into his unconscious conflicts, thus eliminating the re-pressed forces which were incapacitating him. The real world of the individual was considered secondary" (Haley, 1971). In the 1950s, how-ever, a few people saw themselves as breaking away from these established ideas of treatment. "It would be comfortable to assume that such therapists turned to family treatment because they were not getting results with psychoanalytically oriented therapy" (Haley, 1971). In fact, however, traditional concepts of the explanation of behavioral phenomena and techniques for intervention were being challenged by a combination of new theoretical systems. General systems theory, communications theory, and theories of group dynamics and ecology were sparking experimentation with new techniques of intervention: family therapy, encounter groups, and community psychiatry (Minuchin, 1970). In a time in which the heroic ideal of man as the "captain of his ship" was being replaced by the realization that the individual cannot be understood apart from his life contexts, therapists began to broaden their focus to look at those contexts. In family therapy the focus of treatment was no longer on challenging individual perceptions, affect, or behavior, but on changing the structure of the family.

Minuchin (1972) defines structural family therapy as "a body of theory and techniques" that approaches the individual in his social context. Therapy based on this framework is directed toward changing the organization of the family. When the structure of the family group is transformed, the position of members in that group is altered accordingly. As a result, each individual's experiences change. Family therapy, then, is not a method of treatment. "It is a new orientation to the human dilemma" (Haley, 1971). Within this orientation, any number of methods can be taught and used. That is why there are many different schools of family therapy (Minuchin, 1969). Central to all methods, however (as well as to this chapter), is the wider focus than found in the traditional individual therapies.

With such an orientation, individual treatment of alcoholism is at best a partial treatment for many alcoholics. To work with the individual and not try to reach the family simply does not make sense in many cases.

FAMILY STRUCTURE

In family therapy, a family is seen as a system; that is, the family is a natural social group in which transactions have been repeated over time and that have formed patterns which become a governing structure.

Minuchin (1974) suggests thinking of the family structure as beginning when two people join with the purpose of creating a family. Each partner brings his own experiences and expectations to the marriage. These individual frameworks must be reconciled so that each partner can retain his own sense of identity while accommodating and allowing the other partner his.

The transactional patterns mutually evolved become the structure of the spouse dyad. Some transactional patterns are the result of open negotiations and are policed by the couple after having been formulated through discussion and compromise. Others are never recognized.

When a child is born, the spouses must learn new tasks. New responsibilities have appeared and meeting them must become part of the transactional patterns that form the family structure. The transactional patterns that compose the spouse system remain, but the spouse system is now a subsystem of a network which also contains parental transactional patterns.

Any changes in any part of the structure—or any unit of the system—affect the other units. The reactions of others, in turn, affect the first (Scherz, 1970). Throughout the life of the family, there will be other changes that call for accommodations. The family must have the flexibility to adapt to these changes while maintaining the continuity that gives its members a stable reference group.

Families develop their own values as well as rules and it is in families that people learn to love, care, and satisfy their own and other's needs. Individual development and growth depends on this primary social system.

THE INFLUENCE OF ALCOHOLISM ON FAMILY STRUCTURE

In the family afflicted with alcoholism, alcoholism has often been a factor from the very beginning. The transactional patterns of the spouse subsystem may be built around one partner's drinking problem and this skew may also be built into the parental and executive subsystems. Because of one adult's alcoholism, the children may take over executive responsibilities inappropriately early. The nonalcoholic parent, in effect, is an "only parent," and may cede parental responsibility inappropriately to an older child. Role models are distorted, individual "turf" is encroached upon, and nurturing closeness may be impossible.

The children, finding their own needs unmet, may find satisfaction in their roles as pseudoparents. They may encourage the younger children to remain immature so as to secure these roles. Ultimately, as they grow and form their own families, they may become alcoholics themselves and/or marry alcoholics which perpetuates the only patterns they are familiar with. This is an environment with little room for learning how to trust and how to be appropriately close to another person.

By the time a family comes to therapy, alcoholic behavior may be a factor built into the family's equilibrium. Removal of that behavior, however desired, actually becomes a threat. There are all the problems of helping the individual alcoholic change his behavior, plus the problem that, if such change does occur, the family system may respond with homeostatic transactions that encourage the reappearance of alcoholic behavior. Only structural change will remove the unacknowledged pressure on the alcoholic to remain an active alcoholic.

FAMILY THERAPY IN CASES OF ALCOHOLISM

Many therapists working with alcoholics have been grounded in individual studies. Therefore the trained therapist approaches the alcoholic with the expectation that he is dependent, immature, and manipulative. Like the alcoholic's family, the therapist must learn to expect him or her to be an adult who can and must take on adult responsibilities. Expecting the alcoholic to act like a sick person will keep him or her in that role. Both therapist and family must relate to him or her as competent, so as to reinforce competent behavior whenever it appears.

Alcoholics may enter treatment as individuals. In other cases the family may come into therapy with another problem, denying the alcoholism until it is uncovered by or "revealed to" the therapist. Whatever the presenting problem, however, the family should be brought into treatment and become the therapeutic focus. The target is not only the alcoholic individual but also the problem of alcoholism.

Some therapists would focus on the presenting problem, reasoning that alcoholism may clear up as a result of change in the functioning of the family. In my experience, however, alcoholism is such a serious illness, and its impact on the family is so great, that little can be accomplished unless alcoholism is part of the therapeutic contract. This is particularly true when alcoholism is chronic in one of the executive family members. In some families with hidden alcoholism, however, the therapist does have to work with the presenting problem until a relationship of trust and hope has been established. At this point the contract becomes like that reached with families where alcoholism is the presenting problem.

Therapeutic goals will differ according to each family's circumstances and wishes and therapeutic strategies must be tailored to those individual family goals and possibilities. There are, however, a few general precepts which can help guide the therapist as he plans goals and methods for the individual family (Dulfano, 1982). The therapeutic contract will include: (1) focus on helping the alcoholic stop the drinking, making him responsible for it and by doing so removing alcoholism from its central place in the family; (2) at the same time target for change those family transactional patterns that are trapping all family members in growth-curtailing roles; (3) stimulate individual growth of family members which is *not* based on the family disability created by alcoholism.

The first family interview is a time for assessing each member's position in the family. The therapist will then start working on moving each member in a way that will start correcting the structural skews caused by alcoholism. The therapist will work with the spouses on their relationship. There will be work with them in their roles as parents. There will be work with the children, helping them cede parental and executive roles they have prematurely assumed, and helping them find compensations for this change in age-appropriate ways. In essence, therapy is a matter of creating a basis from which the family will be able to grow.

Much work is done with subsystem sessions. Sessions with the spouses may focus on what they want from each other, how they can start giving to each other and satisfying each other's needs. The therapist must help the couple look at each other and at their interactions.

Sometimes it is helpful to model different behavior for the couple. The therapist can function as one member of the couple, making sure when he finishes that the one "replaced" is aware that although the therapist took over his role, he will have to experiment himself with doing things differently. Sometimes it is possible to set up a situation by modeling and then directing the partner whose role you have played to enter and take over. At other times it may be useful to direct the couple to exchange roles. For example, working with a couple in which the woman, an alcoholic, was hypersensitive and easily upset, the therapist directed the pair to change roles, then reenact the argument they were describing. Mary was to be John, and ask "her" to take his shirts to the laundry. John was to be the delicate Mary and get very upset. Seeing one's partner enact one's own behavior can make a person very aware of that behavior in himself.

The focus of therapy is on interactions in the present. Family members often bring historical material, of course, and this is dealt with. But it is dealt with in the present. What is important is how the patients participating in the session are behaving now. It may be useful to know what aspect of the present interaction is causing the historical material to surface, but the only thing that is actually available for therapeutic change is the present. The family must become aware of how the way they act toward each other continues their usual behavior patterns, and how changing those patterns can help them change their lives.

It is often useful to assign tasks that will make the family members try new ways of interacting. For example, in one family the father, a sobered alcoholic, was trying to prove to himself and his children that he was a "good father" by concentrating on earning extra money and repairing the house. The children, however, wanted him to act as their father emotionally. Therefore the therapist assigned a task. On Sunday afternoons the father was not to work on the house. Instead, he and the children were to plan activities that would involve them together—taking the younger children to the park, taking the older son to a ball game, and so on. The task created an opportunity for father and children to practice being father and children and experience the rewards of these new interactions.

This kind of structural modification can create the possibility of new transactional patterns—patterns that reinforce competence and sobriety rather than drinking. It can also perform a valuable preventive function. Children of alcoholics often become involved in their parents' problems to such an extent that their own development is disastrously handicapped.

One example of this situation was a 26-year-old woman who entered therapy because of severe depression. This woman was living in her own apartment and holding down a good job. Yet her problems related back to her mother's alcoholism, on which the patient had been focused since the age of 15. Her father had in effect moved out years ago, but she continued to see his daily contacts with her mother as a sign that her parents' marriage was still viable. She blamed her father for the onset of her mother's illness, but she still saw herself as a go-between vital to the continuation of that relationship.

Because she was almost wholly unable to relate to people, the therapist insisted that she join a group-therapy program. She was unable to talk in the group for many months. Eventually, therefore, the therapist scheduled sessions for her with her mother and separate sessions for her with her father. The mother, still an active alcoholic, was unable to realize her daughter's feelings. Her father, once he realized the extent of his daughter's investment in an empty relationship, told her frankly that he was involved in making a new life for himself with another woman. He kept in touch with his wife only to make sure that she was physically safe.

After 11 years of investment in holding her parents' marriage together, as she thought, the woman found this shattering. Continued therapy focused on helping her accept that her mother's drinking problem was not under her control and on changing the role she had assumed for years. She started to build a life of her own, but this will be at best a long process.

Alcoholism does more than damage the individual alcoholic. It causes fundamental skews in his/her family's organization and functioning. Only structural modification will help the family affected by alcoholism develop functional mechanisms for dealing with problems and for supporting its members as they grow and function in the extrafamilial world.

CASE HISTORIES*

Case 1. The Williams family was a case in which both parents were alcoholics, with a 20-year history of problem drinking. Separated for four years, each spouse had worked individually on his own drinking problems through AA and treatment with different individual therapists. A few months before beginning family treatment, the couple had reconciled for the sake of their children. At this point Paul had been sober for a year and a half, and Janet for eight months. But sobriety was not enough. The couple felt unable to integrate their individual growth into their relationship as spouses, and this difficulty was hampering their individual work. Janet felt she needed a man in the house to be her co-parent, but she did not want to relate to Paul sexually or to fulfill his other demands as a husband in a relationship that did not include drinking.

Both Janet and Paul, however, were willing to work at becoming better parents. Consequently, a family session was arranged.

In family therapy the patient is the family, whatever the individual problem or presenting problem may be. In the first session, therefore, the therapist began to assess the family's existing structure.

The younger children, Jean, 13, and Bob, 11, complained in the session that their brother Fred, 18, bossed them around. The therapist inferred that Fred had become the substitute father in the family, a structural skew typical in families afflicted with alcoholism. Thus, one treatment goal was immediately obvious: to help Fred step down from

---

* All names and circumstances have been changed to protect the privacy of the families interviewed.

his role as substitute father and to help Paul establish himself in that role. This was not interpreted to the family, but the therapist mentally formulated three steps to that goal. In therapy the family would need (1) to recognize the existing family structure, which included Fred's displacement of his father, (2) to see that displacement as a problem, and (3) to understand that this confusion of roles was a result of a long period of parental drinking, but that the parents were now capable of being parents.

The therapist raised the subject of alcoholism. Everyone denied that this had ever been a problem (a typical reaction in families afflicted with alcoholism). Fred, acting as the family spokesperson, said "You have the wrong idea about drinking. There was never any lack of food in the house." The therapist, persisting, said, "Who took care of the household chores, like cleaning?" Paul, Jr., 15, grimaced and pointed at himself. This was another example of a child's stepping into an executive role as a direct consequence of the behavior of the alcoholics who had become, while drinking, in effect absent members of the family.

As the session continued, the position of each member of the family became clearer. Fred, at 18, acted as family spokesman. He was a parental child, whose authoritarian behavior had been endorsed by his mother. Paul, Jr., who had assumed some of his mother's tasks in doing the household chores, was referred to by her as "the good boy in the family." The two youngest children were withdrawn, emphatically playing the role of children. Jean, at 13, had closed off communication with her family in order to avoid their overwhelming expectations that she be a diligent and neat young lady. Bob, at 11, presented himself as a 7- or 8- year-old by using baby talk. During the session, Janet corrected Jean's and Bob's behavior, telling them to speak up or sit straight, and remarking, "You should have washed your hands before we got here," and "Tie your shoes." It became evident that Janet kept Jean and Bob as "the babies" so that she could keep herself busy in the role of a mother with young children who needed constant care.

The father was an outsider, only now beginning to relate to his family, but doing this mostly as a disciplinarian. His attempts to be a good father were sincere but tended to be confined to lecturing.

But at the end of the session, it was Paul, Sr., who pointed out that this was the first time in years the family had been able to sit together and talk "without yelling and screaming." The family left the session with a feeling of hope. Lines of communication had been reopened. Two of the children were beginning to realize that their parental functioning was inappropriate because no longer necessary, and the parents were recognizing that their drinking had pushed the children into these roles.

The therapeutic goal with the Williams family was to change the interactions that kept the children in executive positions and the parents as incompetents. In particular, Paul, Jr., and Fred would have to return executive authority to their parents and find developmentally appropriate compensations for this loss of power.

Paul and Janet had to learn to support each other in the role of parents. One approach to this problem was spouse sessions, in which the therapist encouraged the couple to work on their relationship. Part of the problem was Paul's long and irregular working hours. Supported by the therapist and by Janet's statement that she needed him at home, Paul was able to confront his boss and tell him he would no longer be available for unlimited overtime. As he began to spend more time with his family, he was able to practice supportive ways of acting as a husband and father.

Naturally this change did not come easily. The homeostatic mechanisms that keep a family functioning in its usual manner have great power. For example, when Janet and Paul had been drinking, the family had had no regular mealtimes. One of the things the couple wanted to establish—a ritual which symbolized their new life—was a regular dinner time. But almost every night one of the children was late. Still, the improvement in the spouse relationship was supporting change. Janet was learning to express anger openly, instead of covertly punishing Paul by rejecting him sexually. Gradually the couple were working their way toward mutual support as they resumed their roles as parents.

Bob was the first to react visibly to this family change: he ran away from home. Bob had been very close to his mother, so close that the growing relationship between his parents meant, to him, loss.

Formerly, Paul and Janet would have used alcohol to alleviate the anxiety caused by such a crisis; and they would have reacted autonomously instead of as a parental team, contradicting each other and increasing the confusion until Paul, Jr., or Fred had stepped into the vacuum. This time, Paul was away at work when Janet learned that Bob had run away. In this crisis, she turned first to her AA sponsor. She explained that she had turned to her sponsor rather than to her husband because she wanted to be sure of getting support and had not felt that her relationship with Paul was strong enough for her to lean on him. She felt that if she were not supported in this stressful situation, she might jeopardize her sobriety. She was afraid of regressing to her old pattern of drinking to resolve problems.

The therapist framed this crisis as an opportunity for Paul and Janet to practice problem-solving together. An emergency session was arranged with the couple so they could discuss how they would deal with Bob when he returned.

For perhaps the first time in this couple's relationship, they were able to sit down together and make decisions about their children's problems. The therapist encouraged them to support each other without blaming themselves for the incident.

Alcoholics should not be pushed to take responsibility too soon. Experimenting with a new way of living, they have to learn to trust themselves and the people around them. In this situation, Janet, feeling the need of support, had turned to her AA sponsor. Paul was wounded, but after talking over the present stage of their relationship with the help of the therapist, he was able to accept Janet's reluctance to depend on him. Thus, the situation posed an opportunity, not only for better parental functioning, but for further progress in the spouse subunit.

Paul's reaction to Bob's running away had been rage. In the session with the spouses, the therapist helped him calm down and understand the dynamics of the incident. By running away, Bob was giving a message to his family which he could not verbalize. Together, therapist and parents set a therapeutic goal. When Bob came back, they would help him verbalize his reasons for leaving home. When the couple left they felt united and ready to deal with their son.

Bob was found in the evening, and a session was immediately arranged for the following morning. At first Bob was unable to talk, but by the middle of the session, with the help of the therapist and both his parents, he was able to say, "I had to go. There isn't enough room in the house for Daddy and me."

Janet told Bob, "I need both of you. I care for both of you." This statement, coming on the heels of rejection by both his wife and son, brought tears to Paul's eyes. Watching his rigid father showing feeling and listening to his mother, Bob realized, for perhaps the first time in his life, that his parents were responsible and responsive adults to whom he could talk. Everyone agreed to work further on the problem of helping Bob talk to his parents. The therapist also alerted Bob's Alateen counselor to the need to help Bob find age-appropriate peer-group compensation for the necessary distancing from his mother.

Bob's problem talking with his parents was another direct result of their alcoholism. Children cannot experience a drunk adult as a rational, approachable, possible guide to the child's problems in growing up. This therapeutic session may well have been Bob's first opportunity to talk to his mother and father. He, as well as the other children, had to learn that the parents were no longer people the children had to protect, but responsible adults who could help and guide them.

Later the therapeutic focus shifted to Fred, who was, the younger children said, drinking and smoking far too much. It is, unfortunately, common to find the children of alcoholics becoming alcoholic themselves, but the family focus in this case made preventive work possible. The fact that the alcoholism was now discussed openly allowed the parents to share some of their own experiences with drinking while they were teenagers. Because Janet and Paul were able to share the memory of their own emotions directly, these discussions had a profound effect on Fred.

In some family sessions the therapist urged the family to role-play a family scene in which drinking behavior had been present. This proved quite useful in helping the children share what they had experienced during the years when their parents were drinking and in making the parents aware of the impact their behavior had had on their children.

At the same time, the Williams family had to learn to detach from alcoholism. When old behaviors were used and blamed on the time the parents were actively using alcohol, the therapist made the family aware that the alcoholism was not there any more—that the problem was to deal with the situation in new terms. Specifically, Janet and Paul had to learn to support each other without blaming and to make demands on each other without the fear that making demands would drive the partner back to drinking. The children also had to learn to stop protecting both parents for fear of making them resume drinking.

After seven months of therapy, the Williams family decided to stop treatment. Paul and Janet were maintaining sobriety, and the family members agreed they felt comfortable with the changes that were happening. The therapist agreed with them, but impressed on them the fact that help would always be available if the family felt unable to cope with further changes.

Termination of family therapy should always be open-ended. The family will have more problems, for problems are part of living. In the future they may find that they cannot deal with a change brought about by family modification or external circumstances. If that happens, they must feel free to reenter therapy.

Even during the course of treatment it may be valuable to stop sessions for a time, giving the family the opportunity to experience the results of their growth without the therapist's intervention. A therapist, as Lutham and Kirschenbaum (1974) have pointed out, has to trust a family's commitment to their own growth. But the family must know that the therapist is available to help with any problems they cannot cope with by themselves.

These interventions illustrate the all-important goal of therapy in these families, namely, to go beyond the maintenance of sobriety and toward the development of a supportive system for sustaining the individual growth of the alcoholic member(s) and encouraging positive changes in other members who have been affected by the alcoholism.

When we began therapy with the Williams family, we chose to focus on the alcoholism, although we knew that sobriety had already been achieved. Thus, the current problem of Paul's and Janet's inability to deal cooperatively with the children was purposely related to the period when the parents had been drinking, because the dysfunctional structures had largely been established then.

In other cases, however, like that of Mary McCarthy, below, family treatment may start with an "unrelated" symptom. It is then the function of the therapist to uncover the alcoholism and help the members deal with it before trying to accomplish any other changes in the family.

Case 2. Mary McCarthy was a 20-year old divorcee and mother of a 2-year-old daughter. When she and her husband separated, she returned to her parents. She was their only child. A few months after her divorce, she was hospitalized for a serious depression. It was known to the staff that she had been abusing drugs for years, but she was not using them when she entered the psychiatric ward. After admission, she became completely withdrawn and refused to talk to the staff or to other patients on the ward.

A family session was arranged with the participation of Mary, her parents, and Mary's daughter. As the session progressed and it became apparent that Mary insisted on mutism, it was decided to split the family group by sending the father out to an adjacent room where he could observe the proceedings through a one-way mirror with a second therapist. This technique, frequently used in family therapy, allows the therapist to create an environment in which the "removal" of one family member can allow other members to relate to each other in different ways. In this case we wanted to see if the absence of the father would allow the mother and daughter to open up.

But when the second therapist sat next to Mr. McCarthy behind the mirror, she was struck by the strong smell of alcohol on his breath, though it was only 9:15 A.M. Seizing on the possible significance of this clue, the therapist asked Mr. McCarthy to rejoin the session, and immediately confronted him with the question: had he been drinking before the session?

With this confrontation a dramatic change took place. Mary suddenly opened up and started to talk about her own experiences with drinking and her strong resentment toward her father for having used her as a drinking partner during her early teens. At this point the focus changed from Mary, the depressed, uncooperative patient, to the family, and particularly to the alcoholism in the family. It became apparent that this subject, which was being covered up by all the members, constituted a significant problem which had to be dealt with.

An alcoholic frequently tries to recruit the spouse as a drinking partner. The nonalcoholic spouse will often agree in the hope that this will help control the alcoholic's intake. In Mary's case, since Mrs. McCarthy had not made herself available for this role, Mr. McCarthy had taken his teenage daughter along on his trips to the bar, and she had become alcoholic herself.

When the presence of alcoholism was recognized in the family session, the father and daughter started to blame each other for the drinking problem. The mother got up, left the group, and went to the corner to pick up Mary's baby, who had been busy playing. When challenged by the therapist about her withdrawal, Mrs. McCarthy said she did not have anything to contribute to what was going on. But she returned to the group and sat there, holding Mary's baby on her lap. As her mother returned, Mary sat down next to her and caressed her baby—the first sign of affection she had been able to show in the session.

Families with alcoholism are often found to lack the normal maintenance of generational boundaries between parents and children. In the McCarthy's case, moreover, the marriage bond had probably been weak from the beginning. Both spouses had looked elsewhere to satisfy their needs for companionship. Mr. McCarthy had made his daughter his companion, and Mrs. McCarthy had accepted being displaced. But a child cannot substitute for a parent and still grow up into a full human being.

What we saw in the session reflected years of family interactions: Mary and her father heavily involved, and Mrs. McCarthy separated from them, with "nothing to say."

Family treatment would have been the best method for the McCarthys. Therapy could have helped Mary extricate herself from the partner relationship with her father. Concomitantly, the therapist would have worked to strengthen the spouse relationship, so the void left by Mary's departure could be filled by Mrs. McCarthy. Unfortunately, the parents refused to enter therapy. The therapist spoke to Mrs. McCarthy and recommended Al-Anon (Ablon, 1974). Mrs. McCarthy felt she was not ready for that. Mr. McCarthy could not be reached.

Consequently, Mary had to be seen individually. The therapist referred her to AA to work on her alcoholism. Early sessions also focused specifically on helping her to separate from her parents. Without this separation, the pressure to satisfy her father's needs would have hindered her sobriety and healthy functioning.

The McCarthy family was typical of many families afflicted with alcoholism: the need to deny this problem superseded all other considerations (Dulfano, 1977). But when there is alcoholism in a family, whether it is the cause of the problem or a symptom of other problems, and whether it is presented as a problem or not, it must be dealt with.

Case 3. Kate O'Connor was 14 when she was referred to a specialist in alcoholism by the psychiatric hospital where she had been admitted by court order. Kate was not addicted as yet, but her father was known to be an alcoholic and she was abusing both drugs and alcohol; she was definitely considered at risk.

The therapist met a very angry young woman. Kate wanted to go home; she considered it outrageous that she could not get anyone to give her a definite date for discharge. She admitted that she had been hospitalized at her mother's insistance after she had physically attacked her mother, but she still wanted to go home.

The home life Kate described was chaotic at best. Her father had left home when she was nine. Out of the home he was able to stay sober, but when he returned, he began drinking again. Her mother then left the home for a period of about eight months.

Kate considered this conclusive proof that her father's drinking was her mother's fault. She complained that her mother blamed her for everything that happened in the family and confided that she was terribly afraid of repeating her family history by becoming an alcoholic or perhaps marrying one.

Kate's parents were attending a "parents' support group" that focused on how to parent and Kate was being seen in individual therapy. The consultant suggested a family session.

The first session was attended by Kate and her parents. Mr. and Mrs. O'Conner, both in their early 40s, and who seemed depressed and angry. Mr. O'Conner expressed concern about Kate, but he was very quiet. The mother was extremely angry. She said Kate was totally out of control and repeated the story of how Kate had attacked her. Mrs. O'Conner also repeated some of the family history—how the father, "a drunk," had left her. The father sat listening and said nothing at all.

Seeking to broaden the focus, the therapist asked whether the O'Conners had other children. Mother answered that Patrick, 20, Michael, 18, and Johnny, 15, were all living at home. Were there any problems with them? Mother said Johnny was a good boy, but she conceded that the other two "drank quite a bit."

The consultant moved toward a discussion of alcoholism. The father admitted he was still having problems: He had been intoxicated the previous weekend. He was in AA and was "working on it." The mother was heavily involved in AlAnon; she said she'd learned to detach herself from her husband's drinking. The father managed to make the point that he was very concerned about Patrick and Michael, who were drinking "pretty heavily."

The consultant asked why this wasn't seen as a problem. Why weren't the boys here?

Because they weren't the problem, the mother rejoined angrily. Kate was the one who made trouble. The boys were holding down jobs and leading their own lives. If they drank, what did anyone expect, with their father setting the example? Father began to reply, but Kate shut him up with the angry comment that he just had no guts at all.

By now the therapist had formed the picture of a family with a highly central and very angry mother and a father who wanted to rejoin the family but was given no space. Accordingly, the therapist insisted that the entire family attend the next session and made it the father's job to see that the boys got there. Mother was to support him, silently. After an extensive discussion of the difficulties—the long drive, the loss of time from work, and so forth, a time was agreed on.

The consultant saw the three boys sitting with their parents in the waiting room before the next session. In the elevator she met Kate and mentioned having seen them. Kate gave an angry laugh—her mother had told her that Father had threatened to kick them out of the house if they did not come.

The boys had not seen their sister for three weeks. But as the family met in the therapy room only Mother spoke to Kate. Everyone was hostile and the boys were furious—they were losing pay to come here and for what? It was Kate's fault. Patrick was bleary eyed and his face was swollen from a beating he had gotten over the weekend. He complained that he had not been able to come home—Mother had imposed a new rule: If you drink, don't come home.

Michael seized the floor and maintained that Kate was the problem.

She was a liar and a thief. He and Kate got into a furious argument about a sleeping bag Michael said she'd stolen. The rest of the family listened in silence until Kate burst into tears and ran out of the room. The therapist followed Kate and tried to get her to return. Kate refused, but did promise to return to the ward.

Now the entire family joined in telling the therapist how much of a problem Kate was. In the atmosphere of angry accusations, Patrick began to complain about the mother. She just had to control them all. Look at the way she treated the father. Driving down here she had not let up on him for one minute.

Mother's response was an angry statement: She was filing for a divorce.

In the silence that followed the phone rang. It was the hospital. Kate, still hysterical, had to be placed under restraints. She was asking for her mother. The therapist decided to take the entire family over to see her.

Kate was restrained on her bed. The boys stood immobile at the door. Mother and father entered, but only Mother approached and she barely touched Kate's hand. The youngest boy had tears in his eyes, but no one was able to respond as Kate began to scream that this was all her mother's fault.

The family was virtually in shock. The consultant decided against trying to make them talk then, but suggested a session with the parents alone on the following day and one with the full family on the day after. Everyone agreed without argument.

The meeting with the parents focused on setting an agenda. It was agreed that the parents must take charge to bring some order into the family situation. Rules must be set by the parents, agreed to by the children, and followed by everyone.

At the full family session the next day everyone expressed himself as feeling better. Patrick began to attack the mother's treatment of the father, but the consultant stopped him to ask about the drinking. Father said he had definitely decided to stop. The boys said they had both made weekend plans that did not include the local pub.

The family outlined changes which obviously had already been discussed. They had agreed to stop battling over meals and a procedure for absences had been worked out. The yardwork had been apportioned. In general, they were agreed that each family member must be responsible for his own life, with privacy to be maintained, although many of the specifics remained to be worked out.

Kate's reaction to the family's exchanges was highly positive. She looked as if a burden had been lifted from her.

The family used the session to continue to discuss changes and ways of communicating. Obviously they had a formidable task. The parents must decide upon the divorce and do it not as a result of Kate's acting out, but because they were unable to work out their relationship.

Kate was referred to group therapy as an adjunct to family work. The family itself was referred to a mental health center closer to their home for continued sessions. Each member of the family expressed strong commitment to continuing the work begun during these sessions.

The O'Conners were a family in which alcoholism ran from generation to generation—we later learned that the father came from an alcoholic family and mother's father had died of alcoholism. If Kate, the identified patient, had been seen only individually, the pattern would have continued.

DISCUSSION

Therapists may overlook alcoholism, either through lack of familiarity with its symptoms or through lack of training in how to cope with them. When therapists treat families with presenting problems like schizophrenia or depression, they have access to a body of information about the disease. Too often a therapist may lack an equivalent knowledge about alcoholism, and he may therefore ignore it or fail to uncover it. But untreated alcoholism can only continue to perpetuate the structural skews that are affecting the family and the life of each family member.

The therapist should beware, however, of the dangers of focusing too much on the search for the original cause of alcoholism (Berenson, 1976). The search for cause during therapy is likely to be fruitless, and even countertherapeutic, since it offers the patients a way to avoid dealing with the alcoholism's present consequences. One of the advantages of the family-therapy approach is its orientation toward the present. Therapy focuses on actions and structure which exist now. They can be observed directly and brought directly into the consciousness of the family members by the therapist during the sessions.

In the cases presented here, the alcoholics were young adults. But alcoholism in other family members also has great impact on a family. The growing problem of adolescent alcoholism may have enormous family implications.

Work with adolescent alcoholics is usually done in group therapy, since teenagers may start drinking because they cannot cope with peer-group pressures. Group therapy can give them a positive experience in which they can learn to cope with such situations. In addition, it is important to include their parents in therapy to help them avoid focusing exclusively on drinking in dealing with their child. After educating the parents about alcoholism, it is necessary to work to change the family structure. We assume in such cases that peer pressures created a need, but it is also common to find that the family environment has fed into these pressures.

Finally, when working with families with alcoholism, it is important to take each family's cultural patterns into account. A problem seen as very serious in a lower-class family might have little impact on an upper-class family. By the same token, the family's view of itself and its wishes must be taken into account. Families are not all the same, any more than individuals are. There is no rubber-stamp treatment for alcoholism on either the family or the individual level.

CONCLUSION

Alcoholism is very much a family disease, and many professionals are beginning to deal with alcoholism on the family level (Ablon, 1976; Bowen, 1974; Ewing and Fox, 1968; Meeks and Kelly, 1970; Steinglass, 1976; Ward and Faillace, 1970). As yet no comprehensive theory of family approaches to alcoholism has been developed (Pattison, 1977), but it is hoped that increasing experience with the practical advantages of this approach will encourage professionals to work toward the integration of the two fields.

Alcoholism is often unacknowledged by families who enter therapy. Nevertheless, if the therapist senses its presence, he must help the family articulate the problem. Ideally, the openness developed about alcoholism can encourage openness about other issues and perhaps facilitate communication, which may have been stifled for years.

If treatment begins with an individual who is recovering from a drinking bout, family sessions should begin as soon as the alcoholic is detoxified. In this sort of crisis situation, a family's equilibrium/homeostasis has already been disrupted, and the family may be particularly amenable to contracting for therapeutic help. If the alcoholic member is already in treatment and there is no crisis situation, however, it can be difficult to involve the family in therapy. Family members are usually quite satisfied with seeing the alcoholism as the drinking member's problem rather than as the entire family's problem, and they are reluctant to confront their own participation in the problem. The alcoholic member, who has been receiving support from the therapist, may not want to risk this support by letting the therapist see how his family blames and derides him.

One way of approaching this problem is to pose removal of alcoholism as a central factor for the whole family. If it becomes accepted that the goal of therapy is change in the entire family, it becomes possible to deemphasize the drinking problem in family sessions. Individual sessions and participation in AA can proceed concurrently with family sessions, and the focus in the family sessions can be shifted to a wider formulation of the problem.

It is essential for the individual drinker and for the family to acknowledge alcoholism as a problem, and it is important that they learn about this illness and its part in their life. But they must also be freed from making alcoholism the scapegoat for every problem and be helped to develop healthy ways for dealing with the other problems of life.

References

Ablon, J. Al-Anon family group. *American Journal of Psychotherapy*, 1974, *28*, 30–45.

Ablon, J. Family structure and behavior in alcoholism: A review of the literataure. In B. Kissin and H. Begleiter (Eds.), *The biology of alcoholism.* Vol. 4. New York: Plenum, 1976.

Bacon, S. D. Excessive drinking and the institution of the family. *Alcohol, Science, and Society* (Quarterly Journal of Studies on Alcohol Education). New Haven: Yale Summer School of Alcohol Studies, 1945.

Bailey, M. B. *Alcoholism and family casework.* New York: The Community Council of Greater New York, 1968.

Bailey, M. B., Haberman, P. W., and Sheinberg, J. Distinctive characteristics of the alcoholic family. In *Report of the Health Research Council of the City of New York.* New York: National Council on Alcoholism (mimeo), 1965.

Berenson, D. Alcohol and the family system. In P. J. Guerin, Jr. (Ed.) *Family therapy: theory and practice.* New York: Gardner Press, 1976.

Bowen, M. Alcoholism as viewed through family systems theory and family psychotherapy. *Annals of the New York Academy of Sciences*, 1974, *233*, 115–122.

Cork, M. R. *The forgotten children.* Toronto: Addiction Research Foundation of Ontario, 1969.

Dulfano, C. Alcoholism in the family system. In T. Buckley (Ed.), *New directions in family therapy.* Oceanside, N. Y.: Tabor Science Publications, 1977.

Dulfano C. *Families alcoholism and recovery—ten stories.* Center City, Minn., Hazelden Publishing House, 1982.

Edwards, P., Harvey, C., and Whitehead, P. C. Wives of alcoholics: A critical review and analysis. *Quarterly Journal of Studies on Alcohol*, 1973, *34*, 112.

Ewing, J. A., and Fox, R. E. Family therapy of alcoholism. In J. Masserman (Ed.), *Current psychiatric therapies.* Vol. 8. New York: Grune and Stratton, 1968.

Finlay, D. G. Effect of role network pressure on an alcoholic's approach to treatment. *Social Work*, 1966, *11*, 71–77.

Haley, J. A review of the family therapy field. In J. Haley (Ed.), *A family therapy reader.* New York: Grune and Stratton, 1971.

Jackson, J. K. The adjustment of the family to the crisis of alcoholism. *Quarterly Journal of Studies on Alcohol*, 1954, *15*, 562–586.

Lutham, S. G., and Kirschenbaum, M. *The dynamic family*. Palo Alto: Science and Behavior Books, 1974.

Meeks, D. E., and Kelly, C. Family therapy with the families of recovered alcoholics. *Quarterly Journal of Studies on Alcohol*, 1970, *31*, 339–413.

Minuchin, S. Family therapy: Technique or theory? In J. Masserman (Ed.), *Science and psychoanalysis*. Vol. 14. New York. Grune and Stratton, 1969.

Minuchin, S. The use of an ecological framework in the treatment of a child. In E. J. Anthony and C. Koupernik (Ed.), *The child in his family*. New York: Wiley, 1970.

Minuchin, S. Structural family therapy. In G. Caplan (Ed.), *American handbook of psychiatry*. Vol. 3., revised ed. New York: Basic Books, 1972.

Minuchin, S. *Families and family therapy: A structural approach*. Cambridge: Harvard University Press, 1974.

Pattison, E. M. Ten years of change in alcoholism treatment and delivery systems. *American Journal of Psychiatry*, 1977, *134*, 261–266.

Price, G. M. Alcoholism is a family illness. *Casework Papers*, 1960.

Scherz, F. H. Theory and practice of family therapy. In R. W. Roberts and R. H. Nee (Eds.), *Theories of social case work*. Chicago: University of Chicago Press, 1970.

Smith, B. *A tree grows in Brooklyn*. New York: Harper & Row, 1943.

Steinglass, P. Experimenting with family treatment approaches to alcoholism, 1950–1975, a review. *Family Process*, 1976, *15*, 97–123.

Ward, R. F., and Faillace, L. A. The alcoholic and his helpers. *Quarterly Journal of Studies on Alcohol*, 1970, *31*, 684–691.

9

Intervention Techniques and Married Couples Group Therapy

Donald M. Gallant and David B. Mallott

Introduction

The teaching of skills for treating alcoholics must consider the different ways in which patients may come to the attention of the therapist. These ways may include those individuals who identify themselves as alcoholics and are seeking assistance voluntarily; (2) cases who are detected by skilled clinicians in the course of their work (because the alcoholic presents more or less indirect evidence of excessive use of alcohol); and (3) those patients who are so labeled by a third person who, in turn, makes the initial therapeutic contact without the subject's willing participation in that decision. It is the last manner of referral that is detailed in the first section of this chapter.

All therapists concerned with the treatment of alcoholics should be exposed to the techniques of early intervention therapy. In many cases this may save years of hardship for the family and friends, as well as the patient. Early intervention with an alcoholic compresses the past crises caused by misuse of alcohol into one dramatic confrontation in order to penetrate the defense mechanism of denial so that the patient will agree to get help. This type of intervention approach is a radical departure from the classical Alcoholics Anonymous (AA) view which

Donald M. Gallant • Professor of Psychiatry and Adjunct Professor of Psychopharmacology, Tulane University School of Medicine; Psychiatric Consultant to Southeast Louisiana Hospital, New Orleans, Louisiana.   David B. Mallott • Assistant Professor of Psychiatry, Tulane University School of Medicine, New Orleans, Louisiana.

infers that the patient must reach the depths of his own personal crisis before he is ready for help. This approach is also a philosophical departure from the Al-Anon approach which concentrates on the spouse's emotional detachment from the alcoholic's drinking behavior. This step-by-step procedure, which involves education of the spouse, family members, friends, and sometimes employers uses a number of carefully planned sessions for information and training before the formal confrontation is a technique that all alcoholism counselors should acquire. There are two points regarding intervention techniques that should be stressed: first, it is a potent therapeutic tool to be used only after careful training; second, the ethics of intruding on the privacy of the alcoholic with this technique are still questioned by some individuals.

The second section of this chapter details the married couples group therapy technique that the authors use in their consultation with state and private alcoholism agencies. This type of group process is a natural consequence of a successful intervention with the alcoholic spouse of a husband or wife. Group therapy with married couples enables the alcoholic and the spouse to develop personal freedom and decrease defensiveness in their relationship, eliminates minor bickering within a group, and helps the alcoholic and the spouse decrease their distortions of each other by observing similar behavior in other alcoholic couples. In addition, the initial neurotic needs that may have attracted the partners to each other in hopes of gratifying their own dependent or narcissistic tendencies can now be faced and treated in an open manner. It is the opinion of the authors of this chapter that married couples group therapy is the treatment of choice for married alcoholic patients. The defense mechanisms of denial and projection, exaggerated in the alcohol-marital problem, are more easily approached and treated within a group setting.

The Basis of the Therapeutic Relationship

In all modes of psychotherapy, trust is the essence of the therapist–patient relationship, and indeed, of all human relationships. Without this trust, the most intense efforts of a therapist may be useless when it comes to helping a patient. As this trust develops during the relationship, patient compliance will assuredly increase. This basic element of therapy should be emphasized for all psychotherapists who practice individual, as well as group therapy, techniques. Unfortunately, the theme of trust is not discussed frequently enough between the therapist and the patient. Often, even the most experienced psychiatrists are surprised by all expression of distrust from a long-term patient who has never before shown a lack of trust in the therapist.

A sensible division of the three important elements of a therapeutic relationship has been described by Truax and Carkhuff (Truax and Carkhuff, 1967). The concepts of non-possessive warmth (or the ability to show the patient that you care without "suffocating" him or her), accurate empathy (the ability to convey to the patient that you understand his or her feelings), and genuineness (conveying honesty to the patient and being able to admit your mistakes in an appropriate manner) are the foundation for the therapeutic relationship. The authors of this chapter would add a fourth element, the ability to convey the impression to the patient that you are professionally competent. When the therapist is able to incorporate these four elements into his relationship with the patient, a bond of trust is established and true therapy begins. However, without the factors of caring, empathy, honesty, and an ability to convey professional competence, the patient's symptoms may worsen. When these four factors are present to a high degree, the patient should show greater evidence of constructive personality change, whether in individual or group therapy. It is essential for all therapists to develop and improve these traits as long as they are practicing psychotherapy. These elements of the therapist–patient relationship are the most important concepts that we incorporate into our attempt to help each of our patients with the problem of alcoholism.

TECHNIQUES OF EARLY INTERVENTION AND TREATMENT

Early intervention with an alcohol abuser telescopes and compresses the past crises caused by alcoholism into one dramatic confrontation. This is done in order to overwhelm the mechanism of denial so that the patient will agree to get help. It is a therapeutic maneuver designed to help the patient *now* rather than to wait interminably for the alcohol abuser to "hit bottom," to lose or destroy his or her family, health, or job; if we wait, it may be too late. For example, it is not unusual in the field of alcoholism, to treat a severe, chronic alcoholic successfully and then have him hemorrhage to death from esophageal varices 6 to 12 months after he stopped drinking. The help, although initially successful, came too late.

Some AA and Al-Anon members are reluctant to recommend this method because they hold the opinion that the patient should "hit bottom" and make the decision for themselves while the family stays detached. They also are not exposed to intervention techniques. However, when early intervention is used with adequate preparation and sensitivity, it may save the patient and the family many years of suffering, and in some cases, prevent the marriage from breaking up. There are a number of different intervention approaches (Johnson, 1973; Gallant, 1982). For example, in the Johnson Institute technique, the patient is usually given a choice between hospitalization or temporary separation from his family or other significant relationships. In our intervention approach at Tulane Medical School, the available options are inpatient or outpatient therapy with disulfiram used as needed or, alternatively, temporary separation from the family. The varied options attempt to heavily influence the patient to select a therapy without "boxing him into a corner." Each therapist chooses an option according to the available human resources, treatment facilities, attitudes about confrontation techniques, and experience with alcoholics.

Adequate preparation, sensitivity, and experience are required for this early therapeutic intervention technique. The following steps describe the approach adopted by the authors. It is the spouse of the alcoholic who usually calls feeling upset and hopeless because the alcoholic spouse refuses to see that there is a problem or the need for help. An initial interview should be arranged with the spouse to obtain a history of the problem and to identify the key people in the environment who have the most influence on the alcoholic individual. The therapist should explain to the spouse that she or he is a patient as well and, thus, the confidentiality of the alcoholic is not involved. The next meeting should include the teenage or adult children and possibly one or two close friends whose attendance is requested in order to validate the spouse's history. They are also educated about the disease of alcoholism. All these people become the intervention team. They are asked to assume a nonjudgmental attitude and make a list of three to five painful or embarrassing events, avoiding labels, associated with the *behavior* demonstrated by the alcoholic while intoxicated. During this exploratory session with these people, three key attitudes for intervention are emphasized: (1) always express genuine concern to the alcoholic; (2) be nonjudgmental; (3) be honest.

Since the specific goal of the intervention is to have the alcoholic come in to see the therapist at least once, the spouse is asked to inform the alcoholic person about each meeting and to invite him or her to attend. It would then be the job of the therapist to convince the alcoholic patient to enter therapy. The spouse should also explain to the alcoholic that the children and friends were interviewed at the request of the therapist and not by the spouse's choice. Thus, some of the anger in the patient will be directed toward the therapist in order to avoid additional anger in the household. Nothing is to be done behind the back of the alcoholic during this phase of the intervention. By keeping the patient informed of this process, it is less likely to precipitate unexpected tragic events such as a sincere or manipulative suicide attempt.

Having prepared their list of "significant events," the team should stage a practice session for the intervention. This is helpful in: (1) identifying unexpected problems; (2) enhancing the ability to be concise and work together; (3) exploring resistance; (4) increasing the confidence of the treatment team. Part of the confrontation should be rehearsed with the therapist in order to avoid any gross disagreement and to eliminate individuals who may overprotect the patient. If some members of the team cannot carry out their roles, they should be excused and offered the opportunity to help in the future. A chairperson is selected to serve as coordinator so as to keep the team united and focused. The chairperson may be a professional in the field of alcoholism, a family physician, one of the significant members of the family, a friend, or the employer. The time of the actual confrontation must be carefully planned to be sure that the patient will be alcohol free. A confrontation with an intoxicated patient will be ineffective. This is the only session that is conducted without warning the alcoholic patient. At the confrontation meeting with the patient, the problems caused by the drinking are presented by all the members of the team. The patient is told that he must enter treatment for the alcoholism and is given several treatment options that include inpatient and/or outpatient treatment.

Usually, the authors enlist the aid of another couple who has had a successful intervention. This couple joins the intervention meeting. Their presence helps to defuse the situation by offering the alcoholic an opportunity to identify with someone else who has gone through the same painful process.

Finally, there *has* to be a commitment by the entire intervention team that a great deal is at stake if the alcoholic refuses the treatment options offered. It is unusual for a patient to reject the confrontation and the treatment options, but the intervention team should be prepared for this possibility.

Each team member must have thought out what he or she is prepared to do if the person refuses to see the therapist. The power of this strategy is consolidating all of the consequences into a single time frame and making it very clear that the only remedy is treatment as defined by the team (e.g., "If you refuse to see Dr._____, you can't come home."). Each team member must be ready to present the ultimatum in a clear and unyielding fashion. If a team member falters on the commitment, the team must rally to hold that member to the commitment. Because of this possibility, it is very important that each member has thought out what he or she is prepared to do and has communicated this decision to the other team members. Rash but empty threats will be of no use in the intervention process. These threats only increase the denial.

With the scales weighted so inequitably (separation versus one visit to the physician), it is easy to see that it would be difficult for the person to refuse. One of the possible reasons why this type of technique rarely fails is that the alcoholic patient has not been pushed into a corner without alternatives. Nonetheless, the threat of separation is quite severe compared with having to see a physician for one visit. Another reason for the success of this type of approach is that before the massive intervention the patient was able to deny his problem. Angry individual accusations about the drinking behavior only made the patient more defensive. Now he has been forced to look at the effects of his drinking behavior on the people that he loves and to abandon at least a small piece of the denial mechanism. Even if the patient refuses to return to the therapist for a follow-up session, he still has had the denial penetrated and the entire family problem can now be handled in a more realistic and open manner.

The technique of intervention is summarized in the following: (1) A concerned person seeks help for a problem related to the alcoholism of the person he or she cares about. (The concerned person is usually a spouse, but may be a child, employer, or friend.) The process is kept open and the spouse informs the alcoholic about the meetings. Be sure the alcohol abuser is informed that the therapist (not the concerned person) has invited the participants. This procedure describes the reality of the situation and directs the anger away from the concerned person. (2) This person is enlisted to gather other significant persons into a meeting about the intervention process. This group will be organized into an intervention team. (3) Team members are educated about the alcoholism, the treatment, and the intervention process. They are told about the denial of the alcoholic, symptoms of the illness, prognosis, and so forth. (4) Each team member is asked to make a list of 3 to 5 significant events in the relationship in which he or she was hurt in some way by the alcohol-dependent person. The list should be specific as to time, place, and circumstances, as well as nonjudgmental and without the use of labels; just detailed descriptions and reactions to the behavior. (5) Each event should be presented in a nonjudgmental way and emphasize the connection between the use of alcohol and the event (e.g., "You came late to my school play. You were drinking and made a scene in the audience. The Principal finally asked you to leave. I was so embarrassed, Dad."). Note that the statements should include the team member's feelings, "I felt helpless, scared, frustrated, angry," etc. (6) All team members are cautioned to temporarily suspend past quarrels among themselves for the benefit of the team effort. It is important to present a united front with a consistent message: "We are concerned about your drinking and its effect on your behavior. We can no longer stand helplessly in the wings while you destroy yourself and us. You need treatment." (7) A chairperson is selected to serve as coordinator. (8) Treatment options are discussed, selected, and arranged prior to the intervention.

It is also important to understand the use of treatment contracts with the patient in association with this intervention approach. During the confrontation, the alcoholic can be offered the choice of a visit with a physician for an initial interview, to ongoing outpatient treatment, or referral to an inpatient service. In the great majority of the cases, the patient will select the choice of seeing the physician for one visit. The patient–therapist contract offers the patient a sequence of treatment modalities, including Alcoholics Anonymous, with each one leading to a more controlled treatment setting if the patient fails in the initial arrangement. During the initial visit, a contract regarding disulfiram (Antabuse) use can be made stipulating that the alcoholic patient agrees to take the medication if he drinks again. In this manner, the patient is not backed into a corner with no way out except an angry use of denial. It should be emphasized again that it is highly unusual for a patient to totally reject this confrontation and very rarely does the alcoholic refuse the contract options that are offered (Gallant, 1982).

A special point should be made about adolescent alcohol abusers. In this group the effect of peer pressure is immense, far more powerful than the effects of the therapist, the school, or the home environment. Therefore, it is essential to have one or two reliable alcohol-free peers of the young alcohol abuser available for the intervention. It is also important to find one or two healthy adult models with whom the adolescent alcohol abuser can have a positive identification. Such individuals may have a greater influence on the adolescent than the family. It is also essential for these adolescents to change their peer groups after the intervention treatment has been initiated. It is almost impossible for them to stay free of alcohol if they return to their former alcohol-using peers who will have a greater influence on the young alcohol abuser than the therapist no matter how experienced he or she may be. With the adolescent, helping the youth find and assimilate into new peer groups is one of the most important elements of therapy.

The obvious goals of the intervention are to bring the alcoholic into treatment by using a dramatic confrontation to help penetrate his or her denial. In most cases the family and/or friends have previously tried without success to have the alcoholic person cutdown or stop drinking. Usually these attempts have failed because: (1) the approach was made in an inflamatory and accusatory fashion that placed the alcoholic person on the defensive and increased existing denial; (2) the concerned persons were uninformed about the diagnosis and proper treatment of alcoholism; (3) each attempt was made at a different time and in an uncoordinated fashion. Consequently, the alcoholic was able to use denial in an effective manner and, at times, an available person may have enabled further resistance to professional help (e.g., after his wife threw him out of the house, his best friend took him in). This type of person is called an *enabler* because such friends or relatives permit the alcoholic person to continue the pattern of alcohol abuse.

The concept behind the intervention technique is that alcoholism is a progressive illness and very rarely goes into remission without outside help. The intervention technique attempts to telescope or compress the events associated with alcohol abuse into an early therapeutic confrontation in order to precipitate a crisis. This occurs in the present rather than waiting for years of suffering, risking loss of family, job, or health. One of the natural concomitants of this intervention is married couples group therapy for the alcoholic and the spouse. This type of group therapy is described in the second section of this chapter.

CASE HISTORIES OF INTERVENTIONS

Case 1. In this case, one sees a middle-class, 38-year-old woman married to an alcoholic who has tried Al-Anon but without change in the drinking pattern of her husband or in the deteriorating relationships within the family.

A 38-year-old wife called to say that her family was in a desperate situation. She is married to a 40-year-old contractor whose drinking had progressed steadily to the point where he was totally intoxicated by the time he reached home at the end of the day. He had a 16-year-old son who had been doing well at school and on the football team. However, in the past six months his grades had decreased in a significant manner and he had quit the football team. In addition, he developed a slight tick over his left eye and barely talked to either his father or mother. The second child was a 13-year-old daughter who apparently was depressed and walked around the house sulking. She was described as negative and rebellious. It was becoming increasingly difficult for either the father or mother to control her behavior, especially when she returned home during evening hours after having been with her friends. An initial appointment was scheduled with the wife.

During our first meeting, in addition to the above information, she related that the early years of their marriage had been quite good. She said that her husband was a successful contractor in the building of homes and apparently did most of his drinking while at work. During lunch time and toward the end of the day, he would increase his intake of beer. At the end of the day, he would invite a majority of the men who worked for him to a local bar where he continued to imbibe until he reached a state of severe intoxication. He then developed a habit of stopping off at the homes of one or two of his best friends in an attempt to sober up before arriving home. He did very little drinking at his friends' homes but still was not able to reach a sober state by the time he arrived at his house. There would be very little conversation on arrival and the patient would quickly undress, eat very little, if at all, and then retire to the bedroom where he went to sleep. He was described as not being physically or verbally abusive, but the relationship between him and his family was practically nonexistent. Occasionally, he would become quite curt and irritated if any friends of his children were visiting or if they were playing records or engaged in other adolescent activities. We suggested to this woman that we next have a session with her and the two children.

During our second session, the children validated the wife's history and related several embarrassing situations that had occurred as a result of their father's drinking. One typical incident, graduation from ballet class, was described by the daughter. The graduation of the ballet class took place in a local auditorium where a bar had been set up in the back area. The father had been steadily drinking at the bar while the dancing had proceeded and by the end of the graduation ceremony, he was totally intoxicated. When his daughter attempted to introduce some of her friends to him, he made some obscene remarks which she found difficult to forget. She was intensely embarrassed as she related this episode which had occurred more than six months earlier. On the next day, when she confronted her father at home, he could not remember the event and it was obvious that he had an alcoholic blackout during that period. The son discussed the discouragement that he felt about the family situation. He talked about his father never attending any of the football games and never giving him approval for how well he had been performing in school or on the football field. He was embarrassed that his father was one of the few fathers that never attended any football games and he never knew what to tell his friends about why this was so. He said that the few times that he saw his father was shortly after his arrival home from work and in the morning just before he left for school. After this session, it was decided to have the next meeting with the two best friends of the father, the two children, and the mother in order to identify key members of the intervention team. Prior to each of these sessions, the alcoholic had been notified about the meetings and was told that he was welcome to attend if he agreed to treatment. It was made clear to him that treatment would consist either of inpatient therapy for 4 to 6 weeks or outpatient therapy with the use of disulfiram and regular attendance at married couples therapy. Each time the father was notified about this invitation, he would become very angry and say, "What business does this shrink have in butting into our family affairs?" The wife replied that she was the patient and the evaluation showed that the husband's drinking was affecting the spouse's emotional state. That was the reason for the invitation to attend the meetings. The alcoholic showed a usual response after this angry episode by never mentioning it until the next meeting. His denial was intensified during subsequent weeks but he also decreased his drinking for the several days after such an invitation. This is not an unusual sequence of events during preparation for the confrontation.

During the third meeting with the wife, two children, and two best friends, we reviewed the drinking history. The two friends were surprised that the wife's husband was drinking so much. However, consensual validation by the children both convinced them and refreshed their memories. They then started to recall some of the events when her husband would arrive slightly intoxicated at their house and wondered why he was drinking so early in the day. During this meeting, the wife stated that she was ready to leave the husband unless he did something about the drinking problem. The children supported her statement and all five persons agreed to have a confrontation with the patient. We then arranged a fourth meeting to prepare the list of embarrassing events that were associated with the husband's alcoholism and to rehearse the intervention.

During the fourth meeting, it was emphasized that the confrontation should consist of the attitudes of nonjudgment, caring, and honesty. Each person was asked to list the episodes that caused them to become angry, embarrassed, or anxious. Since no evidence of severe depression or suicidal intent could be detected from the history obtained from the wife, children, and friends, it was decided to allow the wife to arrange the confrontation on a Saturday morning at home shortly after her husband awoke. We were available at the phone in case the intervention caused unexpected reactions.

The intervention meeting took place at the alcoholic's home on Saturday morning at about 8:00 A.M. It went quite well. Each one of the participants read their list from sheets of paper to avoid any angry "eyeballing." We find this technique much more comfortable for all the parties involved. The entire motive is to have the patient come in for help and not to make him angry. He agreed to come in to see us as long as his friends were no longer involved. We arranged the meeting with the alcoholic, the wife, the two children and one of our couples who had successfully terminated therapy. We use this couple as an auxiliary therapeutic team in order to draw off some of the anger from the therapists.

During the follow-up session, we presented further educational material to the children, the alcoholic, and the wife. We reviewed the genetics of alcoholism (which was quite strong in his family), discussed the meaning of the alcohol blackouts, and the loss of control of drinking. The auxiliary couple subsequently did most of the interviewing with the husband, attempting to have this new alcoholic patient identify with them. The husband of the auxiliary couple said that he had gone through the same type of denial, developed a great deal of anger as people had requested him to seek help, and was able to present the denial process as being a normal accompaniment of alcoholism. In this manner, we attempt to diffuse the anger that many of the alcoholics bring into therapy following an intervention. The alcoholic was then given the choice of entering our inpatient service for 4 to 6 weeks or entering our outpatient married couples group therapy while taking disulfiram on a daily basis at breakfast with his children and wife, or having the wife and children separate from him at this point in time. He chose married couples group therapy on an outpatient basis with the disulfiram and attended regularly for the next 12 months. At that time, he requested to have the disulfiram discontinued and asked to be terminated from group therapy as he believed that he had made sufficient progress. In that period of time, his son had returned to the football team, had lost his nervous tick, and was performing well in school. The daughter had blossomed and was relating in a very comfortable way. The group was asked to give an opinion as to whether or not they thought he was ready for discharge and the decision was almost unanimous that he had shown significant progress in therapy. He was now relating more openly and directly with his daughter and son, was more involved in their school and extracurricular activities, and was confiding in a more intimate way with his wife. The wife confirmed the fact that the marriage had improved in many areas and the patient was then told that he was discharged. However, both the patient and his wife were also informed that if there was any sign or tendency toward relapse concerning either behavior or alcohol intake, they should immediately call the therapist and arrange a follow-up meeting. At this time, the alcoholic patient, his wife, and children are still doing quite well.

Case 2. This case presents a patient who was 69 years of age and shows that one is never too old for an intervention.

A 72-year-old physician called to say that he wanted to come for an interview concerning his wife. Upon arrival at the office, he related that his wife had been a controlled social drinker for many years until she reached middle age. At that time, her children were grown, had moved out of the house and married. She had never planned adequately for this environmental change and started drinking by herself. Since that time, the alcohol intake had steadily increased to the point where she was intoxicated on a daily basis and was frequently found drunk on the floor at home by the husband when he arrived back from his office. All of their three grown children were aware of the situation, as was her best friend who happened to be a nurse in the doctor's office. One of the children was slightly retarded and married to another mild mental retardate. They lived next door to the doctor and his wife. The physician explained that this daughter was becoming extremely upset because she did not know how to handle her mother when she arrived in the mother's home and found her in a stuporous state. This daughter would develop acute anxiety attacks and panic, calling several of the neighbors to help her place her mother in bed. As a consequence of this situation, the entire neighborhood was very much aware of this woman's drinking problem. It may be interesting to note that the doctor and his wife were members of several highly regarded social organizations and the alcoholic wife had placed a great value on appearances.

A second meeting was conducted with the doctor, the three grown children, and the wife's best friend. Part of the session was devoted to education on alcoholism including the subject of denial, alcohol blackouts, psychologic consequences of prolonged alcohol intake on both the patient and the family, and the possible hereditary aspects of the problem. It was suggested that each of the participants draw up a list of embarrassing or painful events associated with the wife's drinking episodes. The doctor was told to go home and inform his wife about this meeting and ask her if she wanted to attend the next meeting. As is usual, she became extremely angry at him, decreased her drinking, but absolutely refused to come in and see the psychiatrist.

During the third meeting, the list of drinking episodes was reviewed and it became quite apparent that the wife had had numerous blackouts, some of them endangering her life as well as the lives of others. She had driven a car during an alcohol blackout and not remembered where she parked it, had cursed out one of her children over the phone (which she would never do in a sober state), and had locked her mentally retarded daughter out of the house when the daughter had become upset about the woman's drinking. It did appear that there was some depression present in this 69-year-old female alcoholic and we were concerned about an exacerbation of this depression during the intervention or even a subsequent suicide attempt. Therefore, it was thought advisable to have the intervention at the medical school in the psychiatrist's office. This was the only time that total honesty was not used with alcoholic patient. Her husband told her that he wanted her to come to the medical school to see a physician about the evaluation of high blood pressure and to possibly investigate the cause of the hypertension. Although there was some truth behind this distortion (since it did appear that excessive alcohol intake was responsible for the hypertension), it was our opinion that she would have never arrived for the intervention session if the truth had been told to her.

Of course, she was quite surprised at seeing her children and her best friend in the physician's office at the medical school and the initial part of the intervention started with a great deal of anger on the part of the alcoholic wife. The psychiatrist took full blame for arranging the situation and did say that her husband had come to him because he was very upset, nervous, and distrubed about the future of their marriage which had been such a good one for so many years. The children were very supportive and reviewed their lists of her drinking behavior in a very benign manner while her friend was somewhat more direct and blunt about the alcohol blackouts that had been embarrassing to a number of people, as well as to the husband. This intervention session was a more upsetting one than that described in Case 1. The wife started to cry, became angry, defensive, and finally after about one hour started to listen to the children and her friend, as well as to her husband. The husband, in a very dramatic manner, said that he and the children were going to cut off all communications with her unless she agreed to start treatment at this time. By the end of the session, the major uncomfortable feeling that the patient expressed was severe embarrassment associated with her need for appearance and false pride. Depression was not a significant problem and there was an agreement to have her follow-up as an outpatient with her husband administering the disulfiram to her. She readily agreed to this compromise situation as she could never picture herself as ever going to "an alcoholic place." She also agreed to go to married couples group therapy with her husband on a regular basis while taking the disulfiram.

After the second married couples group therapy, she asked to see the psychiatrist in private with her husband. She said that she felt totally humiliated having to expose herself at the age of 69 in front of so many young people regarding her drinking. She did not want anyone to find out about her drinking problem and she urged us to make a contract with her as follows. She said that she would continue to take the disulfiram on an indefinite basis from her husband as long as she never had to go to married couples group therapy again or see the psychiatrist. She said that her drinking had caused her severe humiliation and that she did not want to have to continually be reminded about this humiliating part of her life. We then agreed to abide by her request for the contract and to this day, the patient has remained totally abstinent and the husband describes the marriage as a very happy one.

In this particular case, the intervention method apparently not only halted the patient's drinking but literally turned her on the road to behavior changes without having to use long-term follow-up psychotherapy.

Married Couples Group Psychotherapy

Outcome evaluations of married couples group therapy have shown the technique to be quite efficacious (Gallant, Rich, Bey, and Terranova, 1970; Blinder and Kirschenbaum, 1967; Leichter, 1962; and Sager, Grundlach, Kremer, and Linz, 1968). In one study of 118 couples, the success rate during an 18 month follow-up, which included significant economic and social gains, as well as total abstinence, was approximately 60% (Gallant, 1970). The success rate in this particular follow-up would have even been higher if decreased or controlled drinking would have been included in the success group. The most significant part of the follow-up period in this particular evaluation appeared to be during the first three months after discharge from the inpatient service, when the majority of failures occurred. One other encouraging fact that was observed in the follow-up evaluation of these 118 couples was that only three couples were considered to be permanently separated at the time of the 18th month evaluation, which is less than expected with the national average divorce rate.

In the treatment of patients with alcohol abuse or alcohol dependence, it is absolutely essential to incorporate all of the human resources that are available to the patients within the treatment setting. Thus, it would be wrong to ignore the spouse of the alcoholic patient or minimize the use of the spouse in treatment. Each one of us sees the world through our own eyes and it would not be wise to totally accept the alcoholic's view of the world that he or she presents in the therapy sessions. The goals of the group psychotherapy technique with married couples are: (1) penetration of the patient's severe denial in association with the goal of abstinence; and (2) helping the couples develop a satisfactory living experience and improve their interpersonal relationships.

The couples groups meet every week for 2 hours or every 2 weeks for 4 hour meetings. The group that meets once every two weeks includes patients whose work schedule does not permit them to visit the clinic every week. Each group consists of 6 to 7 couples and is open-ended. Duration of time in the group lasts from 1 to 3 years, depending on the severity of the intrapsychic and interpersonal problems that each couple brings to the group. In the group meetings, "the here and now" approach to treatment is greatly emphasized. Honest, direct impressions and opinions of other patients in group are consistently requested of the couples. Opinions of improvement in behavior, character deficits, constructive or destructive behavior, attitude toward spouse, and so forth, are constant foci of therapy in the treatment sessions.

Some of the following are possible reasons that may account for the success of the marital couples group approach: (1) The spouse of the patient helps to keep "pulling" the patient back to treatment, and drop-out rate is lower as the result of the spouse's cooperation. The patient cannot say, "I'm the only one who is trying in the marriage." (2) There is a common goal of abstinence to unify the group. The primary goal is really to start the couple working on their marriage problems, but sobriety is required for this goal. (3) In some cases, the therapist utilizes the spouse to administer disulfiram to the patient when it is considered to be psychologically sound and absolutely necessary if we are to maintain the patient in a sober state while working on the intrapersonal, as well as the interpersonal, problems. (4) The therapist obtains a more realistic view of the home life of the patient by seeing some of the marital interactions in the group which force the patient to use less denial and distortion. Habitual psychomotor or nonverbal communications between the partners (smirks, grimaces, etc.) allow the therapist and the group to see the feelings and mood which are behind the verbal interchanges. The noncontent presentation of the patient and the spouse are readily visible in relation to motor mannerisms and manner of speech. Thus, the therapist and the group can refuse to accept the distortions of both husband and wife and thereby aid in the correction of the neurotic interaction. (5) The initial neurotic needs that may have attracted the partners to each other in hopes of gratifying their own dependent or narcissistic tendencies now can be faced and treated in an open manner. (6) The marital couples group approach enables the alcoholic patient to develop personal freedom and decrease the defensiveness (e.g., giving permission to an extremely dependent alcoholic wife to speak up to her dominating husband in the group). In other situations, the unhealthy guilt of the spouse and symbiotic acceptance of the alcoholic can be decreased (e.g., enabling the wife of the patient to set limits and to force him to give up his denial and to realize in a direct and honest manner that this is the "last time around"). This development can be therapeutic. (7) With both partners present, minor bickering is eliminated in the group and the important essential problems of the couple are directly faced. In couples therapy, the minor bickering can persist, with each mate forever complaining to the therapist about the spouse.

These patients must be treated together to prevent a recurrent neurotic disequilibrium. For example, as the male alcoholic makes progress in therapy and decides to resume his appropriate responsibilities, the wife must be aware of this change and allow him to resume his role in the home. If the wife is deprived of the opportunity of participating with her husband in treatment, then the therapist, as well as the patient, could misinterpret her attitude and classify her as a castrating, dominating, or controlling wife. This distortion by the therapists, as well as by the patients, has already filled the literature with the classical picture of the alcoholic's wife as one who has a need to keep her husband in a submissive role. This generalization, on closer examination and upon treatment of these couples, is usually untrue and misleading. Most wives of alcoholics are only too happy to give up inappropriate roles that were thrust on them by an alcoholic husband who could not sustain his responsibilities. Another example that demonstrates the need for the spouse of the patient to participate in the treatment situation is the case of the wife who resolves some of her intrapsychic emotional problems and becomes more sexually aroused. If she is married to a man who has symptoms of relative impotency, his excuse for faulty performance is now gone and complete impotency can develop.

Most of the couples attending group therapy also use AA and Al-Anon for help with abstinence. If the alcoholic does resume drinking, a contract is then drawn up with the agreement that the patient will then have the spouse administer disulfiram, suspended in water, on a daily basis. The agreement states that the disulfiram is a symbol of the alcoholic's commitment to his family as well as to treatment. Thus, the patient is taking disulfiram in order to decrease the spouse's daily anticipatory anxiety about the patient's drinking and to eliminate false accusations of having "sneaked a drink." It is then emphasized that disulfiram is an insurance policy rather than a "crutch." The patient's reaction to this suggestion, after having had a "slip," is one way of estimating the degree of his denial and noncompliance in therapy.

There are exceptions to using married couples group therapy as a routine technique. If one of the spouses is overtly psychotic, the mental illness will become quite conspicious in the married couples group and further alienate the couple. If there are serious secondary psychological problems in the children, it would then be necessary to use a family therapy approach in addition to the married couples therapy sessions. If there are acute, embarrassing sexual problems that are threatening to disrupt the marital relationship within the immediate future, then it would be absolutely necessary to see the couple in private sexual counseling sessions as well as in the married couples group since the group may not be at a stage where such personal problems could be explored in front of relative strangers. Outside of these few exceptions, we routinely prepare the married couples for couples group therapy and have them start the group sessions as soon as the orientation has been completed.

CASE HISTORIES OF COUPLES GROUP THERAPY

Case 1.   A 42-year-old alcoholic woman was a very passive, dependent individual married to a dominating, aggressive man. At the time of the marriage, she was an extremely attractive woman and her appearance was one of the reasons her husband wanted to marry her. He was a very aggressive, hard-driving businessman who put too much value on appearance. His value system included possession of a beautiful wife, driving foreign cars, wearing expensive clothes, and being seen in the best restaurants. Whenever his wife attempted to assert herself in an appropriate manner, he would clamp down rather aggressively which only increased her nonassertiveness that she had developed during childhood with an overbearing father and a weak mother.

In the married couples group therapy sessions, she did quite well as far as her abstinence was concerned but still had difficulties in asserting herself with her husband. In a series of several sessions, some of the female spouses in the couples group expressed direct opinions to him which he had accepted in a rather appropriate manner, much to the patient's surprise. In addition, there was a free discussion of his value system on appearances which only undermined his wife's confidence. She was 42 years of age and could not keep up the young attractive appearance that she presented at the time of their marriage. During a couples therapy session, one of the other wives asked her to directly tell her husband about her needing to have him give an opinion concerning her personality characteristics as well as her appearance.

Much to her surprise, he started to talk about her honesty and sincerity with people, something he had never done in private. The use of the "here and now" was of definite help in having her speak directly to her husband. The task was much more easily accomplished than if one had asked her to go home and question him about his value system. Success within the present group setting helped to create immediate positive reinforcement from other members of the group and also enabled the patients to see that the spouse can respond to appropriate direct comments, thus overcoming some of her unfounded fears of an angry reaction by her husband.

During another session, one of the other wives in the group directly disagreed with the husband concerning his opinion about one of the political figures in the area. Much to the wife's amazement, her husband did not respond in an angry way to this confrontation but rather appeared to be somewhat flexible in his thinking. Some of the other members in the group pointed out that she was allowing past neurotic habit patterns between her and her husband to influence her behavior in the present. It is these advantages of the "here and now," use of consensual validation, correction of neurotic distortions between the couple, and available modeling experiences within the group setting that appear to add psychotherapeutic efficacy to this particular technique.

Case 2. The following case emphasizes the need to have the spouse of the alcoholic patient involved in the same therapy setting in order to understand the changes the patient is undergoing during his abstinence.

A 48-year-old alcoholic male had been married for 20 years to a woman who originally had been relatively appropriate in the way she asserted herself with both family and friends. However, over the years, as her husband's drinking increased, she had to assume more responsibility, not only for raising the children, but for managing the family finances as well. The alcoholic husband, although an extremely conscientious accountant, would become very irresponsible and squandered financial resources during his episodes of drinking. Not only did he gamble more money than he could afford, but he would also go off on buying sprees which the family could not afford. Finally, although he originally would not agree to discuss his drinking, he did allow his wife to take over the financial purse strings for the household. As the years went by, she assumed more and more responsibility for the checkbook as well as for the savings account and other financial holdings of the family.

Prior to entrance into married couples therapy, the alcoholic husband had completed an inpatient alcoholism treatment program and was already taking disulfiram on a regular basis during the family dinnertime in order to allay some of the anxiety of the children and wife about the drinking problem. In the married couples group setting, the subject of sharing the responsibilities of the discipline of the children and the managing of the finances in the household came up in the group. The wife expressed some natural anxiety about turning the checkbook over to the husband, particularly in view of his past history of financial irresponsibility. Some of the other wives in the group talked about their experiences and about how difficult it was for them once again to start sharing the financial responsibility with their husbands once they had become abstinent. One of the wives said to the spouse "as long as he's taking the Antabuse, there should be no realistic worry. Also, if you're going to trust the marriage, you might as well trust it all the way until he proves you wrong. How long can you go on questioning the situation without undermining your own confidence in him as well as his confidence?" Similar comments from other spouses of alcoholics in the group helped this wife to make a decision about sharing responsibilities for the checkbook with the husband. She was able to see behavior changes in her husband not only at home but within the group setting and was able to understand that her anxiety about giving up some of the responsibility was quite normal.

One month later in the married couples group therapy session, this same spouse started talking about how wonderful it was to "not have to carry the world around on your back." She went on to say that on looking back, "I'm only too happy to have someone share all these troubles with me and it's actually a pleasure to have someone worry with you." These types of modeling experiences are constantly available in married couples group therapy. These techniques enable the spouse and the patient to correct past neurotic distortions that develop in the marriage and also help the spouse of the alcoholic to understand the changes that the alcoholic patient is currently undergoing within the therapy setting. She can see these changes happen in front of her eyes and not depend on the verbal reports that the patient may bring home from traditional group therapy where the spouse is not included.

SUMMARY

Techniques of early intervention are therapeutic maneuvers designed to help the patient in the present rather than to wait interminably for the alcohol abuser to "hit bottom"; if we wait, it may be too late for the patient as well as for the family. The concept behind the intervention technique is that alcoholism is a progressive illness and very rarely goes into remission without outside help. The intervention technique attempts to telescope the events associated with alcohol abuse into an early therapeutic confrontation in order to precipitate a crisis in the present rather than waiting for years of suffering to take place with the risk of the future loss of family, job, friends, psychologic health, or medical health. One of the recommended types of follow-up therapy after this type of intervention is married couples group therapy for the alcoholic and the spouse.

There are many reasons for treating the marital partners in the same group in an honest and open manner. If there is any relationship where direct honesty and openness is essential, it is the marital experience. In fact, treating the husband and wife by separate therapists can magnify the distortions and misunderstandings between the partners, thus possibly bringing about a separation or divorce because of the unrealistic treatment structure. With different therapists, each one is encouraged by the experience to discuss marital problems outside the marriage without the partner being present. This can be interpreted by some outsiders as "acting out" in relation to the marriage. Projection of blame and responsibility, which is a neurotic pattern in many marriages, can be treated only with both parties present at the same time. With the exception of the specific exclusions mentioned previously in this chapter, marital couples group therapy with alcoholics who are living with a spouse is the treatment of choice with these authors.

REFERENCES

Blinder, M. G., and Kirschenbaum, M. The technique of married couples group therapy. *Archives General Psychiatry*, 1967, 17, 44–52.

Gallant, D. M. *Alcohol and Drug Abuse Curriculum Guide for Psychiatry Faculty*, DHHS Pub. No. 82–1159, ADAMHA, 1982, 19–22.

Gallant, D. M., Rich, A., Bey, E., and Terranova, L. Group psychotherapy with married couples: A successful technique in New Orleans alcoholism clinic patients. *Journal of Louisiana State Medical Society*, 1970, 122, 41–44.

Johnson, V. E. *I'll quit tomorrow.* New York: Harper & Row, 1973.

Leichter, E. Group psychotherapy with married couples: Some characteristic treatment dynamics. *International Journal of Group Psychotherapy*, 1962, 12, 154–163.

Sager, C. S., Grundlach, R., Kremer, M., and Linz, R. The married in treatment. *Archives of General Psychiatry*, 1968, 19, 205–217.

Truax, C. B., and Carkhuff, R. R. *Toward effective counseling and psychotherapy: Training and practice.* Chicago: Aldine, 1967.

10

Use of the Social and Family Network in Individual Therapy

Marc Galanter

Introduction

In this chapter I will discuss an innovative treatment approach for the alcohol dependent patient. Although this approach may be used specifically with the alcoholic patient, it is equally useful for many drug-abusing patients. It is important that the clinician have access to an effective format for rehabilitation of these patients, because traditional approaches may have limited impact on addictive illness (Vaillant, 1981; Steinglass, 1976). A treatment approach will therefore be outlined, based on the author's experience, with the use of a social support network as an integral part of the therapy. In this way I will illustrate some of the themes of social therapy which may be used in a practical approach to treatment. The origins of this approach lie in both network therapy as developed by Speck and others (Speck, 1967) and in more widely used family therapy techniques.

This approach can be useful in addressing a broad range of addicted patients. These patients are characterized by the following clinical hallmarks of addictive illness, relevant to this treatment model. First, when they initiate consumption of their addictive agent, be it alcohol, cocaine, opiates, or depressant drugs, they frequently cannot limit that consumption to a reasonable and predictable level; this phenomenon has been termed *loss of control* by clinicians who treat alcohol- or drug-de-

Marc Galanter • Professor of Psychiatry, Albert Einstein College of Medicine, Bronx, New York.

pendent persons. Second, they have consistently demonstrated relapse to the agent of abuse; that is, they have attempted to stop using the drug for varying periods of time but have returned to it, despite a specific intent to avoid it.

This treatment approach is not necessary for those abusers who can, in fact, learn to set limits on their alcohol or drug use; their abuse may be treated as a behavioral symptom in a more traditional psychotherapeutic fashion. It is also not directed at those patients for whom the addictive pattern is most unmanageable, such as long-term intravenous opiate addicts, and others with unusual destabilizing circumstances such as homelessness, severe character pathology, or psychosis. These patients may need special supportive care such as drug substitution (i.e., methadone maintenance), inpatient detoxification, or long-term residential treatment.

In reviewing this material, the reader should focus on those aspects of the treatment outlined here which are at variance with his usual therapeutic approach. Whereas it is essential to rely on acquired clinical judgment and experience, it is equally important with the substance abuser to be prepared to depart from the usual mode of psychotherapeutic treatment. For example, activity rather than passivity is essential when a problem of drug exposure is suggested; the concept of therapist and patient enclosed in an inviolable envelope must be modified; immediate circumstances which may expose the patient to drug use must take precedence over issues of long-term understanding and insight. These principles are applicable within the technique outlined here. Other approaches, too, such as the use of couples group therapy and other techniques discussed in this book (Gallant, Rich, Bey, and Terranova, 1970) may incorporate most of these principles.

THE INITIAL ENCOUNTERS

The patient should be asked to bring his spouse or a close friend to the first session. Drug-dependent patients often do not like certain things they hear when they first come for treatment and may deny or rationalize even if they have voluntarily sought help. Because of their denial of the problem, a significant other is essential to both history taking and to implementing a viable treatment plan. A close relation can often cut through the denial in the way that an unfamiliar therapist cannot and can therefore be invaluable in setting a standard of realism in dealing with the addiction.

Some patients make clear that they wish to come to the initial session on their own. This is often associated with their desire to preserve the option of continued substance abuse and is born out of the fear that an alliance will be established independent of them to prevent this. Although a delay may be tolerated for a session or two, there should be no ambiguity at the outset that effective treatment can only be undertaken on the basis of a therapeutic alliance around the drug issue. This includes the support of significant others and it is expected that a network of close friends and/or relations will be brought in within a session or two at the most.

Not only are patients sometimes reluctant to establish a network, their relatives may also be resistant. For example, it may be necessary to develop a strategy for engaging a resistant spouse into a cooperative role:

Case 1. A 40-year-old lawyer came for treatment of his drinking problem primarily because his marriage was doing poorly. He secured his wife's agreement to come to the initial session and hoped that the therapy would serve as a bridge for improving their failing relationship. She was actually reluctant to establish closer ties to him and told me that she preferred not to be involved in the treatment. She came a half-hour late for the second conjoint session, citing heavy rains along the route from their home in an outlying suburb. She was in an angry mood, throwing out that she could not come again as she had to tend to their four children and organize their after-school activities. Rather than retreating from my position, I expressed considerable regret that she was being compromised by the plan and stated my own appreciation that she had gone so far out of her way to help out. I pointed out to her how valuable she was to the plan (never noting in fact she was being much less than positive to date), and that I needed her to support my own imperfect ability to help her husband achieve sobriety, underlining the serious limitations of the individual therapist who alone treats the alcoholic. I agreed to her skipping a session the next week, giving acknowledgment to a relatively unimportant conflicting appointment, in exchange for her agreement to come the week thereafter. After a month it became clearer to her that it was in her interest—on a pragmatic level—to participate.

Therapists are used to thinking they are right and expecting (or at least hoping for) a good measure of respect for their views. This example is given to underline the strategic importance of generating whatever understanding may be necessary to achieve a viable relationship with a network member, even at the risk of feeling rejected. This may also take a good measure of cajoling and even manipulation at the outset of treatment.

The weight of clinical experience supports the view that abstinence is the most practical goal to propose to the addicted person for his rehabilitation (Gitlow and Peyser, 1980; Zimberg, 1982). For abstinence to be expected, however, the therapist should assure the provision of necessary social supports for the patient. Let us consider how a long-term support network is initiated for this purpose, beginning with availability of the therapist, significant others, and a self-help group.

In the first place, the therapist should be available for consultation on the phone and should indicate to the patient that he wants to be called if problems arise. This makes the therapist's commitment clear and sets the tone for a "team effort." It begins to undercut one reason for relapse; the patient's sense that he will be on his own if he is unable to manage the situation. The astute therapist, though, will assure the patient that he does not spend excessive time at the telephone or in emergency sessions, and therefore the patient will develop a support network which can handle the majority of day-to-day problems. This will generally leave the therapist only to respond to occasional questions of interpreting the terms of the understanding between himself, the patient, and support network members. If there is question about the ability of the patient and network to manage the period between the initial sessions, the first few scheduled sessions may be arranged at intervals of only one to three days. In any case, frequent appointments should be scheduled at the outset of a pharmacologic detoxification (as with benzodiazepines for alcoholism), so that the patient need never manage more than a few days medication at a time.

What is most essential, though, is that the network be forged into a working group to provide necessary support for the patient between the initial sessions. As will be discussed below, membership ranges from one to several persons close to the patient. Larger networks have been utilized by Speck (1967) in treating schizophrenic patients. Contacts between network members at this stage typically include telephone calls (usually at the patient's initiative), dinner arrangements, and social encounters, and should be preplanned to a fair extent during the joint session. These encounters are most often undertaken at the time when alcohol or drug use is likely to occur. In planning together, however, it should be made clear to network members that relatively little unusual effort will be required for the long-term, that after the patient is stabilized, their participation will come to little more than attendance at infrequent meetings with the patient and therapist. This is reassuring to those network members who are unable to make a major time commitment to the patient, as well as to those patients who do not want to be placed in a dependent position.

TECHNIQUES IN SOCIAL AND FAMILY NETWORK THERAPY

Introducing AA and Disulfiram

Use of self-help modalities is desirable whenever possible. For the alcoholic, certainly, participation in Alcoholics Anonymous (Zinberg, 1977) is strongly encouraged. Groups such as Narcotics Anonymous, Pills Anonymous, and Cocaine Anonymous (in some communities) are modeled after AA, and play a similarly useful role. One approach is to tell the patient that he is expected to attend at least two AA meetings a week so as to familiarize himself with the program. If after a month he is quite reluctant to continue and other aspects of the treatment are going well, his nonparticipation may have to be accepted. This acceptance, as illustrated below, may sometimes be used as one "chip" in the game of securing compliance with other aspects of the treatment.

For the alcoholic, disulfiram (Antabuse) may be a useful tool in assuring abstinence, but becomes much more valuable when carefully integrated into work with the patient and network. For example, it is a good idea to use the initial telephone contact to engage the patient's agreement to be abstinent from alcohol for the day immediately prior to the first session. The therapist then has the option of prescribing or administering disulfiram at that time. For a patient who is in earnest about seeking assistance for alcoholism, this is often not difficult, if some time is spent on the phone making plans to avoid a drinking context during that period. If it is not feasible to undertake this on the phone, it may be addressed in the first session. Such planning with the patient will almost always involve organizing time with significant others and therefore serves as a basis for developing the patient's support network.

Disulfiram is typically initiated with a dose of 500 mg, and then 250 mg. It is taken every morning when the urge to drink is generally least. Particulars of administration in the context of treatment should be reviewed (Ewing, 1982).

Anticipating the Recurrence of Drug Use

Most individual (Hayman, 1956) and family (Steinglass, 1976) therapists see the alcohol or drug abuser as a patient with poor prognosis. This is largely because in the context of traditional psychotherapy, there are no behavioral controls to prevent the recurrence of drug use and resources are not available for behavioral intervention if a recurrence takes place—which usually does. A system of impediments to the emergence of relapse which rests heavily on the actual or symbolic role of the network, must therefore be established. The therapist must have assistance in addressing any minor episode of drug use so that this ever-present problem does not lead to an unmanageable relapse or an unsuccessful termination of therapy.

Preventing Relapse

How can the support network be used to deal with recurrences of drug use, when, in fact, the patient's prior association with these same persons did not prevent him from using alcohol or drugs? In answering this question, it is necessary to clarify what the therapist must do to construct an effective support network. The following examples illustrate how this may be done. In the first case, a specific format was defined with the network to monitor a patient's compliance with a disulfiram regimen:

Case 2. A 33-year-old public relations executive had moved to New York from a remote city three years before coming to treatment. She had no long-standing close relationships in the city, a circumstance not uncommon for a single alcoholic in a setting removed from her origins. She presented with a 10-year history of heavy drinking which had increased in severity since her arrival, no doubt associated with her social isolation. Although she consumed a bottle of wine each night and additional hard liquor, she was able to get to work regularly. Six months before the outset of treatment she had attended AA meetings for two weeks and had been abstinent during that time. She had then relapsed, though, and became disillusioned with the possibility of maintaining abstinence. At the outset of treatment, it was necessary to reassure her that her prior relapse was in large part a function of not having established sufficient outside supports (including a more sound relationship with AA), and having seen herself as having failed after only one slip. I realized, though, that there was basis for concern as to whether she should do any better now, if the same formula was reinstituted in the absence of sufficient reliable supports, which she did not seem to have. Together we came upon the idea of bringing in an old friend whom she saw occasionally, and whom she felt she could trust. We made the following arrangement with her friend. The patient came to sessions twice a week. She would see her friend once each weekend. On each of these thrice-weekly occasions, she would be observed taking disulfiram, so that even if she missed a daily dose in between, it would not be possible for her to resume drinking on a regular basis undetected. The interpersonal support inherent in this arrangement, bolstered by conjoint meetings with her and her friend, also allowed her to return to AA with a sense of confidence in her ability to maintain abstinence.

The ensuing example illustrates how an ongoing network may be used to abort an emerging relapse. A high index of suspicion for signs of trouble was important, as was a clear understanding with the network members that they would be mobilized when necessary. Also illustrated, however, is the serious vulnerability of a network whose members may deny or rationalize because of their own drug use.

Case 3. A 34-year-old cameraman became addicted to cocaine and used it heavily on a daily basis. He acquired a considerable amount of capital by extensive dealing, primarily among friends and acquaintances, to support his habit. After a point, though, his wife moved out of the house and took their baby, saying she could no longer tolerate his heavy drug use. Ironically, she had been using cocaine herself, but to a lesser extent. The couple was reunited in the context of a therapy predicated on the patient's abstinence (and secondarily, on hers, too). It was supported by a network consisting of the wife, the patient's brother, and a good friend. The issue of relapse arose in an interesting context, one which illustrates how the subtleties of attitude among network members influence the patient's attitudes. Each network member had a contributing role. The wife, seeing her husband's boredom and disillusionment at the contraction of his successful but illicit drug sales career, suggested that he might be able to sell cocaine, although not use it himself. His friend had previously experienced difficulties with cocaine and had stopped on his own, but still used it occasionally. The brother, a staunch advocate of abstinence from all drugs (and all other human frailties, for that matter), was feared by the patient as unable to empathize with his problems, although the patient did feel considerable affection toward him. No network member provided a suitable model for comfortable abstinence, given these circumstances. Difficulties gradually emerged when the patient had been in treatment for six months, with only one occasion of use of a small amount. I was away on vacation for a month and returned to find that he had again taken cocaine on two occasions. On a third, he had brought some over to the home of his friend from the network and was fortunately persuaded to return it to the supplier. Although he had not taken the drug on this latter occasion, it seemed essential to seize on the circumstance to reverse his orientation toward intermittent use. I therefore summoned the network for weekly meetings, three in all, during which the risks inherent in the patient's occasional use of drugs were examined in a nonjudgmental way. The group affirmed what had seemingly been clear, but had not been fully adopted, the need for total abstinence in order to avoid the vulnerability to serious relapse. In this situation it became necessary to explore the ambivalence of the wife and the friend. The brother's rigidity was also addressed to underline that a judgmental attitude was not constructive in this situation.

The Network for Treatment Monitoring

The administration of disulfiram under observation is a treatment option which is easily adapted to work with social networks. A patient who takes disulfiram cannot drink; a patient who agrees to be observed by a responsible party while taking disulfiram will not miss his dose without the observer's knowing. This may take a measure of persuasion and, above all, the therapist's commitment that such an approach can be reasonable and helpful. Here is one example of how this can take place.

Case 4.   Ted is a 55-year-old musician who, like many colleagues in his field, has a successful career in the context of alcohol addiction. He is a man whose discomfort with dependency and compliance leads him to disregard some of the most routine of social norms; he drives without a license, for example. Although he acknowledges no responsibility or concern for those who hold authority over him, he is in fact solicitous and responsible toward those who rely on him. It is because of this that he decided to take action about his drinking when his wife was soon to deliver their first child, even though he had paid little attention to her concern previously; the two had a tacit understanding that they would not place "demands" on each other. The patient presented saying he wanted to have disulfiram prescribed and made it implicitly clear that he was not too interested in a great deal of professional advice. I was concerned, though, since I had little faith that he would continue taking his disulfiram for a day longer than it was his *own* intention to do so, and that his intention might not be too long-lived. Whereas compliance based on trust was hardly his style, it seemed necessary to corral him into an arrangement whereby he would agree to be monitored for at least the initial months of abstinence. The network began with his wife alone. I had pressed him to attend AA meetings and to bring his college age daughter from a previous marriage into the network. It seemed feasible to stage a negotiation in which I would concede some points to him so that he could save face; he might then agree to having his wife observe him taking disulfiram: I conceded that the daughter's involvement should be a matter for his own decision, thereby making it clear that there was room for his own decision-making in defining the therapeutic contract. I then said that the odds on his maintaining stable abstinence were significantly decreased if he did not go to AA meetings (it was clear to me he never would, anyway). I told him, though, that I could not in good conscience treat him if he neither went to AA nor participated in the observed disulfiram regimen. The odds of the treatment having a meaningful impact under such circumstances were not very good. I was in earnest and this seemed to be a fair test of his commitment to treatment, anyway. He agreed to comply to observation by his wife for a year, but not long-term AA attendance. He continued with this disulfiram regimen with good reliability, as agreed, thus allowing him to get through his most vulnerable period. He then, subsequently, took the disulfiram on an *ad hoc* basis, while remaining abstinent and continuing in therapy.

Some patients are more easily convinced to attend AA meetings. Others, although no more interested than the patient just described, may be more compliant. The therapist must use this compliance, mobilizing the support network as appropriate, in order to continue pressure for the patient's involvement with AA for a reasonable trial. It may take a considerable period of time, but ultimately a patient may experience something of a conversion, wherein he adopts the group ethos and expresses a deep commitment to abstinence, a measure of commitment rarely observed in patients who experience psychotherapy alone. When this occurs, the therapist may assume a more passive role in monitoring the patient's abstinence and keep an eye on his ongoing involvement in AA.

TECHNICAL CONSIDERATIONS

Defining the Network's Membership

Establishing a network is a task which requires the active collaboration of patient and therapist. The two, aided by those parties who initially join the network, must search for the right balance of members. This process is not without problems and the therapist must think in a strategic fashion. For example:

Case 5. A 25-year-old graduate student had been abusing cocaine since high school, in part drawing in funds from his affluent family, who lived in a remote city. At two points in the process of establishing his support network, the reactions of his live-in girlfriend (who worked with us from the outset) were particularly important. Both he and she agreed to bring in his 19-year-old sister, a freshman at a nearby college. He then mentioned a "friend" of his, apparently a woman whom he found attractive, even though there was no history of an overt romantic involvement. I sensed that his girlfriend did not like the idea, although she offered no rationale for excluding this potential rival. The idea of having to rely for assistance solely on a younger sister and two women who might see each other as competitors was unappealing. I therefore finessed the idea of the "friend." We then fell to evaluating the patient's uncle, whom he preferred to exclude, but his girlfriend thought appropriate. It later turned out (as I had expected) that the uncle was in many ways a potentially disapproving representative of the parental generation. In this case, I encouraged the patient to accept the uncle as a network member so as to round out the range of relationships within the group and spelled out the rationale for this. In matter of fact, the uncle turned out to be caring and supportive, particularly after he was helped to understand the nature of the addictive process.

The therapist must carefully promote the choice of appropriate network members, just as the platoon leader selects those who will go into combat with him. The network will be crucial in determining the balance of the therapy.

Defining the Network's Task

As conceived here, the therapist's relationship to the network is like that of a team leader rather than that of a family therapist. The network is established to implement a straightforward task, that of aiding the therapist to sustain the patient's abstinence. It must be directed with the same clarity of purpose that an organizational task force is directed to build more cars, open a branch office, or revise its management procedures. Competing and alternative goals must be suppressed, or at least prevented from interfering with the primary task.

Unlike those involved in traditional family therapy, network members are not led to expect symptom relief or self-realization. This prevents the development of competing goals for the network's meetings. It also assures the members protection from having their own motives scrutinized and thereby supports their continuing involvement without the threat of an assault on their psychological defenses. Since network members have—kindly—volunteered to participate, their motives must not be impugned. Their constructive behavior should be commended. It is useful to acknowledge appreciation for the contribution they are making to the therapy. There is always a counterproductive tendency on their part to minimize the value of their contribution.

The network must, therefore, be structured as an effective working group with good morale. This is not always easy:

Case 6. A 45-year old single woman served as an executive in a large family-held business—except when her alcohol problem led her into protracted binges. Her father, brother, and sister, were prepared to banish her from the business, but decided first to seek consultation. Because they had initiated the contact, they were included in the initial network and indeed were very helpful in stabilizing the patient. Unfortunately, however, the father was a domineering figure who intruded in all aspects of the business and often evoked angry outbursts from his children. The children typically reacted with petulance which provoked him in return. The situation came to a head when both the patient's siblings angrily petitioned me to exclude the father from the network two months into the treatment. This presented a problem because the father's control over the business made his involvement important to securing the patient's compliance. The patient's relapse was still a real possibility. This potentially coercive role, however, was an issue that the group could not easily deal with. I decided to support the father's membership in the group, indicating the constructive role he had played in getting the therapy started. It seemed necessary to support the earnestness of his concern for his daughter, rather than the children's dismay at their father's (very real) obstinacy. It was clear to me that the father could not deal with a situation where he was not accorded sufficient respect, and that there was no real place in this network for addressing the father's character pathology directly. The hubbub did, in fact, quiet down with time. The children became less provocative themselves, as the group responded to my pleas for civil behavior.

The Frequency of Network Sessions

At the outset of therapy, it is important to see the patient with the group on a weekly basis for at least the first month. Unstable circumstances demand more frequent contacts with the network. Sessions can be tapered off to biweekly and then monthly intervals after a time.

In order to sustain the continuing commitment of the group (particularly that between the therapist and the network members), network sessions should be held every three months or so for the duration of the individual therapy. Once the patient has stabilized, the meetings tend less to address day-to-day issues. They may begin with a recounting by the patient of the drug situation. Reflections on the patient's progress and goals, or sometimes on relations between the network members, may then be discussed. In any case, it is essential that an agreement be made that network members contact the therapist if they are concerned about the patient's possible use of alcohol or drugs, and that the therapist himself contact the network members if he becomes concerned over a potential relapse.

Confidentiality

This raises the issues of confidentiality and the nature of the therapist's commitment to the patient. The overriding commitment of the therapist to the patient is that he support him in maintaining the drug-free state. Open communication on matters regarding alcohol and drugs should be maintained among the network, the patient, and the therapist. The therapist must set the proper tone of mutual trust and understanding so that the patient's right to privacy not otherwise be compromised. It is also made explicit that absolute confidentiality applies to all other (nondrug-related) communications between therapist and patient and that network members should not expect to communicate with the therapist about any matter which does not directly relate to alcohol or drug problems.

Intrusive Measures

Certain circumstances may necessitate further incursions on the patient's autonomy so as to assure compliance with treatment. This is particularly true when the patient has begun treatment reluctantly, as with overt pressure from family or employer or when the possibility of relapse will have grave consequences. Options include the possibility of financial constraints, a spouse's moving out, and urine monitoring. These, of course, can only be undertaken with the patient's agreement, based on the fact that greater or more immediate loss is being averted. Such steps may also provide greater certitude against relapse to all concerned, including an uneasy therapist and family.

Case 7. A 35-year-old man had used heroin intranasally for two years and then intravenously for eight months; he had previously used other drugs. He was stealing money from the family business where he worked. The patient underwent ambulatory detoxification, but relapsed to heroin use, and finally underwent a hospitalization which lasted 5 weeks. He was then referred to me on discharge and was to continue with meetings of Narcotics Anonymous. His network consisted of his mother and his wife, and the following family members involved in the family business: his father, his younger sister and brother, and his uncle. His family was very concerned about allowing him to get involved in the business. We therefore agreed to do two things so that he might be included with less concern on everyone's part. The patient agreed to have his urine spot-checked on a regular basis, and he and I, along with the network, discussed his financial circumstances in the firm, clarifying what consequences might emerge should he return to active addiction. An informal, but explicit, agreement was reached in this matter, thereby helping the patient understand the constraints under which he was operating and leaving the family more comfortable about his returning to work. Since this agreement was undertaken with the network, it became a part of the treatment plan.

Adapting Individual Therapy to the Network Treatment

As noted above, network sessions are scheduled on a weekly basis at the outset of treatment. This is likely to compromise the number of individual contacts. Indeed, if sessions are held once a week, the patient may not be seen individually for a period of time. This may be perceived as a deprivation by the patient unless the individual therapy is presented as an opportunity for further growth *predicated* on achieving stable abstinence assured through work with the network.

When the individual therapy does begin, the traditional objectives of therapy must be ordered so as to accommodate the goals of the substance abuse treatment. For insight-oriented therapy, clarification of unconscious motivations is a primary objective; for supportive therapy, the bolstering of established constructive defenses is primary. In the therapeutic context which we are describing, however, the following objectives are given precedence.

Of first importance is the need to address exposure to substances of abuse, or exposure to cues which might precipitate alcohol or drug use (Galanter, 1983). Both patient and therapist should be sensitive to this matter and explore these situations as they arise. Secondly, a stable social context in an appropriate social environment—one conducive to abstinence with minimal disruption of life circumstances—should be supported. Considerations of minor disruptions in place of residence, friends, or job, need not be a primary issue for the patient with character disorder or neurosis, but they cannot go untended here. For a considerable period of time, the substance abuser is highly vulnerable to exacerbations of the addictive illness and must be viewed with considerable caution and in some respects, as one treats the recently compensated psychotic.

Finally, after attending to these priorities, psychological conflicts which the patient must resolve, relative to his own growth, are considered. As the therapy continues, these come to assume a more prominent role. In the earlier phases, they are likely to directly reflect issues associated with previous drug use. Later, however, the tenor of treatment will come to resemble increasingly the traditional psychotherapeutic context. At this point the therapist is in the admirable position of working with a patient who, while exercising insight into his problems, is also motivated by the realization of a new and previously untapped potential.

Summary

An approach to the office treatment of alcohol and drug dependent patients is described in which a social network is used to bolster the integrity of the therapeutic alliance. It is drawn from persons close to the patient, typically members of his immediate family or close friends, and is used for social support in assuring compliance with the treatment regimen and in undercutting denial. Its specific function is explained to the patient and network members: (1) to assure that the patient's abstinence from the outset of treatment; (2) to mitigate against the occurrence of slips; and (3) to support reintegration into treatment should relapses to alcohol or drug use occur.

References

Ewing, J. A. Disulfiram and other deterrant drugs. In E. M. Pattison and E. Kaufman (Eds.), *Encyclopedic handbook of alcoholism*. New York: Gardner Press, 1982.

Galanter, M. Cognitive Labelling: Adapting psychotherapy to the treatment of alcohol abuse. *Journal of Psychiatric Treatment and Evaluation*, 1983, 5, 551–556.

Gallant, D. M., Rich, A., Bey, E., and Terranova, L. Group psychotherapy with married couples: A successful technique in New Orleans Alcoholism Clinic patients. *Journal of Louisiana State Medical Society*, 1970, 122, 41–44.

Gitlow, S. E. and Peyser, H. S. (Eds.), *Alcoholism: A practical treatment guide*. New York: Grune & Stratton, 1980.

Hayman, M. Current attitudes to alcoholism of psychiatrists in Southern California. *American Journal of Psychiatry*, 1956, 112, 484–493.

Speck, R. Psychotherapy of the social network of a schizophrenic family. *Family Process*, 1967, 6, 208.

Steinglass, P. Experimenting with family treatment approaches to alcoholism, 1950–1975: A review. *Family Process*, 1976, 15, 97–123.

Vaillant, G. E. Dangers of psychotherapy in the treatment of alcoholism. In M. H. Bean and N. E. Zinberg (Eds.), *Dynamic approaches to the understanding and treatment of alcoholism*. New York: The Free Press, 1981.

Zimberg, S. *The clinical management of alcoholism*. New York: Brunner Mazel, 1982.

Zinberg, N. Alcoholics anonymous and the treatment and prevention of alcoholism. *Alcoholism: Clinical and Experimental Research*, 1977, 1, 91–102.

Treatment of the Significant Other

DONALD P. HOWARD AND NANCY T. HOWARD

INTRODUCTION

In our practice and experience over the years, we occasionally become so removed from the ordinary world in our work with alcoholism, the family, and the problem drinker and with our treatment staff that we forget that not everyone believes that alcoholism is a family problem. We become acclimated to our world, busily developing newer, always more interesting methods of training counselors, when all of a sudden, "whomp," we are brought down to earth by someone asking: "Do you think there is anything you can do before the alcoholic hits rock bottom?" or "What can you say to the client whose husband won't stop drinking?" The questioners may have read that alcoholism is a family affair, but they have not seen treatment offered to anyone other than the alcoholic. They may know that programs exist that counsel the family while the problem drinker is in treatment, offering one or two sessions, but they have not believed you can really approach a program of treatment for alcoholism as a family problem.

The field of alcoholism has traveled a great distance, yet we remain pioneers, particularly in this area working with the family of the problem drinker while the problem drinker is actively drinking. (We use the term problem drinker and alcoholic interchangeably, as we see no difference except ease of acceptability by the client with the former.) We follow the trailblazing of Kellerman (1969), Jackson (1954), and Cork (1969), people who pushed the boundaries of alcoholism outward to include

---

DONALD P. HOWARD AND NANCY T. HOWARD • The Howard Institute Family Counseling Center, Columbia, Missouri.

the significant others in the treatment of alcoholism. Our approach gives it one more shove, in that we work with the family before the problem drinker stops drinking.

The Al-Anon Family Groups patterned after Alcoholics Anonymous were for many years the sole source of assistance for the family and friends of the alcoholic. The Al-Anon traditions and guides for living provide a safe environment for sharing and caring. Al-Anon members can relate their personal experiences within the group and find a release in the commonality of their problems and the understanding that has been so long absent in their lives. Family members and friends can, by working within the Al-Anon program, learn how to work for self-improvement.

The traditions of Al-Anon prohibit its members from actively seeking membership at a public level or employing early intervention techniques within the community. A counseling center such as ours, involved in early intervention, must take actions that would violate these traditions that are so valuable for the continuing success of the Al-Anon program.

Our counseling center utilizes Al-Anon groups in a program of mutual referral and enjoys the presence of members as volunteers. Our counseling program differs from Al-Anon in that we develop an individual treatment plan for each client and follow a definite educational scheme. A counseling session differs from the self-help program of Al-Anon.

Not every significant other will choose Al-Anon, being reluctant to get involved; some do not understand their purpose or their own problems. Alcoholism is still misunderstood by many people, who associate Al-Anon with late-stage alcoholism; their spouse, parent, son, or daughter may not fit their erroneous image of the alcoholic. A counseling center may provide in many instances a more comfortable entrance and method of defining "the problem." Al-Anon is a supportive group which can complement a counseling program for the family and friends. We recommend Al-Anon to all clients and provide contacts to escort the person to their first meetings.

Significant other is a good term, one which immediately engages the social worker and counselor. We have adopted this term into the therapeutic jargon because it relates a certain meaning to practitioners—a significant other being any person who has developed emotional ties to the alcoholic. Yet, when we use the word often, we risk stripping the flesh and blood from those very alive persons: mother, husband, sister, son, dear friend. When you read *significant other*, try not to skim the word, but think of a living, breathing person, someone you can visualize as being involved in the day-to-day struggles with the problem drinker. The significant others are the folks who pour liquor down the drain, clobber the drinker on occasion or want to clobber him, beg God on their hands and knees while they hold his head up above the toilet to deliver them from this misery, kiss the alcoholic and listen to his promise to change and believe that he can, simply by wishing, praying, and moving out of the house for the night. Way down deep inside, when they let themselves be aware of their inside, they know it is beginning to look hopeless.

GETTING INSIDE THE FOUR WALLS

You and I think we can recognize the family with a drinking problem by relying on our traditional criteria for identification. Alcoholics are the people whose children run around half-dressed, come to school unprepared; they sleep a lot during class; they hug the sidelines during recess; they are sullen and withdrawn; or they are the hyperactive ones; they are the ones constantly wanting attention. How many of us are receiving referrals from the school system because a teacher or principal identifies a child whose family has a drinking problem?

If you work in a poverty program, you don't need any help identifying the families with drinking problems. You know their names and addresses, but nobody can do anything anyway but hope the old man dies or runs away and leaves them all in peace at least for a few weeks.

The family with a drinking problem is not the average, the median, or the mode. They are just as apt to be wealthy as middle-class or poor. They are large families, small, and medium-sized. From the outside looking in, they may be difficult to identify unless they have reached the later part of the middle stage when the lawn goes uncut and the paint peels off the shutters—but if there is money or an industrious wife, they will have the lawn cut and the house painted, and then you are back where you started. Besides, who has the time to ride around neighborhoods in order to identify families with drinking problems?

One thing that all these families have in common is that they are emotionally disturbed, and we can identify the emotional disturbance in people. Our problem is in educating families and persons working in the helping professions to identify families with a drinking problem and then, once identified, in referring children and parents for assistance. Our problem is dispelling the myth that the alcoholic must "hit bottom" before treatment can be initiated. We cannot drive around subdivisions or over country roads looking for houses with peeling paint or unkempt lawns, but we can initiate community alcohol awareness programs to reach the people living within those four walls. We have identified the problem drinker by using the Jellinek Scale (1960) and the Twenty-Question Questionnaire (developed by Johns Hopkins University, Baltimore, Maryland, 1955). We, too, use a questionnaire (Howard and Howard, 1976), but it is directed to the family or friend of the problem drinker. Our method of reaching is called the *touch system*, and is described later in the chapter. We send our information behind the four walls by slipping it in through the electric wires via radio and TV, into the mailbox via letters addressed to the recipient of a citation for Driving While Intoxicated and his or her family, we place it into their pockets via matchbooks, into their cars via litter bags, into their children's hands via balloons, in front of their noses via bumper stickers, and countless educational programs in churches, schools, and civic groups, and by distributing literature at shopping centers and football games. On one Saturday during the year, we boldly knock at their doors and leave them literature letting them know that there is a service available in their community and that the family members can seek help for a drinking problem even before the problem drinker stops drinking. We want the people living and maybe dying inside those four walls to think about help and where it is located the next time they are holding that inebriated head above the toilet, or letting themselves be aware of their inside messages that all is hopeless; we want them to know that we are in the community and believe there is hope.

The People Living inside the Four Walls

The people who live with the problem drinker are like clocks slowly ticking, but there is no way to know whether they are going to run down and stop or are attached to explosives—time bombs ready to explode. The people who live with the problem drinker progress through a debilitating process as markedly as the alcoholic progresses through the early, middle, and late stages of alcoholism. As the condition of the problem drinker deteriorates, the family suffers through lack of, or distorted, communication and decreasing levels of self-worth; the family atmosphere becomes less nurturing and more disturbed (Figure 1).

These disturbances within the family invariably become set in patterns of cyclic behavior: poor communication that results in emotional problems; unresolved conflicts on repeated themes that result in frustration; guilt felt that results in blame given; unrealistic expectations that reflect perceived inadequacies; for each cause a result that produces the cause that produces the result, *ad infinitum*, tick, tick, until explosion or silent emotional death.

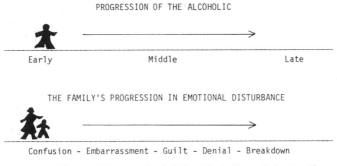

Figure 1. Progression of the Alcoholic and the Family.

The family members over a period of a few years adopt a distorted reality. Each member aids in helping the problem drinker handle reality by stopping it at the front door, shaping it into some more acceptable form they know the problem drinker can handle, or picking up the reality themselves and taking care of the consequences for the problem drinker. In essence, the significant others become enablers acting as a buffer zone between the problem drinker and the "real world." All must accept the music the problem drinker plays. The family moves in rhythm to the drinking behavior and its resultant behaviors. The dance steps become familiar and are learned quickly by the newest and oldest members of the troupe.

A need to cover up and maintain a balance of harmony demands a choreography born of necessity: conflict slides to accommodate; guilt leads to blame; embarrassment swings into cover-up; reality spins the denial; love tangos with hate; round and round they go and where they stop nobody knows. But we do know, for without assistance the family becomes set in its defenses and offenses, unable to break its own cycle of negative reinforcement. It develops its rules and conspiracies: If Grandma calls and Mom is drinking, tell Grandma that she's sleeping. If Dad comes home drunk, go to your room. If he smiles when he comes in the door, then we're safe. If I go to bed, then they'll leave me alone. Oh, Mary, it looks like we won't be able to make it after all . . . Tommy's running a fever . . . you know how it is . . . so sorry.

The family members do the fast shuffle or the soft shoe. They cover up for the problem drinker by rationalizing his or her behavior: "If only he weren't under such stress at work." "If only we hadn't married so young and had finished school." The "if only's" are a list of rationalizations that, if laid end to end, would circle the globe three times over and are growing daily.

And so as dusk settles over and around the four walls, we find the wife peeking out behind the curtains, searching the darkness for familiar headlights—she has learned to recognize the headlights and can estimate the number of beers he has had from the sound of the car pulling into the driveway. A sixth sense? No, just the spouse of a problem drinker, who has watched many nights the headlights pass by the house, watched the car's speed vary in its attempts to maneuver the curve—repeated and predictable behaviors for this family.

A sense of hopelessness settles in with the darkness. And it is Dad's turn to repeat the predictable as he puts his intoxicated wife into bed, covers up the kids and wonders what he did . . . or maybe what he didn't do . . . or, God, just what to do?

The conspiracy of silence keeps the cycle turning, the people isolated from each other and from seeking treatment. The cycle turns, a smooth ride enforced by the supporting spokes of the enabler's reactions to the problem drinker: If there's a problem, I'll fix it. If there's embarrassment, I'll hide it. If there's worry, I'll conceal it. If there's a feeling, I'll bury it. Tick, tick, tick, is it a doomsday clock or an exploding bomb?

THE TREATMENT PLAN: A CHANGE IN THE DANCE STEPS, OR STOP THE CLOCK

If the reader is to remember only one sentence from this chapter, let it be this: *The person who seeks assistance becomes the primary client.* The significant other (remember flesh and blood) is not involved just as a mechanism for treating the alcoholic. Early intervention in the cycle of alcoholism is often a concomitant benefit when family members engage in counseling. Traditionally, the significant other has been regarded as a "bridge," a means of getting the alcoholic to consent to treatment.

We broaden our approach to the significant others. The person who walks into our agency or calls for an appointment becomes our primary client, our first concern. Nine times out of ten, it is the female spouse of the male alcoholic. She realizes that drinking creates problems, and she needs to learn about alcoholism. She will present an irrational world, and she needs to become reality-oriented. She knows her husband needs help, her family needs help, and she needs assistance for her very important self. We view our job in counseling and hold as an ultimate goal to help this person become better prepared to live life and become a mentally healthy individual, whether or not the alcoholic recovers. No matter the outcome for the alcoholic, the spouse and family members need assistance to stabilize.

Initial Evaluation. The first time the client enters the office, we have her fill out an application that automatically identifies the problem drinker (Figure 2). Ninety-three percent of the families we have counseled over the years instituted treatment while the problem drinker was still drinking. Again, this negates the myth that the alcoholic must be motivated to seek help before assistance should be sought. Denial is a living part of alcoholism and of the family. We cannot wait for the alcoholic to stop drinking before we initiate treatment for the family members; we cannot wait for the problem drinker to quit denying the problem before we initiate a program of help. A promise for treatment of a disease whose most prevailing symptom is denial in both the victim and the family members cannot wait for the motivation of the alcoholic. Remember this key factor, an alcoholic cannot continue to live with a healthy, reality-oriented spouse. The alcoholic will have to make the choice to seek assistance for relief from the stress from living with a healthy person or continue to drink. Either way we are preparing the problem drinker for entrance into some form of treatment (inpatient, AA, outpatient).

Instead, we approach counseling with a program that includes a number of essential elements: First, we educate the client about alcoholism, its effects on both the alcholic and the family. This education brings some clarity into the situation she is facing and enables her to start relinquishing some guilt and blame. Certain attitudes and myths detrimental to treatment can be examined and discarded during the

---

Are you coming to Howard Family Institute because you or someone close to you has an alcohol problem: Yes, myself _____

Yes, someone else _____   No _____

If you are coming because of concern for someone else, please complete the following:

Name of Problem Drinker: _____

Address: _____

                                           Street   City   State   Zip

Place of Employment: _____

Address of Employer: _____

                                           Street   City   State

How long employed: _____

Religious Preference: _____

Is this person presently drinking: _____

Figure 2. Client Application.

process of acquiring adequate information. The client becomes more comfortable discussing the drinking problem, actually forming the words with her own mouth and hearing her voice say the words "drinking problem," and this comfort helps to break through distortions and denials.

This initial session with the client is geared toward client comfort. We review the sequence of events that led to the appointment. We ask what expectations she has regarding the counseling situation. Sound simplistic? Bear in mind that a long sequence of occurrences has led to this counseling appointment, incidents that have developed certain expectations and fears about this moment. The counselor's initial responsibility is to assist the client in being as comfortable as possible about requesting help. Your concern can be demonstrated in countless small ways: in not sitting behind a desk, but in chairs grouped in a conversational manner, in making an ashtray and coffee available on a small table along with a handy box of tissues.

We use the Family Questionnaire, consisting of 20 questions, as a counseling tool (Figure 3), making copies available for both the client and the counselor. Many spouses do not know if the problem drinker is really an alcoholic or a social drinker. They are confused by the many different patterns of behavior exhibited by the problem drinker. And even though she knows inside that he has a drinking problem, she would like to be more convinced that it is not true and everything is all right. Some spouses are more ready than others to break through their own denial of the drinking problem. Others may take a longer time to be able to look at reality for more than 20 or 30 minutes at a stretch. Answering the 20-question Questionnaire will help define the problem, determining once and for all if the drinking problem does exist. It is important for the client to have help in being able to say, "Yes, he is an alcoholic. Yes, there is a drinking problem in our family." Breaking through denial will lay the foundation for treatment.

The five areas are the "demythification process" (Figure 4), which is a checklist used in educating the client. Figure 4 occupies the upper left hand corner of the summary sheet above the circle (Figure 5). The counselor refers to this list during the session to ensure that certain information is discussed with the client. We illustrate for the client the progression of the problem drinker from early to middle to late stages, pointing out that this path will inevitably be traveled if the drinking persists. We review the disease concept with her, and the denial aspect. We define an alcoholic as a person who continues to drink, even though the drinking is creating problems at home, at work, or within the community. Finally, we explore the "let's wait till he's ready" myth, the

		Yes	No
1.	Do you worry about your spouse's drinking?	___	___
2.	Have you ever been embarrassed by your spouse's drinking?	___	___
3.	Are holidays more of a nightmare than a celebration because of your spouse's drinking behavior?	___	___
4.	Are most of your spouse's friends heavy drinkers?	___	___
5.	Does your spouse often promise to quit drinking without success?	___	___
6.	Does your spouse's drinking make the atmosphere in the home tense and anxious?	___	___
7.	Does your spouse deny a drinking problem because your spouse drinks only beer?	___	___
8.	Do you find it necessary to lie to employer, relatives, or friends in order to hide your spouse's drinking?	___	___
9.	Has your spouse ever failed to remember what occurred during a drinking period?	___	___
10.	Does your spouse avoid conversation pertaining to alcohol or problem drinking?	___	___
11.	Does your spouse justify his or her drinking problem?	___	___
12.	Does your spouse avoid social situations where alcoholic beverages will not be served?	___	___
13.	Do you ever feel guilty about your spouse's drinking?	___	___
14.	Has your spouse driven a vehicle while under the influence of alcohol?	___	___
15.	Are your children afraid of your spouse while he or she is drinking?	___	___
16.	Are you afraid of physical or verbal abuse when your spouse is drinking?	___	___
17.	Has another person mentioned your spouse's unusual drinking behavior?	___	___
18.	Do you fear riding with your spouse when he or she is drinking?	___	___
19.	Does your spouse have periods of remorse after a drinking occasion and apologize for behavior?	___	___
20.	Does drinking less alcohol bring about the same effects in your spouse as in the past required more?	___	___

The staff of the Family Training Center has served thousands of families in the past several years and based on these experiences suggest the following scale in answering the above twenty questions.

If you have answered YES to any two of the questions, there is a definite warning that a drinking problem may exist in your family.

If you have answered YES to any four of the questions, the chances are that a drinking problem does exist in your family.

If you have answered YES to five or more, there very definitely is a drinking problem in your family.

Figure 3. Family Questionnaire.

	CHECK OFF
DEMYTHIFICATION	
PROGRESSION	
DISEASE CONCEPT	
RESPONSIBILITY	
"NO NEED TO WAIT"	
STEREOTYPE MYTH	

Figure 4. Demythification Process.

notion that the alcoholic must "hit bottom" before he will be ready for assistance. The counselor also may ask the client to describe her impressions and thoughts on who is an alcoholic.

On our summary sheet there is a circle (Figure 5). In the middle of that circle we place the problem drinker's name, writing the names of the significant others in the problem drinker's life—Mom, Dad, children, employer, drinking buddy. Every individual possesses a different set of significant others. These persons, by their responses to the alcoholic, reinforce his behavior and act as a buffer zone between the alcoholic and reality. Often they rescue the problem drinker from uncomfortable and painful predicaments in an attempt to help. The counselor draws a line from each significant other on the edge of the circle to the problem drinker in the middle and writes on the line words that

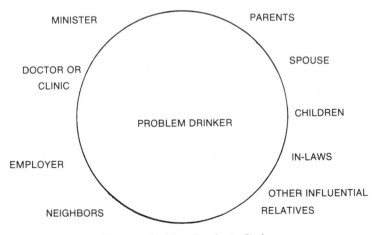

Figure 5. Problem Drinker's Circle.

describe how each person supports the drinking behavior. These actions are like supporting spokes as the cycle revolves. Some of these supporting behaviors are subtle and most are recurring patterns. Usually the role of the significant other is that of a reactor rather than an initiator of action. The summary sheet adds another dimension to the counseling session: it visually engages the client in the education process by allowing her to see how alcoholism is affecting the family and how the significant others reinforce the drinking behavior. The counselor makes a copy of the summary sheet and the 20-question Questionnaire for the client to keep.

The client may then be moved into familiarizing herself with the problems arising within the family system. For this purpose we use a handout (Figure 6). Our paperwork has a purpose. Over a period of time it is desirable for the client to collect educational materials to reinforce what she is learning about alcoholism's effects on the alcoholic, herself, and the family members. The family-system chart helps the client examine various aspects of the family relationship—communication, rules, the self-worth of individual family members, and their ability to relate outside the family unit.

During this exercise it is helpful for the client to explore the origin of these behaviors. They are not the sole result of the drinking problem, but are rooted in their backgrounds as well. How was communication

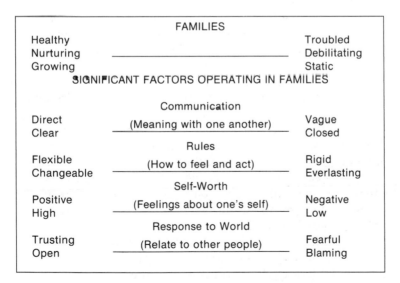

Figure 6. Significant Factors Operating in Families.

in their family of origin? What were the rules? The patterns they had established earlier carried into the marriage, and often the expectations each marital partner had for the other had never been verbalized. The failure to communicate these expectations appears early in the interviews.

Usually the client is a person with low self-esteem. She has undergone intimidation and manipulation and as a result has come to believe that she is not very attractive, physically or mentally. Low self-esteem is frequently the result of burying her emotions and feelings. Usually the spouse feels victimized and has been experiencing some level of depression.

If, during the initial interview and screening, the counselor identifies a serious psychiatric disorder, for example, manic depressive symptoms, schizophrenia, alcoholic psychosis, severe paranoia, the best action is to suggest to the client that further evaluation is necessary for a thorough diagnosis.

A counselor should become acquainted with the psychiatric services within the community and have a liaison for referral established. The referral should be made while the client is in the office so a definite time and date can be arranged. Whenever a referral is made, whether it is a change or a supplement to your services, the client should be given specific names and appointments. He or she is experiencing emotional stress and to leave the client to find his or her own way is insufficient and irresponsible counseling.

Treatment-Plan Contract. After the initial interview and screening period, it is important for the counselor to sit down with the client and form a treatment-plan contract. The informal procedure reviews the client's expectations for the counseling sessions; the counselor must be prepared to keep the contract reality-oriented. A woman may claim she wants her husband—a 40-year-old alcoholic who's been drinking for 22 years—to be sober within a month. Carefully review the individual's situation: How long has the disease taken to progress in this family? What are some realistic expectations of therapy?

Our first contract would probably be for a period of one month. From there the counselor is encouraged to plan a program of self-development and intervention. The goals the client hopes to reach through counseling are broken down into very short-term goals that can be incorporated into daily situations.

If the client has not informed the problem drinker that she is seeing a counselor, a barrier is presented to therapy. It is important that the counselor and client explore and role-play the methods by which she can inform her spouse about the counseling. The client should approach her husband about her concern for herself, for him, and for their relationship. She is seeking professional assistance for the drinking problem in their family as she or he would if a family member had any other health problem. Reality with concern is the approach to be used in forming her approach to her spouse.

Intervention Techniques.   The educational aspect of the counseling program broadens from alcoholism and its effects on the family to the second area of the communication processes in the relationship between the client and the problem drinker and between the client and other persons in the family or her immediate circle. The client can consider the ways that family members act and respond within the family and in other relationships. Independent of the alcoholic and the alcohol-related problem, a person exists whose identity has become clouded.

Self-esteem is enhanced through reading, through the short-term goals, and through homework assignments that help the client to refocus energies from the negative to the positive. Thus, our third guideline is to introduce alternatives for action. The client and her family experience a sense of direction rather than confusion and hopelessness.

Instilling hope in the family's future is one of the greatest of the counselor's responsibilities. Our primary goal is a mentally healthy client. Many times, as mentioned under Treatment-Plan Contract, the family has distorted expectations about improving the situation. Living with the problem drinker produces a habit of denial and leads to a distorted sense of reality in the family members. Often the family members try to isolate the effects of alcoholism, to separate the effects into those only directly related to incidents involving alcohol use or abuse. But the drinking problem manifests itself in many areas: the children's grades, relationships with the parents, poor job performance, accidents at home or work, financial problems, health problems, decrease in sexual desire and activity. The effects are measurable and identifiable.

As the illness progresses, the client may find herself picking up more of the daily family responsibilities. She disciplines the children. She pays the bills. In treatment we encourage her to let the problem drinker know why she is assuming these responsibilities in a clear, straightforward manner, rather than screaming and yelling. She makes plans to return these responsibilities to the problem drinker.

The spouse may become the martyr, a victim, all the while filling her duty sack with resentment of the problem drinker and the world at large. At some point or other, you may want the client to empty her duty sack, listing all the ways she has carried the burden and how she has hated every minute of having to do it. Otherwise the trap is that you will have these resentments creep out and take over during a counseling session, with war stories about how miserable he has been and what she has had to take. Be sure to discuss the fact that she is to empty the sack at this session so you can get rid of it, once and for all.

As the client develops more positive self-esteem and becomes more responsible in the relationship, the problem drinker becomes more uncomfortable with the conflicts this behavior creates at home. The problem drinker finds it more difficult to control the atmosphere in the home—to control the family and the spouse. As more reality is brought in, "as is" and with no special shaping, it becomes more uncomfortable for the problem drinker. He looks for ways to bring back the old balance. As the spouse becomes healthier, the problem drinker's behavior stands out and he or she becomes vulnerable to intervention. The spokes that kept the cycle rolling smoothly are being altered or removed and the ride is becoming wobbly.

One of the mistakes made by the family members and the counselor is to deal with the problem drinker as a rational person and to expect rational reactions. The problem drinker's perceptions are confused and focused on survival, on the only way he knows how to survive. As the atmosphere of reality is created around the problem drinker, he becomes more tense, more anxious, more nervous, more upset. You cannot expect rational reactions from the problem drinker. The most important thing for the significant other to be doing is to be giving caring feedback, leveling, and breaking down the conspiracy of silence.

The significant others slowly change their responses and begin initiating reality-oriented actions, no longer allowing the problem drinker to control their attitudes and behaviors. These responses are not presented in a method of "showdown" or antagonistically. The significant other presents his or her "self" in an assertive manner: "These are my feelings about your behavior. I give you your responsibility and this is mine." We call this *tough love*.

Many times during the counseling sessions we have a rehearsal of the leveling: How the spouse can tell the problem drinker that she cares for him but she cannot continue to tolerate his behavior. As counselors, we are teachers. We teach family members how to communicate and we have a list of guidelines that family members learn in order to give feedback. When the entire family comes into a counseling session, we may have a practice session on giving feedback by doing role-playing between two members. This gives each member a chance to role-play another family member. We review how members have done since the last session in giving each other feedback. How can they improve? You may ask one person to tell the other members how they would like to be reminded not to do something or to do something desired. After all, who knows better what will work for us than ourselves?

An example of a situation needing some rehearsal before opening night is the person who does not want to ride with the alcoholic when he is drinking and driving. Perhaps the spouse could role-play the alcoholic and the counselor will be the spouse. Now you are leaving a party and the alcoholic is intoxicated. How does he react to your announcing that you are not getting into the car? He hits you in the head. A loud argument ensues. He obediently gives you the keys. All of the above? Or none of the above—he wildly drives off, faster than ever, practically running you over on the way. Now how can we plan to break the news ahead of time, before there is an evening out? Again, use your creativity and imagination to help the person learn how to plan her leveling.

This approach may seem too simple and we are not saying that as soon as the spouse learns different responses all will change. But altering this pattern is significant. You are beginning to break the cycle of reinforcement practiced by the significant others. Other methods are encouraged that have been nagging at the family members' sense of values, such as not calling the employer with an excuse, not picking up bad checks. These new behaviors are a key to treatment, along with having the spouse level and let the problem drinker know that she cares but cannot continue certain practices. The removal of the spokes promotes a sense of independence and self-respect in the significant other. Havoc has reigned in the family for many an unknown reason; if all hell breaks loose this time, at least the family members will know what it is for and that it is in the name of progress and of freedom and hope for all of them.

In discussing the cycle of reinforcement, the counselor should be alert to the fact that the key enabler may be someone outside of the immediate family. It may be the employer. Often it is the parents of the alcoholic, whether they live in the same community or miles away. With the permission of the spouse, and for the price of a stamp, we contact the person(s) and explain the program, enclose literature, and encourage them to enter the treatment program with the family. These persons can become important in the process of intervention; the letter is one of the most effective communications tools the counselor and client possess. In the security of their own home, these people can read your message in its totality, save face, get red-hot mad, jump on your words, tear them up, mull them over, then tape them together, consider them for the tenth time, and through a private process begin to accept the truth of the situation.

We have found letter writing essential to our business. A letter to a significant other far away can bring a response of encouragement and support and grateful acknowledgment that someone has broken the silence. A letter from the counselor to the client after the first and second visits telling her that you are glad she came in to see you, that you know it took courage, and highlighting some of your discussion could become your greatest counseling technique. We have decreased our dropout rate considerably by letters of reinforcement to our clients—whether they are individual family members or group participants. The common feedback that we receive is that it felt so good to get a nice letter, to know that someone was thinking about them.

The Problem Drinker Entering Therapy. As counseling with the spouse and/or family members progresses, the problem drinker is more inclined to seek assistance. This is an appropriate time for the spouse to let the problem drinker know that he is welcome to schedule a counseling appointment.

The timing of the problem drinker's entrance into therapy with the family is of primary importance. Generally, the spouse comes in for assistance prior to the alcoholic's receiving treatment. After working in an educational program with the significant other designed to stabilize the family over a period of at least two to three months, we suggest that the family ask the problem drinker if he would like to accompany them. Often we will drop the problem drinker a short note, suggesting he come in for a visit, have a cup of coffee, and talk about the situation. Often the person will respond to the contact from the counselor.

Many people think they have to create a crisis within the family situation to get the problem drinker in for assistance. We believe that you do not have to create crises within the family of a problem drinker—they are happening all the time. Instead, to deal with reality on a day-to-day basis, the significant others inform the problem drinker about the changes little by little before a situation occurs. The most effective way is to change the routine—stop the music if they don't like the tune. When the family members can perceive and accept reality for themselves and learn to present it to the problem drinker, they have defused the ticking bomb.

With sobriety in the family, the significant others have a very important role to play. They are usually very anxious about the problem drinker's sobriety: hopeful, yet fearful. They worry about how long it will last, about what can be said when the problem drinker comes home from work. Should there be liquor in the house? Should they go out to a party? Should they go to a wedding reception? The problem drinker is thinking similar thoughts. He is excited but scared. He does not usually believe he is going to maintain sobriety. He usually does not know how to interact socially without the use of alcohol. Others are expecting him to make mature, rational decisions, although he might have been a practicing alcoholic for as long as 25 years. He needs the encouragement and the understanding of the significant others. Many times this includes the employer. Often the employer is going to expect the person to swing right back. That is why it is helpful as a counselor to get permission to visit with the employer, to let him know the problem drinker is going to be coming in to work and trying to do a good job, to give him a chance. But the employer should be cautioned to treat the problem drinker like any other employee.

The spouse will also have other concerns. What should she do if he has a drink? How should she react if she smells liquor on his breath? These items are vital for the counselor to cover with the client.

If the client is to become a mature, responsible adult, then naturally we have to treat him as one and give him the opportunity to solve his own problems.

CASE HISTORIES

Case 1. Joanne came to the counseling center after reading a brochure on the agency which she found in the reading rack in the back of her church. She was married to a physician and they had three teenage daughters. When she came for the initial interview she was coming just for information and said she knew there was nothing she could do until John became motivated to stop drinking.

During the first two sessions, we traced the drinking history and the family's patterns of reacting to John's drinking in order to find the ways to enact change. After the first session we also began an education program on alcoholism. Joanne did reading assignments and written homework.

Her first assignment was to inform her husband that she was coming for counseling at the center because they had a drinking problem in their family that was affecting her mental health and that of the whole family. We did some rehearsal, with Joanne and me changing roles. First, she reacted to me as she thought her husband would. The role-playing gave her more confidence and she decided to tell him after the first session. She felt it would make her more nervous to think about it. Of course, John was irate, was very worried that his reputation would suffer, and demanded that she discontinue the counseling sessions.

Joanne did not stop coming to the center, and after the first three sessions the education program convinced her that their situation would only get worse if there were no changes. She could see that she had allowed herself to believe that John could do it by himself in the past, while he actually never had been successful at quitting drinking for more than a week or two. The progression of alcoholism is a significant aspect to cover with a spouse; in Joanne's case, knowing that alcoholism is progressive as long as the alcoholic continues to drink allowed her to take more risks.

During the first month Joanne became more aware of the ways the family was denying reality and reinforcing her husband's irresponsible behavior: she canceled engagements because he was intoxicated; the family sat through meals while he fumbled drunkenly, attempting to eat; she and the girls rode in the car with him when he was driving while intoxicated.

She began to level with John about the reality of their life. She informed him that she would no longer ride in the car with him if he had been drinking. She also told him she would no longer make up stories to explain their absence at engagements. Of course he tested her and it was extremely difficult for Joanne to follow through because it was embarrassing. However, we discussed the fact that she was embarrassed often anyway. John no longer asked her to cancel any appointments and managed to be sober for engagements. Joanne began attending Al-Anon on a regular basis and gained support from its philosophy and members.

The girls and Joanne discussed how to handle the dinner problem and decided that she would tell John that when he came to dinner too intoxicated to eat in a polite manner, they would move to another room to complete their meal—and they did. They informed him why they were leaving the room. They did not respond to his goading and antagonism, but picked up their plates and left.

The children gained more confidence when they saw Joanne become less nervous and begin to plan activities without waiting to see how John would feel. The older two children talked to their father about his drinking, telling him that they loved him, they liked to be around him when he was not drinking, but when he was drinking he hurt their feelings and embarrassed them.

The key to this family's situation was consistency in handing John the reality and responsibility for his behavior. The initial changes were uncomfortable for all the members of the family, but as Joanne said: "We should be used to being uncomfortable. At least now I know why he is angry."

From time to time during her struggle, when she wanted to slip back into the old habits, we would review the changes, no matter how small, that she had made. We would talk about the decisions she was making for herself and write a list of positives about herself or her life. The list grew as the weeks went by and she became healthier. After a three-month period of once-a-week sessions, Joanne, the children, and I agreed that they would present John with an ultimatum. They told John that they were worried about his drinking and the effects it had on all of them. They loved him and wanted him to see the counselor. If he did not, they were considering other alternatives, that is, separation.

John had observed the changes and the self-confidence of Joanne's actions over the three-month period and believed she would follow through. Joanne had gained control of her life in these months and John knew he could no longer control her.

John came in for counseling. They also became involved in marital counseling and John was referred to Alcoholics Anonymous. John has maintained sobriety since entrance into the program.

Case 2. Grace and Ben are both 52 years old and have been married for 30 years with six children ranging in age from 12 to 24. Four children are married and live away from home. Ben works as a foreman in construction.

Grace came to our counseling center after hearing an announcement on the radio regarding our Family Forum, a structured educational program on alcoholism, and seeing the Family Questionnaire and a bus sign advertising the agency. She had been a member of Al-Anon and had been to her minister for counseling. Her minister told her that Ben would have to decide to quit on his own. He thought Ben was improving since he was drinking beer instead of hard liquor.

Our first step was for Grace to attend the Forum. Through the education program she began to see how her husband and his drinking controlled the psychological atmosphere in the home. Nobody in the house was dealing with the drinking problem. We reviewed the demythification of alcoholism (Figure 4). Grace informed Ben she was coming for counseling, provoking a violent reaction in him. He took the car keys away from her and Grace began to take a cab to the Center.

As part of Grace's treatment plan, she decided to take the following actions:

1. She would openly talk about his drinking problem with the children.
2. She would not ride with him when he was driving while intoxicated.
3. She would set any bottles she found on the kitchen table.
4. She would write to the married children and ask them to attend a counseling session when they came home for Thanksgiving and to write to their father. They agreed to tell him they cared for him and they wanted to have a nice holiday. They hoped he would not drink over the holiday because if he did they would have to leave. Grace and the children agreed to the plan. Two of the couples traveled quite a distance.

The families arrived the day before Thanksgiving, and a co-therapist and I held a conjoint session with the entire family of eleven. We reviewed the disease concept of alcoholism, the progression of the disease, and the reinforcing behavior, as well as the fact that they did not level with their father about his drinking, that the family "walked on eggshells," and that they could help create an atmosphere of reality around their father even though they lived miles away.

Thanksgiving day Ben started drinking. The children sat down with him and told him they were unhappy he chose to drink. They assured him they loved him and were very worried about him. They told him they were leaving—and they did. Ben yelled insults at them and told them they didn't care.

When the children arrived home, they wrote to Ben. His daughters-in-law wrote to him too. They asked him please to see a counselor and emphasized that they loved him. Ben came in for counseling three days later.

The same agreement was made regarding the Christmas holidays. The children came home and Ben did not drink, so they stayed and enjoyed their first sober family Christmas. Ben claims it was his first sober Christmas since age 14. We had another family counseling session over the holiday with the entire family, including Ben. The children are continuing to write letters of reinforcement. Ben and Grace have a long way to go but they are making a beginning.

Another aspect of this family is that one of Ben's sons and his wife identified a drinking problem in their family as a result of the education and counseling session. Ben's son has a drinking problem and the couple is coming for counseling. A more extensive discussion of sexual problems in alcoholics can be seen in Chapter 12.

REEXAMINATION OF GOALS

Perhaps the outcome of counseling will be separation and divorce. Our goal is not preset that the family will remain intact, but our goal, as mentioned earlier, is to assist the family members to become healthy, responsible persons capable of meeting and enjoying life to their capacity with or without the problem drinker. A decision of divorce should not terminate the counseling relationship for any significant other or the problem drinker, but should be a good reason for continuing. The family members, including the problem drinker sober or not, will need support for this decision.

We reevaluate the treatment plan and update the short- and long-term goals periodically. We caution ourselves to make a program that fits the needs of the individual and family rather than our goals and our view of the family.

Sexual Problems. Most problem drinkers and alcoholics have a variety of sexual problems, including premature ejaculation, impotence, and fear of rejection. In the area of sexuality, many myths exist and many individuals do not know how to talk about their own sexual needs, expectations, desires, and fears. Usually both the problem drinker and spouse have a fear of intimacy.

Most problem drinkers have learned during their late teens and early twenties to use alcohol to relieve anxieties. Many times they turned to alcohol when they were worried about poor grades or problems at school. As a result, the alcoholic or problem drinker has not learned to solve everyday problems in life by the trial-and-error method. He has not learned to be a responsible adult nor how to maintain an adult relationship. The inability to initiate and form intimate relationships is the single most important sexual problem for the alcoholic and the significant other (Howard and Howard, 1977a,b).

The alcoholic is filled with myths and fears and with sexual needs that have no way of being communicated and understood. These problems will grow progressively worse with the drinking problem. This holds true for both the alcoholic and the spouse of the alcoholic. In marriage, the alcoholic becomes isolated, depressed, and alienated from the spouse and from himself as he forms an intimate relationship with alcohol. As the disease progresses, the alcoholic is lonely and has feelings of low self-worth and low self-esteem. The problem drinker is very skillful at covering up these feelings of inadequacy, thus preventing himself from recognizing the problem. The problem drinker fears rejection by his spouse to an extreme degree and actually anticipates the event. These feelings of low self-esteem and fear of rejection usually create difficulties in forming satisfying personal relationships, particularly an intimate one with a spouse.

Alcohol releases many of our sexual inhibitions by affecting those cells in the brain that control inhibitions. After a person has used alcohol extensively for a number of years, it affects all aspects of his behavior and his ability to function in a sexual relationship.

We find the spouse very afraid to show affection for fear that intercourse will automatically ensue, often at inappropriate or unwanted times. The spontaneity is taken out of the response and in many ways the persons' sexuality is repressed. This is sad because this is what the problem drinker is reaching out for—an intimate relationship, a sexual relationship.

A person's sexual performance under the influence of alcohol is diminished. It removes the inhibition, but also affects the performance and ability to have an erection. Shakespeare said, "Alcohol provokes the desire, but lessens the performance." Alcohol sedates. It is a depressant. Once a man is unable to achieve an erection, he will worry about his ability to perform. In many ways he becomes spectator to his own intimate relationship.

This condition is not limited to the alcoholic population, but to the male population in general. The man fears impotence. When you add communication problems, the situation seems insoluble. The solution requires open communication and strong egos, which neither the alcoholic nor the spouse usually possesses. It takes an alert, well-trained counselor to be able to work on this problem area.

The alcoholic and spouse will benefit immensely from an educational program on intimacy. Usually the persons' backgrounds along with the myths and misinformation they have collected over the years and during sexual experiences, particularly during the drinking periods, have created blocks to communication and change in this area. The way the couple communicates is linked with their images of themselves, and their sexuality affects and is affected by their self-images and communication. Therefore, education concerning their sexuality and expression of that sexuality is of overall importance in counseling for change. See Chapter 12 in this book on managing sexual problems in alcoholics.

We suggest that a couple write down their own needs, desires, and expectations in their relationship, in all areas including sexuality, and discuss these with their counselor. What does this relationship mean to them? What does love mean to them? What types of foreplay do they enjoy and what type of atmosphere in their bedroom would make it romantic? Counseling can be of assistance to couples by providing a third party to guide them and direct communication. A counselor may have more tools to help further exploration. Weekend programs such as marital enrichment groups can also be beneficial.

TOUCH SYSTEM

All of these counseling techniques are of little value if the community is not made aware that they exist. Therefore we feel it important to explain our "touch system," the method we use to reach the significant other via public education and community awareness (Howard and Howard, 1977b).

The object of the system is to increase the visibility of alcoholism as a treatable disease with a 60–80% recovery rate. Approximately 10%

of the population suffers from alcoholism, with four or five others directly affected by the disease. Consequently, approximately 25% of the total community is affected in a personal way by a person with a drinking problem.

Since denial is such an inherent part of the disease, focus your energies on the significant others, not just on the alcoholic. Emphasize, "Don't *ride* with a drinking driver," rather than "Don't drink and drive." We try to touch the family, believing that if they perceive the message often enough, they will contact us for help.

Over the years, our agency has increased the use of the system so that today our referrals have been touched by our efforts over five times each. Some samples are:

- Bumper stickers for cars reading: "Do you have a family drinking problem? Call 449-2581."
- Matchbooks with much the same message placed in bars, banks, restaurants, and liquor stores.
- Litter bags distributed through grocery and liquor stores at the station where liquor is wrapped.
- Balloons for children at grade schools and junior high schools.
- Agency brochures in the back of every church in the community.
- Displays at the library, shopping centers, annual company picnics.
- Printed college football schedules bearing the message, "Have a family drinking problem? Call for assistance."
- Free public service announcements placed on radio and television and in the newspapers.

All these methods say to the person emotionally involved with the problem drinker, "It's OK to come in for education and information. There is always hope with action. Don't wait." We have to reach out to tell them that *they* have to reach out. This is assertive early intervention.

High visibility may also be obtained by door-to-door community-awareness campaigns. In this low-key approach we divide the community into workable segments, making the campaign possible with the use of our volunteer force. The volunteer gives out an agency brochure at each residence and says, "Hello, I'm a volunteer for Howard Family Institute. We simply wanted you to know that these services are available right here in Columbia."

In-service training provides information to other human service agencies. People who work with people are going to come into contact with alcoholism, and in-service training can help them learn to identify the illness and know where to go for assistance. In effect it enlarges your own staff because these other people become screeners, identifiers, and referrers of your agency. Ministers, doctors, social service agencies, and welfare workers all come into contact with families who have drinking problems. If we help them learn the symptoms, we can touch many more people who need help with the drinking problem. The touch system becomes a multiple referral network.

Summary

The area of counseling families with drinking problems is full of new territories to be explored. We cannot remain satisfied with simply saying that alcoholism affects the family, by writing a chapter of a book on how it happens. We must become active in using our energy and creativity to open new frontiers for treatment of families and for early-intervention techniques in hospitals, treatment units, and outpatient clinics.

Our approach to the significant others, the family with a drinking problem, does not limit all its attention to the alcoholic but emphasizes the ability of each human being to change within a relationship and family. The statement of Satir (1972) that every member of the family can influence every other member has given impetus to early intervention into the cycle of alcoholism through effecting change with the significant others.

Alcoholism, however, stifles growth and fogs issues needing resolution and changes in a healthy family. Therefore we cannot work simply for change, *ignoring* the existence and hazards of a drinking problem because its vaporous, elusive substance will form again and again, causing the family to lose direction—forcing them to choose the well-worn, comfortable paths which reinforce the cycle of alcoholism.

Counseling the family with education about alcoholism may produce a longer and more discouraging counseling situation for the significant others. The exclusion of the educational aspects from the treatment program may not break the denial process, as is so necessary to successful treatment and recovery from alcholism. The counselor is encouraged to work with the significant other seeking treatment as the primary client and to work with and through the family members and other important persons to stabilize the family. It is hoped that this planned program will provide the alcoholic with the impetus to seek help earlier.

Our counseling program is based on the premise that we can not wait for the problem drinker to "hit bottom." We must employ a system for reaching out into the community with programs of education and awareness to change myths that hamper early intervention and treatment for significant others. Our "touch system" is both a necessity and a possibility with a planned step-by-step timetable. These methods will reach within the four walls where the family waits in loneliness and hopelessness, preparing them to seek assistance for a drinking problem.

The success of the family involves the family and you, the helper. You must be the biggest booster and believer in change, particularly where a drinking problem exists. You do not have to cruise the neighborhoods looking for unkempt lawns and houses, nor wipe all the alcoholics off your welfare roles. You can believe that the spouse can change, that the children can change—change measured by their yardsticks and not ours. Education is a primary tool for change, believing that knowledge can light the darkness, that positive information can turn the "I can't" into "I can!"

REFERENCES

Cork, M. R. *The forgotten children*. Toronto, Canada: Addiction Research Foundation, 1969.

Howard, D., and Howard, N. *A family approach to problem drinking*. Columbia, Mo.: Family Training Center, 1976.

Howard, D., and Howard, N. *Touching me, touching you*. Columbia, Mo.: Family Training Center, 1977a.

Howard, D., and Howard, N. *The family counseling model—an early intervention to problem drinking*. Columbia, Mo.: Family Training Center, 1977b.

Jackson, J. The adjustment of the family to the crises of alcoholism. *Quarterly Journal of Studies on Alcohol*, 1954, 15(4), 562–586.

Jellinek, E. M. *Disease concept of alcoholism*. New Haven: United Printing Services, 1960.

Kellerman, J. L. *Alcoholism, a merry-go-round named denial*. Al-Anon Family Group Headquarters, 1969.

Satir, V. *Peoplemaking*. Palo Alto, Calif. Science and Behavior Books, 1972.

"Twenty-Question Questionnaire for the Alcoholic," Johns Hopkins University Medical School, Baltimore, Md., 1955.

12

Management of Sexual Dysfunctions in Alcoholics

DAVID J. POWELL

INTRODUCTION

It is widely believed that alcohol is a sexual stimulant that releases inhibitions and enhances sexual performance. Ogden Nash wrote, "Candy is dandy, but liquor is quicker." This belief is understandable because sexual behavior and alcohol consumption are often combined in society. Many first sexual encounters are associated with drinking, and alcohol seems to lower sexual inhibitions and facilitate sociosexual interaction.

Although alcohol in small amounts does free inhibitions, continued use contributes to sexual concerns, difficulties, and dysfunctions. For the alcoholic, booze and sex become incompatible bedpartners that result in organic and psychogenic sexual dysfunctions.

In this author's 18 years of practice with alcoholics, it has become essential to deal with the client's sexual needs. We talk about treating the whole person, yet too rarely do we deal with sexual functioning. A counselor once asked a client if he smoked after intercourse, to which the client responded, "I don't know. I've never looked." If alcohologists do not look, they will not find the relationship between alcoholism and sexual problems. Most admit there is a relationship; few deal with it because of a lack of scientific knowledge about sexuality and ignorance of clinical data and sex counseling approaches. Counselors must be able to deal with the alcoholic's sexual concerns because continued sexual

---

DAVID J. POWELL • President, Education and Training Programs, Inc., Granby, Connecticut.

problems may inhibit recovery as a whole by impairing marital relationships and individual self-growth.

SEXUAL CONCERNS, DIFFICULTIES, AND DYSFUNCTIONS IN ALCOHOLICS

Sexual problems arise due to the interrelationship of sexual and interactional breakdowns. As the marriage deteriorates, the sex life changes. It becomes a vicious cycle: Interactions decline so sex becomes impaired so interactions decline further. In the alcoholic couple, this pattern is most acute due to the complications of the drinking behavior. A number of factors contribute: lack of trust, role reversals, control and power struggles, feelings of hostility and resentment, contractual and communication breakdowns, and loss of self-identity and esteem.

Sexual Concerns.   As drinking clouds one's perceptions of reality, concerns arise about body image. What is normal? Am I adequate? Is my penis too small? Are my breasts too large? Too small? These questions are not unique to the alcoholic except that his thinking is distorted by drinking. Other concerns include gender identity, sexual secrets and fantasies exposed while drinking, and inability to relax without alcohol.

Sexual Difficulties.   There are changes in the frequency of affection and contact. Drunkenness acts as a deterrent to sexual interest for most partners. Displays of affection become intermittent and extinct. There are problems of sexual timing. She is interested when he is sober. He associates sex with drinking. As the alcoholic's world closes in on the family, options for sex also close in. For most alcoholic couples, communication breaks down and sexual foreplay is markedly reduced. Alcoholic relationships are overwhelmed by bedroom power plays, usually masking communication problems. This may increase resentment and add to aggressive/abusive sexual behavior. Heterosexual versus homosexual identity can be a problem, as well as issues regarding sexual preferences.

Sexual Dysfunctions.   Numerous studies have been conducted on drinking and male sexual dysfunctions, fewer on female drinkers. Males experience recurrent bouts with ejaculatory problems, impotence, and inhibited sexual desire (ISD). A number of associated problems also occur: The process of feminization, gynecomastia (breast enlargement, loss of body hair, and muscle tone), and atrophy of the testicles.

Although traditional studies of female alcoholics have indicated a broad range of sexual dysfunctions, including painful intercourse (dyspareunia), being nonorgasmic (anorgasmia), involuntary spasmatic contractions of the vaginal muscles (vaginismus), and inhibited sexual desire, Apter-Marsh (1982) and Smith and Buxton (1982) found no major areas of sexual dysfunction. There is a tendency in the first 3 months of recovery for sexual frequency and orgasmic ability to decrease, but this reverses itself in later sobriety.

Sexual dysfunctions should not be confused with sexual dissatisfaction. The most common complaint for alcoholic women is disinterest in sex due more to intimacy issues and relationship disharmony than to organic etiology.

The time period studied is critical. Dysfunctions noted during drinking years, early abstention, and later sobriety may be markedly different. Too few studies have examined sexual dysfunctions longitudinally.

RESEARCH FINDINGS: MALE PHYSIOLOGICAL FACTORS

Alcohol acts as a causative and implicative agent in male impotence. For men in their 40s and 50s, alcoholism is the most prevalent etiological factor for male secondary impotence, more than any other single factor (Masters and Johnson, 1970). This is due to the direct gonadal effects of alcohol which include decreases in testosterone production, relative and absolute shifts to greater estrogen levels, and impaired sperm production. The male genitals must be supplied with adequate testosterone levels to achieve and maintain erections. Research has shown that male alcoholics experience reduced testosterone levels. In chronic alcoholism, there is an increase in the activity of a liver enzyme that degrades testosterone (Rubin and Lieber, 1976). As blood alcohol concentrations increase, plasma testosterone levels decrease, and luteinizing hormone (LH) levels increase, thus giving the sense of greater libido but resulting in impotence. The peripheral suppression of testosterone by the testes may be a result of enzyme-induced increased hepatic clearance or a more direct effect on testosterone biosynthesis (Powell, 1980).

Increased estrogen levels (hyperestrogenization) are secondary to alcohol-induced liver damage in which the liver converts a higher proportion of androgen to estrogen. The combination of the two mechanisms (plus low levels of luteinizing hormone and follicle stimulating hormone) is the most likely cause of long-term feminization effects, impotence, sterility, and inhibited sexual desire (Akhtar, 1977).

If an alcoholic is experiencing first stage liver disease (i.e., fatty liver), testosterone production should return to near normal levels as abstinence continues. In early recovery (1 to 2 months), the newly sober alcoholic may be unable to perform sexually and may experience disinterest due to physiological changes (Van Thiel, 1977).

If greater liver damage has occurred, irreversible effects on sexual functioning may be noted: testicular atrophy, chronically low sperm count, loss of body hair, and libido. Normal testosterone levels may never return. Extragonadal effects of alcohol include increased hepatic 5 alpha-testosterone reductase levels and an increased percentage of testosterone bound to protein. These effects diminish penile tumescence (rate of erection) and penile diameter. Alcoholism can prevent formation of erectal capacity sufficient for vaginal penetration. Thus, alcohol exerts multiple effects on the hypothalamus-pituitary-gonadal axis in the male. Another physiological factor may be impaired spinal reflexes leading to decreased sensation and enervation for erection. In chronic cases, a degeneration of nerves connected to erectile functioning may result in irreversible organic impotence. Other medical complications such as peripheral neuropathy and anemia may also contribute to sexual dysfunction.

RESEARCH FINDINGS: MALE PSYCHOLOGICAL FACTORS

Sexual self-doubts (performance anxiety) are factors in sexual problems. "Can I do this? Will I get an erection? Will I come too quickly?" These doubts can prevent sexual activity from occurring. If performance anxiety does not affect the alcoholic, relationship conflicts probably will. Alcoholic marriages are overwhelmed by resentment and distress. Sex while drinking may be associated with feelings of rejection, anger, and revulsion. Sexual approaches may be inappropriate, insensitive, or aggressive. The co-alcoholic may be viewed as cold, rejecting, unfeminine, or "frigid." Self-punishment is inflicted; sexual pleasure is avoided.

Henry, an alcoholic, after an evening of drinking, tries to have sex with his wife. Because of excessive alcohol use and a host of other factors (too late at night, tiredness, distractions), nothing happens. He is unable to have an erection. Next night, he decides to show her; He will get the biggest erection possible. To bolster himself, he drinks and the inevitable second "failure" occurs. Now he is labeled himself as impotent. He watches for an erection. This is performance anxiety.

Barbara (nonalcoholic) was married to John (alcoholic). Whenever drinking, he forced her to perform sexual acts she considered repulsive, including sadomasochism and bondage. Barbara would be awakened from sleep in the midst of oral sex. The last thing she wanted was sex with John, whether he was drinking or sober.

After two years of sobriety, Doug (alcoholic) had difficulty resolving for himself his sexual behaviors while drinking. Cross-dressing and exhibitionism were common for him. Ann, his wife, was embarrasssed and resentful of this.

RESEARCH FINDINGS: FEMALE PHYSIOLOGICAL FACTORS

Considerably less research has been done on female alcoholics. Conflicting findings on sexual performance result from the stage of drinking versus recovery studied. Laboratory research on nonalcoholic women while drinking indicates decreased vaginal lubrication but increased subjective perceptions of sexual arousal. The more intoxicated, the more the woman predicted she would be aroused.

Other studies indicated no consistent effects on progesterone, prolactin, or follicle stimulating hormones in alcoholic women. There are apparently no reductions in testosterone or increased luteininzing hormone (LH) levels, probably due to the differing source of testosterone in women versus men (adrenal versus testicular). The lack of LH rise and increased subjective perceptions of sexual arousal seems to indicate there is no connection with increased libido and LH levels, as was indicated for men.

Studies have shown linkages between alcohol-related hepatic disorders and a lack of vaginal lubrication. Vaginismus may occur which prevents penetration by involuntary spasmatic contractions of the pubococcygeal muscle surrounding the vaginal area. Alcohol acts as a direct gonadal toxin in alcoholic women, thus inhibiting sexual performance.

This may cause other associated sexual symptomatology: premature menopausal conditions, menstrual irregularities, breast atrophy, redistribution of body fat, cessation of ovulation, masculinization, and a drying effect of cellular fluids. Apparently, the greater the intoxication, the longer it takes to reach orgasm. Yet, subjects report increased arousal and greater orgasmic pleasure at high blood alcohol levels despite the physiological indices to the contrary.

RESEARCH FINDINGS: FEMALE PSYCHOLOGICAL FACTORS

Sexual problems for alcoholic women occur more in the areas of inhibited sexual desire, which is probably psychogenic rather than organic. The lack of body awareness and sensitivity is exacerbated by drinking. Self-esteem is low, thus there is a tendency to shift the focus from self-pleasure to alcohol. They tend to express themselves sexually in a more direct stereotypical manner using provocative and seductive behavior and approaching sex from a more manipulative stance. Fears of performance are also prevalent. Relationships are marked by resentment toward the rebuffs of one's partner and a lack of communication. Feelings of isolation, depression, and inadequacy are prevalent.

Apter-Marsh (1982) found female alcoholic's behavior with partners showed its greatest activity during the active drinking phase and lowest during the first 3 months of recovery. After this period, sexual behavior tended to return to pre-addiction levels. During drinking, sexual activity was 80% partnered and 20% masturbatory sex versus 60% and 40% during early recovery.

Orgasmic frequency with a partner was higher in recovery than during drinking, although there was a greater level of sexual activity during the drinking phase. Women's orgasmic ability always appears to be greater via masturbation than with partnered sex. Almost half of the women in Apter-Marsh's study had been raped or experienced incest (Wilsnack, 1974).

THE DIAGNOSTIC PROCESS

Alcoholism can coexist with other psychiatric and medical conditions. For example, depression is particularly common in female alcoholics. Since sexual problems can be related to psychiatric problems as well as to alcoholism, a sound differential diagnosis is important. First, one must determine organicity versus psychogenicity of the dysfunction. Of sexual problems, 15% to 25% are physiologically based in the nonalcohol population and undoubtedly higher in alcoholics. A complete physical and lab work-up can determine etiology. Areas of organicity requiring differential diagnosis include: anatomic conditions affecting genital functions (i.e., hymenael abnormalities, Peyronie's disease, infected episiotomy, etc.); endocrine conditions (i.e., diabetes, pituitary, adrenal, thyroid disorders, hypogonadism); vascular factors (i.e., vessel blockage, vasculities, sclerosis, heart disease); neurological factors (i.e., impaired sexual reflexes or sensory pathways, chronic pain); miscellaneous (i.e., liver or kidney disease, malignancy, pelvic infections [vaginitis], endometriosis, dietary and nutritional deficiencies, and urologic disorders).

Differential diagnosis should determine psychogenic etiologic and coexisting psychological conditions such as: dispositional influences, including attachment, separation and loss issues (proceptive concerns), locus of control, mastery, maturity, and narcissism issues, and sexual orientation concerns. Contributing influences include informational factors (lack of knowledge, communication breakdowns), cognitive factors (attending to cues, spectatoring, unrealistic expectations), traumatic factors (rape memory, incest, violence, child abuse), and attitudinal factors (feelings of disgust, dislike, servicing).

Immediate influences to be differentiated include emotional factors (performance anxiety, fears, guilt, apathy), physical factors (exhaustion), and religious orthodoxy. Personality influences include self-image, fears of success/failure, control issues, need to punish self/others, hypertension, depression, mania, hostility to the other sex, intimacy fears (acception issues), inability to let go emotionally, rigidity, obsessive behavior, lack of creativity, and inability to play.

Finally, relational influences to be examined in the differential diagnostic process include egalitarian versus double standards of behavior in the relationship, power plays ("he has the money, she has the sex"), boredom with the relationship, symbiosis, conflict habituation, hostility, independence versus interdependence, destructive transactions, differing value systems, and disparate interests.

TREATMENT IMPLICATIONS

The pain of relationships can stand out in bold contrast to the "new life" found in sobriety. For some alcoholics, recovery can be as problem ridden as was the active drinking stage. Sexual problems can become a major hurdle in the continued recovery process. Dr. G. D. Talbott, Ridgeview Institute (1982) said, "The predominant problem in recidivism in the Institute is unresolved sexual problems."

Treatment resurrects the sexual difficulties masked by drinking. The expectation of many recovering people is that without alcohol sexual activity will return to "normal." Many alcoholic couples, however, have never had a chemical free normal sex life. When a satisfactory sexual life does not occur, anxiety and the pressure to perform grows. Sexual approaches are avoided—no one wants to risk failure.

For the recovering alcoholic, the energy needed to maintain sobriety is crucial. Regular AA meetings, outpatient treatment, alumni groups, drunken driver classes, and so forth, deplete the energy supply. There is often not enough energy left to work on the sex life as well. Throughout recovery, the maintenance of sobriety comes first and supersedes all issues. Yet, as problems arise they should be addressed progressively and in an integrated manner. General treatment implications include the following: developing an atmosphere of openness and comfort with sexual topics; dealing with guilt, anger, hostility, shame, interest, and ability loss; modification of destructive sexual values and beliefs; changing sexual behaviors gradually and teaching appropriate assertiveness; dealing with concerns about intimacy, emotional involvement, and identity; and confronting the unique concerns of the unmarried/unpartnered.

Alcoholics need to know early in recovery that sexual problems may appear, but will likely disappear in time. They need to anticipate the changes that occur in recovery. Fears, feelings and concerns about prior sexual experiences should be ventilated. They need to learn that their sexual identity is not under attack, but that they are merely in the midst of a sexual change.

BROAD TREATMENT PRINCIPLES

Regardless of the treatment setting, sexual issues can be addressed at various stages and in varying degrees. Sexual counseling is a form of psychotherapy that integrates biomedical and psychosocial components in the treatment of sexual problems. This simple definition lays the foundation for demystifying the therapy process. Alcohologists can deal with psychosocial problems without being psychologists, nutritional issues without being nutritionists, and sexual concerns without being sexologists. Although there are limits on what the alcoholism counselor should deal with, sexual issues can be addressed. The key for the counselor, however, is knowing his limits and the therapeutic boundaries within that treatment program.

A premise for sex therapy is that sexual problems are unit problems. The focus should be on the individual's needs within a couple context. No one person should assume full responsibility for dysfunctions. For example, he is not impotent, but the couple is experiencing sexual problems, one of which is that he does not get an erection. Other treatment principles include the following: establishing a neutral environment, and staying in the present, without referencing the past or the future. For a therapist it means not being for or against a client. An atmosphere of acceptance, not blaming for feelings, must be established. Clients should learn to be responsible for themselves. Couples should not analyze feelings or wait for the other to fix them. "I cannot give you an orgasm if you don't want one. I can assist, but you're responsible for you."

Treatment also involves communication building and the teaching of listening skills. Counseling helps to make us aware of inner thoughts, perceptions, and feelings, as well as to develop a language and to overcome defenses in communication. Self-representation ("I" messages) is taught, as well as negotiation skills (whose need is the greatest, and giving priority to the best interest of the relationship). Attending and paraphrasing are taught.

Since many of the dysfunctional symptoms are related to alcoholism which may be ameliorated in time with continued abstinence, a sound diagnosis is the key in determining etiology. Yet diagnostic accuracy is not always possible in early recovery. A "wait and see" approach may be appropriate. Therapists should begin early treatment with a good history, treat symptoms that can be corrected easily, and use the "wait and see" approach for the rest. In time, the problems that are not removed in continued sobriety can be treated.

A helpful step in early recovery is to take the pressure off by giving the couple permission to not have intercourse. Emphasis should be on getting to know each other without alcohol, communicating, relaxing, resocializing, and rebuilding a healthy relationship. They should learn the differences between sexual dysfunctions and dissatisfaction/disinterest. They should be reassured that sexual feelings will return in time. Limiting intercourse initially (1 to 3 months) may be helpful, but the impression that all sexual contact is wrong should not be given.

A number of clinical techniques can be taught to varying degrees. Sensate focus (Masters and Johnson, 1970) is an *in vivo* desensitization massage exercise. It enables the couple to slow down sexual interactions and to focus on components that can be processed one at a time. It presents sex as a natural function and helps people to touch who are "out of touch." Individuals and couples in sensate focus are told to refrain from intercourse and to begin with nondemand, nongoal oriented touching for self for the inherent enjoyment of touch. The sequence suggested by the therapist is as follows:

1. Total body touching, excluding breasts and genitals.
2. Total body touching, including breasts and genitals.
3. Mutual touching.
4. Mutual touching in female astride and genitals touching without insertion.
5. Female astride position with insertion.

These exercises are carried out in the nude for the interest of the massager and the enjoyment of the recipient. The toucher is instructed to do so for his pleasure and not to "turn the other on" so as to become aroused himself. Sensate focus is not a series of "tricks," gimmicks, or games to be prescribed indiscriminately. It is a progressive learning experience incorporated into an ongoing treatment plan by a skilled therapist.

Other counseling applications include teaching the "squeeze technique," a simple exercise used to treat rapid ejaculation and to restore confidence in ejaculatory control. The male can learn to stimulate the penis until he perceives orgasm to be imminent, at which point he stops and sufficiently squeezes the penis just below the rim of the glans to cause him to lose his erection partially. Stimulation is subsequently resumed, interrupted again when ejaculation is near. This technique has been shown to be successful in teaching ejaculatory control. A related approach is "stop-start" developed by Semans (Kaplan, 1974). The male focuses on erotic sensations emanating from the penis while being stimulated. When he feels premonitory orgastic sensations, stimulation is stopped. Before the erection is lost, stimulation is resumed and stopped again just prior to orgasm. This process is repeated 2 to 3 times before stimulation to orgasm continues. The emphasis is on erotic feelings only and exploring the range of sensations.

Many techniques can be used to distract obsessive thoughts, "distracting the distractor." Sexual fantasy building is used via erotic literature and other means to expand imaging ability. Self-pleasuring and relaxation methods are taught, such as showering together, breathing and muscular relaxation approaches, and use of a vibrator. Permission is given to be "selfish"—to abandon oneself to erotic feelings to the temporary exclusion of all else. This does not mean a disregard for the other's needs, but a focusing on exquisite sensitivity and mutual generosity. Many men have become overly concerned with their partner's needs—"giving her an orgasm." They need to learn to enjoy themselves again, to stop spectatoring, to avoid the "dip stick" approach to intercourse, and to use the principle of "taking turns."

Spectatoring is when a person critically watches his own sexual performance as though he were a third person presiding as a judge of his own lovemaking. Persistent thoughts occur: "Will it be hard enough? Will I come?" Spectatoring results in erectile or orgastic problems, since autonomic functions must be free of conscious control if they are to unfold naturally. These obsessive defenses may simply result from a fear of failure due to prior events and not a product of psychopathology. If it is only that, then direct intervention and thought stopping techniques can be taught. If, however, it is the result of deeper characterologic problems, it must be resolved first via traditional psychotherapy. Personality characteristics can include obsessive perfectionism, lack of trust, insecurities, deeply destructive interactions, and so forth. In most counseling, the "tip of the iceberg" should be dealt with since at the end of treatment, the client may still be perfectionistic and competitive in general but not sexually.

Hormone replacement therapy may play a valuable role in treatment of sexual problems. Testosterone treatment may give a temporary physiological boost which serves to interrupt a vicious psychological cycle. It intensifies eroticism and induces a concomitant alteration of psychological mechanisms which in combination serve to improve overall sexual functioning. Hormone therapy should be done by a skilled physician and within the context of ongoing sex therapy.

PLISSIT

PLISSIT is an extremely valuable model for alcoholism counselors. It can be adapted to most treatment settings and provides four levels of approach, each letter representing a method for handling sexual problems. PLISSIT's application to alcoholism treatment is also represented below.

	P = Permission giving	All stages of alcoholism care
Brief Therapy	LI = Limited Information	Recovery and middle sobriety
	SS = Specific Suggestions	Same
Intensive Care	IT = Intensive Therapy	Later recovery, out-patient

Each descending level entails greater degrees of skills, training, and knowledge. It also indicates when to refer. PLISS will be addressed in this section; IT in the following.

Permission Giving. Often alcoholics in treatment want to know if they are normal. Hearing that they are from a professional gives them relief. If permission is given to discuss feelings and actions openly, it is much easier for them to make amends for the past. It helps to receive reassurance that thoughts and fantasies are typical. Differentiating between tactile sensations and covert sexual thoughts is important. For example, a mother may feel guilty about being sexually aroused by breast feeding her daughter if she perceives the arousal as latent homosexual desires. A father may have an erection when his son plays on his leg. He may become anxious about homosexual tendencies although his erection is in all likelihood due to direct penile stimulation. Reassurance that these are normal involuntary reactions can relieve considerable anxiety.

Permission giving can also involve sexual behaviors. For example, somewhere the alcoholic female, on hearing that "normal" women are multiple orgasmic, may feel undersexed. It helps to clarify these myths and to alleviate negativism. The counselor can give permission to clients not to engage in particular behaviors if they do not wish to. The key is to give permission in direct relation to the goals of the individual and couple.

When taking a psychosocial intake history the counselor can give permission to talk about sexual issues. Questions should not be in the form of "How's your sex life?" but "Tell me something about your sexual behaviors. It is common for alcoholics to experience sexual problems like difficulty in getting an erection, ejaculating too quickly, not lubricating sufficiently." General education, couple counseling, and group therapy sessions can all deal with sexuality. Basically the message is "I'm comfortable talking about sex. Feel free to do so."

Permission giving does not mean sanctioning all behaviors, particularly those that are destructive to self or others. Permission cannot be given for incest, rape, persistent and indiscriminate masturbatory activity, and so forth. Clear legal and societal boundaries must be adhered to.

Limited Information. This provides the alcoholic with specific factual information about his difficulties. For example, information about normal genital size can be helpful, as is information about the effects of alcohol on sexual performance. Other topics include: masturbation, birth control alternatives, sexual frequency, sexual identity and preference, intercourse during menstruation, oral-genital contact, and aging and sexual behavior.

Usually, the active alcoholic does not link his sexual problems to drinking. He has assumed that these problems are a result of his personal failure in life. Yet many sexual problems have little to do with personality but are a direct result of alcoholic drinking. Limited information about the relationship of alcohol and sexual problems can be reassuring to the alcoholic. Finally, it is helpful to inform patients in early recovery that many of these problems will be ameliorated during the recovery process.

For example, Ted was a 24-year-old alcoholic with extensive sexual experience. (He reported having 500 partners.) Yet, in his drinking, he never understood how his wife urinated with a tampon inserted. Limited information regarding anatomy was helpful in relieving confusion about sexual functioning.

Myths about sexuality can be dispelled through limited information. Some of these myths are as follows: That the male is the sexual expert, men have greater sexual needs, you are responsible for the other's satisfaction, age does not affect sex, old people do not have sex. Limited information gives the alcoholic a chance to change behaviors, to dispel myths, and to experience some relief from negative feelings. It can be given in most stages of treatment through presentations and discussion groups.

During routine physicals, information regarding alcoholism and sex can be given. Brochures, pamphlets, and articles can be available in the unit library for reference. Patients can be given handouts for reading. Slides and films such as "Sex, Booze, and Blues" can be shown followed by group discussion. When limited information is not sufficient to resolve sexual concerns, referral to further in depth treatment is the next step.

Specific Suggestions. Specific suggestions must be based on client information gathered through a sex problem history. The setting and amount of time available will determine the extent of the history-taking. Based on the history, specific suggestions can be given in a direct, problem and time limited manner.

Two key suggestions are "There's always another time," and "It's what you do with what you have that counts." These phrases relieve considerable self-defeating determinism. Other specific suggestions include: the squeeze technique, resocialization training, thought stoppage techniques, Kegel muscle training, fantasy building, and attitude changing.

With alcoholics, a number of specific suggestions can be presented in group, individual, or couple counseling. Most treatment programs can incorporate specific suggestions into therapy at the later stages of care (the 3rd to 4th week of a 28 day program).

The last stage of PLISSIT, IT, will be addressed in a separate section since it involves highly individualized specific treatment approaches.

Sex Problem History-Taking

The first step in therapy is to get a good history of the problem. The basic premise is if you're not going to deal with it, don't ask about it. Otherwise, it is unnecessary at best and voyeuristic and countertherapeutic at worst. A second premise is that in any sex history there are 3 clients: the patient, his partner, and the two together in the context of reciprocal determinism. This is especially true for the alcoholic involved in a regressive relationship.

Principles of Sex Problem History-Taking

A history is valuable as a diagnostic and therapeutic tool, providing time for learning, reassurance, information sharing, and to clear up myths. The counselor should assume that everyone does everything.

There are three circles about all of us: The outer circle involves information that we want people to know. The middle is what is known to only a few people. The inner circle is information never spoken about and usually involves violence or deeper sexual feelings. In history-taking one derives information by asking and reasking questions in graduated, progressive stages.

Histories are falsified by 3 activities: exaggerations, misremembering, and cover-ups. Therapists must temper their acceptance of truth with the reality of a foggy recall due to these activities.

Procedures for Sex Problem History-Taking. A number of procedures are involved in sex problem history-taking. A "play by play" approach should be used and the minimum needed to reverse the problem should be done. Whatever is expressed in the history should be taken at face value since feelings are facts. The counselor, however, is in control of the interview at all times, using a cognitive, directive style, flowing from nonthreatening to emotion-laden/overt functioning information back to neutral material by the use of open-ended questions.

A basic procedure is that information should not be pursued to the client's discomfort just to attain chronological precision. All relevant data should be covered, giving positive feedback after all questions. This doesn't mean saying, "I approve of this behavior," but "I approve of your talking about that. I accept you as a person."

Since alcoholics' recall may be cloudy, a peg system helps to jar memory by pinpointing relevant places, times, events. "How old were you? Where were you?" If the counselor sees one problem , he should look for another. If one problem is present, so might another. For example, an impotent alcoholic probably experienced rapid ejaculation problems at one point. Here is a senario: he ejaculates quickly so he tries to distract himself to slow things down. He thinks about the weather, work, car accidents, anything to take his mind off what is happening. If he is successful, he will feel nothing, hence, impotence. He does not have to worry anymore about rapid ejaculation. This is obviously an effective, unconscious process.

Finally, the counselor should call it like he sees it and not use euphemisms, argots, or slang like "making love, sleep with," and so forth.

The bottom line in history-taking is to never threaten the precarious emotional stability or sobriety of an individual or couple in recovery. Using the basic assessment issues addressed under diagnostic factors, a problem-oriented sex history should include the following.

1. Sociologic and psychologic data (historic, self-concept, identity, parental and family influences, religious, educational and occupational influences)
2. Sex education data (early experiences, experimentation, traumas, rape, incest, contributors to sex education, contraception background)

3. Heterosexual activity (preadolescent, adolescent, dating, premarital, engagements, marital, extramarital, postmarital, current, first signs of sexual problems)
4. Homosexual activity (same as above)
5. Group sex activity (same as above)
6. Erotic responses (sensory, masturbation, fantasy, dreams)
7. Genital characteristics (male and female)
8. Sexual expectations

Problem-oriented information should focus on descriptions of sexual dysfunctions, erectile patterns, level of interest, ejaculatory/orgasmic patterns, partnered versus masturbatory sex, characteristics of current primary sexual relationship, health history, and medical status.

Depending on time, setting, and skill levels, this history can be used *in toto* or in part. The first 8 items can be condensed into a 5 minute psychosocial history-taking session or expanded to 2 hours. The problem history should be incorporated into the psychosocials of most alcoholism treatment programs.

Due to the frequency of impotence problems in alcoholic males, the following questions should be routinely asked in most treatment settings: When do you have erections/lose an erection? Frequency? Do you have erections with masturbation? Manipulation? Vibrators, etc.? Do you have morning erections? Wet dreams?

If the answer is no to all of these questions, a referral to a urologist should be made since the impotence may be due to congenital abnormalities such as an absence of ejaculatory ducts. Detailed information should also be derived on these drugs: antihypertensive drugs, hormone medications, tranquilizers, sedatives, hyponotics, antihistamines, and anticholinergics. Disulfiram can also contribute to impotence (estimated range of 10% to 50% of males using disulfiram). When an individual is placed on disulfiram, along with other precautions given, he should be informed that he may experience impotence problems as a result of the medication.

TREATING INHIBITED SEXUAL DESIRE

Inhibited sexual desire (ISD) is a major problem in recovery, especially for alcoholic women. Since ISD occurs in approximately 60% of depression cases, and depression as a prognostic factor accounts for a significant number of sex therapy failures, the possibility of depression should be examined before dealing with ISD in the recovering alcoholic. If depression remains substantial after a period of recovery and, hence, cannot be directly attributed to drinking, it is a probable contraindicator for sex counseling for ISD. Other indicators include: (1) when insomnia or anorexia interferes with overall functioning; (2) anhedonia is major; (3) too little energy to interact or carry out therapeutic suggestions; (4) immediate risk of suicide; (5) acute mourning; or (6) hallucinations or delusions are present.

Interventions that can be made by a therapist working with ISD include: Behavioral (which includes increasing positive reinforcers; dealing with learned helplessness; reducing stress; teaching problem-solving skills); affective (which includes dealing with anger, resentment, guilt; reducing passivity, distrust; distinquishing love and sex issues; eliminating self-fulfilling prophecy; dealing with sexual valuing systems; sensory awareness blockage); cognitive (which includes eliminating negative thoughts; teaching thought-stopping techniques; reframing myths, cognitions; dealing with boredom); systemic/relational (which includes modifying relationship roles/expectations; changing destructive interactions; reducing partner pressure for sex; affairs, power struggles, workaholism; unattractive partners).

The following 8-step treatment process can be incorporated into most alcoholism treatment programs; steps 1 to 3 for all components of treatment and steps 4 to 8 outpatient.

Step 1. Reducing anxiety/stress
    relaxation training
    education and information (using PLISSIT)
    desensitization of aversion/phobias
    guilt reduction
    removal of performance demands
    contraception issues
Step 2. Treating depression
    medication
    interpersonal skills training
    assertiveness training
    environmental life factors, that is, work and housing problems, etc.
Step 3. Improving the relationship
    conflict reduction, communication building
    increasing trust, sharing, positive reinforcements
Step 4. Dealing with intrapsychic issues
    fears of intimacy, dependence, independence, loss of control
    other interpersonal conflicts
    reducing anger/resentments from drinking

Step 5. Increasing sensory awareness
    sensate focus training
    fantasy and imagery building
    sensation labeling
    increasing situational awareness
    creating a sensual environment
Step 6. Enhancing erotic responses
    improving body image
    masturbation training
    "letting go" exercises, increasing movement, exposure to erotic
        stimuli
    increasing verbal/non-verbal cues
Step 7. Facilitating sexual activity
    building comfort, initiation
    expanding sexual repertoire
    increasing effectiveness of techniques
Step 8. Hormonal replacement therapy

CASE STUDY: INHIBITED SEXUAL DESIRE

Susan*, a 35-year-old alcoholic, was married for 8 years to Joseph, a 38-year-old nonalcoholic. During the last 3 years of heavy drinking, their sexual relationship had become nonexistent, although Susan had 3 "one night stands," of which Joseph was unaware. These affairs were not satisfying to Susan. They were tests to see if she was as asexual as she thought and they were, of course, self-fulfilling prophecies. The lack of sexual activity was due to a mutual lack of desire. Joseph had no interest in her when she was drunk and Susan was out of touch with her body.

Susan was admitted to a 28-day rehabilitation program. Joseph began Al-Anon and outpatient counseling during her stay. Susan's counselor learned of the couple's sexual inactivity and recommended a more involved sex problem history and laboratory tests. No organic etiology appeared in these tests. The program scheduled sexual issues to be addressed in the last 2 weeks of treatment during family counseling sessions. Susan attended lectures and was directed to read pamphlets on sexuality and drinking. Two group therapy sessions dealt with how alcohol affected their sex lives. Attention was given in Susan's treatment to relaxation training and guilt reduction regarding her affairs. Physical and environmental factors affecting their sex life were discussed in group, such as concerns about pregnancy (they decided not to have

* All case study names are fictitious.

children and were using condoms for birth control), body image (he had gained 30 lbs. in the past 2 years and she found him unattractive), and work stress (Susan was very tired after a day's work).

In the last 2 weeks of treatment, Susan and Joseph met with the family therapist. Joseph attended a spouses group on two weekends where sex was discussed. He was quiet in group (feeling embarrassed about their "sexless" relationship), but felt reassured that he was not inadequate as a male. In the family sessions, the therapist discussed their sexual relationship in the context of their overall conflicts. They worked on building communication and reducing the resentments and anger that had built up over the years. Joseph's weight was discussed but tabled to aftercare. They also agreed to see an Ob–Gyn to develop a more reliable birth control plan.

Although they formerly had long periods of sexual inactivity, the therapist gave them permission to continue, for the time being, to limit sexual intercourse but to be sensual in other ways. The counselor recommended sensory awareness and touching exercises. After discharge, Susan attended AA, Joseph Al-Anon, and both went to outpatient treatment. Group counseling sessions discussed the stages of recovery and the difficulties experienced in all aspects of their lives, including sex. Both were sexually inactive for 2 months, using the recommended touching and communication exercises. With 3 months sobriety, they began couple counseling which addressed the destructive interactions in their relationship and sought to reduce conflicts, anger, and resentments of the drinking past.

Susan dealt with her fears about closeness due to her need for independence. Work represented a self-imposed barrier to intimacy—she was preoccupied with work, thus reducing the time available. Joseph feared losing control of his emotions and restrained himself from expressing affection. The counseling addressed their cognitive and attitudinal barriers. Both believed sexual interest just happened. The therapist sought to modify this expectation to "I can enhance my involvement with specific mental and physical actions."

The therapist prescribed direct, reality-based exercises to enhance communication and sensual and sexual activity, including sensate focus. Both found the intercourse ban liberating since it allowed them to be affectionate without worrying about getting lost in closeness. Touching did not mean intercourse but sharing. Genital and mutual touching was particularly difficult for Susan who feared intimacy and sexual arousal. She seemed to turn off desire and sensations and drifted off mentally to work. The therapist aided the focusing by masturbation and "letting go" training. She was taught to increase her verbalizations and body movement—to get the body in gear even if the mind is not yet. Susan found this helpful as a way of distracting herself from obsessive thoughts; from saying "I don't feel like it" to "Let me see what might happen."

Joseph was asked to create a sensual environment free from distractions. Both learned that sex was not the man's responsibility but both could initiate. After the Ob–Gyn consultation, Joseph agreed to a vasectomy which resolved the birth control issue. With the fear of pregnancy gone, her sexual interest was enhanced. Two issues remained. The first was his weight; he decided to begin a weight reduction and exercise program. The other problem was Susan's guilt about her affairs. The therapist felt the affairs should be kept private and that it would serve no therapeutic value to discuss them as a couple. Susan and the therapist met individually to neutralize the guilt. She was given permission to put the affairs behind her as part of her drinking past.

Finally, the therapist helped them to focus on sexual creativity, to develop options of expression, and to facilitate appreciation of low levels of enjoyment. They did not always have to enjoy a "full course meal." Sometimes they would nibble, or have an appetizer or dessert only. After 4 months of weekly couple counseling and dealing with sexual and nonsexual issues, Susan and Joseph terminated therapy at the counselor's recommendation. They were involved in mutually satisfying regular sexual activity. ISD was not apparent.

TREATING IMPOTENCE

Impotence is a significant problem in alcoholism. Due to the high correlation with organic etiology in alcohol-related impotence, physical factors must first be determined. Drug interactions must be ruled out. A determination is needed if it is primary (never having erections), secondary (infrequent), or situational (at certain times with certain partners).

The first principle is to not treat the symptom of impotence at all and to avoid the direct, expected approach. A natural process cannot be induced by patient or therapist. Rather, the distraught male needs to be sufficiently distracted so as to allow the natural physiological process to occur. This happens by reducing the fear of failure and performance pressure. Sexual "homework" is assigned to create nondemanding sexual ambience—sensate focus training, message exercises, teasing, gentle stimulation, along with the concomitant ban on orgasm and coitus. This usually works as a powerful aphrodisiac for the impotent male and produces spontaneous erections during the pleasuring sessions.

The couple is shown incontrovertible evidence that erections happen naturally under proper circumstances—when they are free from performance anxiety. Erections are a natural physiological response to stimuli.

If rapid ejaculation is present, the squeeze or stop/start techniques can be taught. Spectatoring should be addressed, using thought distracting approaches. For some, judgmental self-observation does not cease until the deeper unconscious sources of this activity are resolved. The male is given permission to be selfish and to take sexual turns. This often evokes a sense of great relief. Fears of rejection, loss, failure/success, feelings of guilt, resentment, jealousy and phobia should be dealt with. Resistance to pleasure must be addressed, as well as gender and sexual orientation confusion. Other masculine notions to be dealt with are as follows: "When I was drinking, I was never unable to have an erection." "It is the male's job to satisfy the female partner." "A real man can have erections rapidly under any circumstances." "The size and firmness of an erection are necessary determinants of female satisfaction." "A male has a limited number of ejaculations in his lifetime."

Female notions that need to be treated include: "It's the male's function to be ready, willing, and able whenever desired." "Lack of erection indicates lack of affection or that he's having an affair.' "A man knows instinctively how to please his partner."

Sometimes a wife is invested in the impotence and does not want him to have erections. "If he has an erection, I will have to be orgasmic." In treatment, one begins with the Masters and Johnson maxim "there is no such entity as an uninvolved partner in a relationship contending with sexual inadequacy."

Rational emotive therapy techniques are also helpful, including cognitive methods: disputing irrational beliefs, myth attacking, antipuritanical teaching, cognitive distraction, imaging methods, use of bibliotherapy, and visual aids. Emotive methods include unconditional acceptance, reassurance, shame-attacking and risk-taking exercises, and emotive self-verbalizations. Behavioral methods involve activity homework assignments, *in vivo* flooding, and assertion training.

CASE STUDY: IMPOTENCE

Hank, 42, was married to Betty, 40, when he admitted himself to an alcoholism treatment program that he had been referred to by his company's employee assistance counselor because of job performance impairment. His psychosocial history indicated some "slight concern" about his sex life. Betty told the therapist that he was unable to have an erection for years. He lost all interest in sex. Betty, by self-report, had no sexual problems, was easily aroused and orgasmic "when given the opportunity."

Hank and Betty were reassured by their therapist that the problem was often a result of drinking. Tests were conducted to determine etiology. Although there were slight reductions in testosterone levels, no other significant organic etiology was indicated. A "wait and see" approach was taken on the testosterone; tests were recommended at 3 and 6 months of recovery. Hank attended inpatient lectures on sexuality and was reassured about his feelings of failure and inadequacy. Other patients spoke of similar sexual problems. He discussed in group his anxiety about satisfying Betty and feelings of incompetence—he could not give his "ready and willing" wife an orgasm. These myths were openly discussed in group.

At the time of discharge, Hank and Betty were referred to aftercare treatment with the recommendation of no intercourse during the first month. Touching, communication, and relationship building exercises were prescribed. In outpatient treatment, the therapist continued with these exercises. She dealt with Betty's performance pressure and the way she absolved herself by blaming their sexual problems on Hank. They discussed concepts such as responsibility for self and blaming as a defense mechanism. One month after discharge, the therapist recommended graduated nondemanding sexual activity, following sensate focus steps. Much to Hank's surprise he had an erection with nongenital touching. He, of course, tried to use it by attempting coitus to please Betty and quickly lost his erection. This, however, was an excellent learning experience: Now he knew he could get an erection when he allowed the physiological process to take over. The performance pressure and servicing was discussed as inhibitors to erections. Betty's overreaction to the erection was shown as a stumbling block.

Touching exercises were successful for Hank in maintaining erections. By the third month of recovery, they had returned to regular sexual activity with no signs of erectile incompetence. Testosterone levels were within normal ranges at the 3/6 month checkpoints. Both reported a high level of satisfaction with their sex life. Most important, Hank was still sober, both were active in AA and Al-Anon, and their overall relationship showed significant improvement.

Success and Failure in Sex Therapy with Alcoholics

As in most forms of psychotherapy, the success rate of sex counseling is greatest when dealing with well-established sobriety, high levels of motivation, commitment to change, less severe psychopathology, earlier stages of alcoholic progression, and interactional patterns that are not destructive.

Cases fail because of either patient or therapist factors. Patient factors can involve individual problems, such as a desire by the client to continue drinking, severe psychopathology, low priority of the relationship over work, church, etc., poor stress tolerance ability, desires to hurt oneself or partner, intentional sabatoging to justify termination of the relationship, and cognitive impairment, perhaps as a result of alcoholic organic brain damage.

Patient factors in failure also include relational issues such as a desire to have the alcoholic continue to drink, symbiosis, severe dependency, a lack of commitment to the relationship, and affairs that cannot be resolved.

Failures also result from therapist factors such as an inability to deal with alcoholism, viewing alcoholism as symptomatic, premature treatment termination, lack of a good medical work-up, countertransference issues, poor diagnostic judgment, misjudging resistance and client progress, pacing errors, counselor's pressure to succeed, and personal fatigue and stress.

Probably the greatest cause of failure with alcoholics involves overestimating the degree of recovery. Therefore, there may be a premature onset of sex counseling before an adequate sobriety period has been established. Most important, a major contributor to the failure of sex counseling with the alcoholic is a lack of understanding of alcoholism. An example of this comes from this author's observation of a recognized sex treatment program that tells alcoholics who are actively drinking prior to therapy to simply stop drinking for the two weeks of therapy. They excuse the disease temporarily and treat a behavior that may be a result of the disease. Unfortunately, too few sex therapists understand alcoholism and too few alcohologists understand sex therapy. Thus, clients fail in some measure because we, as professionals, have failed to be able to treat the dual problem: alcoholism and sexual dysfunction.

ETHICAL CONCERNS

Since most new fields of treatment are often enthusiastic about learning skills at the relative expense of fundamental concerns of ethics, some mention must be made about ethical guidelines on sexually focused clinical work. A number of ethical concerns should be mentioned. (For a more complete review of ethical issues, the reader is referred to Masters, Johnson, and Kolodny, 1977.) The importance of privacy and confidentiality must be clearly understood. The clinician must guard against value imperialism and exploitation in counseling and to be aware of values that interfere with the therapeutic process.

Therapist/client boundaries must be adhered to. It is unethical for clinicians to become involved in sexual relations with clients. Therapists that do so are not only guilty of malpractice, but also statutory rape. Nudity involving the client/therapist in counseling goes beyond established therapeutic boundaries. Clinicians must respect the client's rights to pursue different sexual behaviors as well.

For alcoholism workers, the most important ethical concern is to know the limits of one's competency and not to purport to be able to treat something one cannot, but to not totally avoid sexual issues as well. If one cannot deal with a problem, he should refer to someone that can or learn how to treat it.

WHEN TO REFER AND WHERE

Clear guidelines are needed so that alcoholism programs understand the limits of sex therapy: sexual issues should be progressively addressed throughout the treatment process at the stage and degree appropriate to the client's recovery. In general, in-depth sex therapy should be deferred until the fourth to sixth months of sobriety and should be done by a skilled therapist who understands alcoholism. If a counselor is beyond his skill levels, he should refer. If a patient is dealing with sexual issues beyond his recovery stage, they should be deferred.

To whom should the counselor refer? The American Association of Sex Educators, Counselors, and Therapists (AASECT) certifies sex workers. For a list of credentialed counselors, contact AASECT, 2000 N Street, N. W., Suite 110, Washington, D. C., 20036. The difficulty is finding a therapist who is credentialed and understands alcoholism. This is best done by interviewing individuals and inquiring into their background in substance abuse care.

Due to the limited number of sex therapists with alcoholism background, an alternative approach is for alcoholism workers to become skilled in sex therapy. For additional training, the following resource list is provided.

Journal of Sex and Marital Therapy
Human Sciences Press
72 Fifth Avenue
New York, New York 10011

Journal of Sex Education and Therapy
AASECT
Human Sciences Press
72 Fifth Avenue
New York, New York 10011

Medical Aspects of Human Sexuality
Hospital Publications
360 Lexington Avenue
New York, New York 10017

Sex Information and Education Council
SEICUS
Suite 801–802
80 Fifth Avenue
New York, New York 10011

Also, David Shore's book is recommended: *Educational and Training Opportunities in Sexology*, 1979, care of Sullivan House, Chicago, Illinois, 60615.

CONCLUSION

The treatment of alcoholic individuals and their partners for sexual concerns, difficulties, and dysfunctions is a growing area of exploration and research. The field has been saying for years that alcoholism affects sexuality. We must become active in treating these sexual problems in all components of alcoholism care. Creative and relevant approaches to treatment must be found to incorporate counseling about sexual issues into our treatment programs.

The theories and techniques presented above are relevant to all human beings. With the alcoholic, we must also address the disease of alcoholism, its physiological and psychological impact on the individual and family. Alcohol exacerbates coexisting psychological and sexual issues. We cannot avoid the drinking, as so many sex therapists do by treating the symptoms of the disease. Nor can we avoid the sexual issues and focus solely on the drinking. When troubled, the alcoholic and partner may lose direction and slip into the sexual patterns they are most familiar with and thereby reinforce again the alcoholic cycle. A bad sex life does not necessarily make one drink, but it can contribute to an overall destructive pattern that may result in a return to alcoholic behavior.

REFERENCES

Akhtar, M. M. Sexual disorders in male alcoholics. In W. Madden (Ed.), *Alcoholism and drug dependence*. New York: Plenum Press, 1977.

Annon, J. S. *The behavioral treatment of sexual problems*. Vol. 1 and 2. Honolulu, Hawaii: Enabling Systems, 1974, 1975.

Apter-Marsh, M. *The sexual behavior of alcoholic women while drinking and during sobriety*. Unpublished Doctoral Dissertation, San Francisco: Institute of Advanced Study of Human Sexuality, 1982.

Kaplan, H. S. *The new sex therapy*. New York: Brunner/Mazel, 1974.

Masters, W., and Johnson, V. *Human sexual inadequacy*. Boston: Little, Brown, 1970.

Masters, W., and Johnson, V. *Post Graduate Seminar on Sexual Dysfunction*. St. Louis, October, 1982.

Masters, W., Johnson, V., and Kolodny, R. *Ethical issues in sex therapy and research*. Boston: Little, Brown, 1977.

Powell, D. Sexual dysfunction and alcoholism. *Journal of Sex Education and Therapy*, 1980, Vol. 6, No. 2/Fall, Winter.

Rubin, E., and Lieber, C. *Information and feature service*. Washington, D.C.: NIAAA, 1976.

Smith, D. E. and Buxton, M. E. (Eds.), Sexual aspects of substance use and abuse, Special Edition, *Journal of Psychoactive Drugs*. 1982, Bol. 14, January–June, 1–2.

Talbott, G. D. *Alcohol and Drug Programs*. Ridgeview Institute, Smyrna, Ga.: Personal conversation, March 6–10, 1982.

Van Thiel, D. Testicular and spermatozoal auto-antibody in chronic alcoholics with gonadal failure. *Clinical Imminology and Immunopathology*, 1977, *8*, 311–317.

Wilsnack, S. Effects of social drinking on women's fantasy. *Journal of Personality*, 1974, *42*, 43–61.

non.
Trained
Professional

13

The Folk Psychotherapy of Alcoholics Anonymous

L. A. Alibrandi

acting
as therapist

INTRODUCTION

The sober member of Alcoholics Anonymous (AA) offers his/her journey into sobriety as a message of hope to others. The tradition of one drunk helping another came from the spiritual experience of AA's cofounder, Bill Wilson. In a letter to Dr. Carl Jung, Bill described a vision of a society of alcoholics working together to achieve and maintain sobriety (*The AA Grapevine*, 1963).

Later, on a business trip in a strange city, Bill was overcome by the desire to drink. Several important events occurred. He picked up the telephone instead of a drink. Through that phone call he offered help to another. The drunken plea, "Can you help me?" was changed to "Can I help you?" For the first time, a drunk, the traditional taker, found the ability to give. Bill contacted Dr. Bob Smith, a suffering alcoholic, shared the experience of his sobriety after years of drunkenness, and together they founded the AA fellowship.

The importance of service to other alcoholics is heavily emphasized by the text *Alcoholics Anonymous* (1955) in both the Twelfth Step of the program of AA ("Having had a spiritual awakening as the result of these steps, we tried to carry this message to alcoholics, and to practice

L. A. ALBRANDI • Director, Genesis II Outpatient Dependency Treatment, South Coast Medical Center, South Laguna, California.

This is written
for the physicist

239

these principles in all our affairs," p. 60), and in the Fifth Tradition ("Each group has but one primary purpose—to carry its message to the alcoholic who still suffers," p. 564).

Bateson (1976) described the Twelfth Step as that "which enjoins aid to other alcoholics as a necessary spiritual exercise without which the member is likely to relapse" (p. 333). Madsen (1974) called Step 12 "the missionary step, the pledge to help other alcoholics onto the road to sobriety . . .'Twelfth-stepping' gives a sense of purpose and serves as a constant reminder to the alcoholic of 'where he's been' " (p. 182).

According to AA itself, sponsorship evolves from Twelfth-Step work. Making a Twelfth-Step call on an alcoholic who has asked for help and explaining the AA program to him can be considered the beginning of sponsorship:

> The idea of sponsorship goes back to the early days of our Fellowship. As newcomers were attracted to the AA program, an AA—man or woman— with some sobriety became the new arrival's sponsor. The AA told of his own experience, explained the program as he saw it, tried to help the newcomer over the rough spots by answering questions, arranging for him to get to AA meetings and meet other members. (*Questions and Answers on Sponsorship*, 1958)

Sponsorship, then, is Twelfth-Step work, but the sponsor continues to take an interest in the newcomer's adjustment to a way of life without alcohol. According to Madsen (1974),

> As soon as possible, the newcomer is expected to pick out an AA sponsor. The newcomer thereby becomes the sponsor's "baby" or "pigeon" . . . the close tie between sponsor and pigeon may be brief or last for a lifetime, varying with the dependency needs of the pigeon . . . if identification is made with AA and a sponsor, the newcomer is on the program and his chances for a sober life are excellent. (p. 183)

Although the sponsor takes an interest in the newcomer's progress, he does not, ideally, take responsibility for it. AA members say, "We can share with you, but we cannot share for you." By placing the responsibility for his own recovery on the newcomer, the sponsor is free to enjoy the miracle of new sobriety and be reminded of his own recovery.

The focus of this chapter is a detailed examination of the relationship between the sponsor and the newcomer. In a study by the author, AA sponsors were systematically asked how they help others to achieve and maintain sobriety. Emphasis is not only on getting sober, but also on staying sober. To quote one member, "Drunks get sober every morning, or every time they go to jail or a hospital, but in AA we learn how to stay sober." Other treatment programs for alcoholics concentrate on detoxification and, in some cases, brief therapy. But when the drunk leaves the treatment facility he is on his own to maintain sobriety. If he affiliates with AA he finds other alcoholics who are staying sober and, by following their experience, he learns about the AA way of life.

The AA sponsor may not know the way to go, but he knows the way not to go. Chemical escape has taken from the alcoholic what it once offered to him—freedom. By not drinking, one day at a time, the path out of alcoholism begins. The way to sobriety is well lit by those who have gone before, and narrowed by those who have fallen to the side.

Madsen (1974) emphasized that "birds of a feather" flock together. He pointed out the AA belief "that no one can understand an alcoholic but another alcoholic" (p. 158). This philosophy is enacted by what Madsen (1974) classified as a folk society, and every member of AA acts as a "folk-curer, one who administers therapy outside the formal discipline of medicine" (p. 170). The belief that only an alcoholic can help another alcoholic

> parallels the many curing groups in primitive and folk societies where it is believed that to recover from a disease conveys the power to cure the disease . . . the majority of AA's, however, see their gift as simply the ability to share their experience and knowledge. (p. 170)

> Following affiliation, most alcoholics, especially the high-bottom drunks, begin the long process of AA folk psychotherapy. Its goals are to allow the alcoholic to know himself, define responsible goals, simplify and integrate the jungle of conflicting values within him and develop the precious quality of self-respect. (p. 174)

Even though the members of AA function as folk therapists, Madsen (1974) recognized the importance of the newcomer's active participation in the recovery process. AA is seen as merely a "tool" to aid in recovery, but the tool must be picked up and used. An AA sponsor can say to a prospective member, "Just don't drink today." But the newcomer then makes the decision to follow the advice.

Shortly after the alcoholic comes into AA, he finds that he has been invited to share in his own recovery and the recovery of others as well. He begins to receive an intuitive understanding that is compassionate, but not indulgent. "The 'therapists' in AA already have their doctorates in the four fields where the alcoholic reigns supreme: phoniness, self-deception, evasion and self-pity" (*A Member's-Eye View of Alcoholics Anonymous*, 1970). Newcomers find it difficult to con a former con artist.

Another unique quality of the recovered alcoholic in AA is his

> omnipresent, bottomless, enthusiastic willingness to talk about alcoholism—its ins and its outs, its whys and its wherefores . . . his need for a drink is literally talked to death. It has always seemed exquisitely fitting to me that people who once used their mouths to get sick now use them to get well. (*A Member's-Eye View of Alcoholics Anonymous*, 1970)

express feelings   Carry the message

Heavy emphasis is placed on letting go of old ideas. The newcomer is not asked to learn new ideas so much as to unlearn old and often defeating ones. "One of the major objectives of AA therapy is to help the alcoholic finally recognize these ideas and become willing to relinquish his death grip on them" (*A Member's-Eye View of Alcoholics Anonymous*, 1970).

AA is different from most other therapy for the alcoholic in the way the program is presented. The Steps are "reports of action taken rather than rules not to be broken under pain of drunkenness." In most cases the steps are presented to the newcomer by a member who has taken them himself. The AA member shares his experience more often than he gives advice. Two alcoholics talking about their alcoholism make "for identification at depth, a cardinal AA principle" (*A Member's-Eye View of Alcoholics Anonymous*, 1970).

Madsen (1974) refers to AA in terms of tools to aid in recovery from alcoholism. Sponsorship, the most indispensable tool in the maintenance of sobriety, is hereto explored fully in its various aspects.

THE SPONSOR IN AA

Bill Wilson's first attempts at sponsorship were characterized by proselytizing:

> After failure on my part to dry up any drunks, Dr. Silkworth reminded me of Professor William James' observation that truly transforming spiritual experiences are nearly always founded on calamity and collapse. "Stop preaching at them," Dr. Silkworth said, "and give them the hard medical facts first. This may soften them up at depth so that they will be willing to do anything to get well. Then they may accept those spiritual ideas of yours, and even a Higher Power." (*The AA Way of Life*, 1976, p. 242)

These events and Dr. Silkworth's advice led to the sharing of personal experience by the AA sponsor to help the newcomer to achieve sobriety and, at the same time, maintain his own sobriety. "In other words, if you carry the message to still others, you will be making the best possible repayment for the help given to you" (p. 29).

Another benefit of sponsorship, according to a currently active member of AA, is the reminder of what it used to be like. As he shares his own experiences with the newcomer, he recalls the difficulties alcohol created in his life and the progress he has made in sobriety. This sponsor believes that to forget the disaster of his own drinking is to increase the danger of drinking again.

The sponsor operates mainly by intuition. As another AA member pointed out, "It isn't what the newcomer asks that is important. It's what he doesn't ask. And I know about his hidden feelings because of my own. I have 80% knowledge of what's going on in his head based on my own experience."

Each AA member approaches sponsorship in his own way. He is aware of the deceit, denial, rationalization, and manipulation characteristic of many alcoholics. The newcomer "is not *asked* what he is thinking. He is *told* what he is thinking. No one waits to trap him in a lie. He is told what lies he is getting ready to tell" (*A Member's-Eye View of Alcoholics Anonymous*, 1970).

The AA literature has many recommendations for the sponsor in his work with newcomers:

> For a new prospect, outline the program of action, explaining how you made a self-appraisal, how you straightened out your past and why you are now endeavoring to be helpful to him. It is important for him to realize that your attempt to pass this on to him plays a vital part in your own recovery. Actually, he may be helping you more than you are helping him. Make it plain that he is under no obligation to you. (*The AA Way of Life*, 1976, p. 275)

Possible failures that AA sponsors encounter are also discussed:

> As a matter of fact, the successful worker differs from the unsuccessful only in being lucky about his prospects. He simply hits newcomers who are ready and able to stop at once. Given the same prospects, the seemingly unsuccessful person would have produced almost the same results. You have to work on a lot of newcomers before the law of averages commences to assert itself. (p. 165)

Madsen (1974) has also briefly discussed the sponsor's approach:

> The newcomer is urged to "let go" of the burden of the past and the expectations of tomorrow's consequences. His life is now. Focusing on the now, AA is primarily concerned with techniques to deal with frustration and pain. The newcomer is first brought face-to-face with the fact that his Christian-American dream of a coming utopia when everyone will live happily ever after is a lie, or at least not to happen in his lifetime. (p. 177)

AA sponsors often mention their personal relief from guilt over the past which occurs when they share with the newcomer. A formerly shameful experience gains utility and even a certain amount of dignity when it is used to help another alcoholic.

Experience can be neither right nor wrong. It simply is. The sponsor is not obligated to insist that his protégé "follow his experience," and the newcomer is free to use any portion of the experience offered.

AN EMPIRICAL INVESTIGATION

In a study by the author to gain a better understanding of the AA process, each bit of advice given by a sponsor was viewed as a tool for sobriety. The structure underlying the recovery process as exhibited by the sponsor–protégé relationship was examined.

A series of intensive interviews with AA sponsors was initiated. Each sponsor was asked to remember the last newcomer he had worked with, what questions the newcomer had asked, and how the sponsor had answered them. From these interviews and careful study of the AA literature, including *Alcoholics Anonymous* (1955), *The AA Way of Life* (1967), and *Living Sober* (1975), a list of 100 tools was generated (see Table 1). Tools 1–69 represent suggestions made in the AA literature while Tools 70–100 represent additional advice given by sponsors in interviews.

An anthropological technique used to study subcultures, the free and constrained sorting-task method, was applied. For the free sorting task, each of the 100 tools was key-punched on a computer card. Each subject was given a deck of 100 cards and instructed to sort the tools into piles in any way he/she believed they went together. Subjects were told that they could put any number of tools into any number of piles. They were then asked to give each pile a name to give the investigator an idea of why those tools were put together.

In a constrained or time-phase sorting task, each subject was given a second deck of cards and asked to sort them in a specific way:

> Imagine that you are working with members of AA having different lengths of sobriety. Put those tools you would use for someone with one day to one week of sobriety (Stage I) in one pile, those for someone with one week to 60 days (Stage II) in one pile, those for someone with 60 days to 6 months (Stage III) in one pile, those for someone with 6 months to one year (Stage IV) in one pile, and those for someone with over one year of sobriety (Stage V) in one pile. The last pile (VI) is for those tools you would not use. It is important for you to put each tool into the pile/time where you think it best fits.

Finally, each subject was asked if there were any tools he/she used that were not included in the deck, how long he/she had been a sober member of AA, and his/her age.

Subjects for the intensive interviews were three men and three women, all members of AA who had been abstinent for from 4 to 13 years. Each reported doing extensive work with newcomers to AA and with members of AA at various stages of sobriety.

Data for the two sorting tasks were collected from 22 subjects. Each had been a sober member of AA for at least two years and was currently working as a sponsor to newcomers and to members of AA. All subjects were defined as "good sponsors," that is, active folk therapists, by other members of AA. There were 11 men and 11 women who ranged in age from 25 to 50 with an average age of 37.6. Their lengths of sobriety ranged from 2 to 15 years with an average of 5.9 years.

Most subjects felt, initially, that the free sorting task was difficult because they had no frame of reference for such an exercise. Once they began sorting, however, they did so with very little hesitation.

During the constrained sorting task the investigator was constantly reminded by subjects that the tools would be applied differently to each individual newcomer to AA. To quote one subject: "Each tool can be applied at a different time to a different baby. I'm saying 'in a general way' what I would do."

Over half the subjects indicated that they had no use for Tool 33, "Use your common sense." Their comments: "My 'common sense' got me to AA in the first place." "There is nothing 'common' about my sense. It's gotten me in trouble many times."

Tool 22, "Seek professional help," was often seen as applying only in specific cases. Several subjects felt that they could not use it in a general way. Professional help had seemed a hindrance to some and was seen by them as a part of the problem rather than a solution. One sponsor insisted that the alcoholic achieve sobriety through the fellowship and principles of AA. After a period of sobriety, professional help might be applicable, but not in the early efforts to achieve sobriety.

Other comments included that of a woman who said she could not advise avoiding emotional entanglements (Tool 23) because she had never been able to do so herself. It is often true that members of AA will not ask those they work with to do something they have not been able to do. Another woman said she would use Tool 68, "Seek God's will for you and the power to carry it out," early in sobriety because just trying to figure out what such advice meant would help keep some newcomers sober for a while.

TABLE 1.   THE TOOLS

1. Stay away from the first drink.	36. Try not to test your willpower.
2. Use the 24-hour plan.	37. Try to do a good mental house-cleaning.
3. Remember that alcoholism is an incurable, progressive, fatal disease.	38. Salute the daily progress you make.
4. Live and let live.	39. Cherish your recovery.
5. Get active.	40. Develop the habit of gratitude.
6. Use the Serenity Prayer.	41. Suspend judgment of yourself and others.
7. Change old routines.	42. Look at your whole drinking record.
8. Eat or drink something—usually sweet.	43. Share your happiness.
9. Make use of "telephone therapy."	44. Avoid nostalgic sadness.
10. Find a sponsor.	45. Remember that alcoholism is cunning and baffling.
11. Get plenty of rest.	46. Accept responsibility for your actions.
12. Do first things first.	47. Stay sober for yourself.
13. Fend off loneliness.	48. Try not to place conditions on your sobriety.
14. Watch out for anger and resentments.	49. Respect the anonymity of others.
15. Be good to yourself.	50. When all else fails, follow directions.
16. Look out for over-elation.	51. Try to heal yourself by helping others.
17. Easy does it.	52. Share your experience, strength, and hope.
18. Be grateful.	53. Find the courage to change yourself.
19. Remember your last drunk.	54. Find the serenity to accept others.
20. Avoid all chemical mood-changers.	55. Try to turn your life and will over to a Higher Power.
21. Eliminate self-pity.	56. Be willing.
22. Seek professional help.	57. Come with me to a meeting.
23. Steer clear of emotional entanglements.	58. Admit you are powerless over alcohol.
24. Get out of the "if" trap. ("What if . . . ," "If only . . .")	59. Come to believe in a power greater than yourself.
25. Be wary of drinking occasions.	60. Take a searching and fearless moral inventory.
26. Let go of old ideas.	61. Share your inventory with someone else.
27. Read the AA message.	62. Make a list of those you have harmed.
28. Go to AA meetings.	
29. Try the Twelve Steps.	
30. Find your own way.	
31. Replace old habits with new, sober habits.	
32. Keep an open mind.	
33. Use your common sense.	
34. Live in the now.	
35. Avoid major decisions in early sobriety.	

(continued)

TABLE 1.   (*continued*)

63. Make amends to them when possible.	82. Try to become a part of the world you have rejected.
64. Continue to take a personal inventory.	83. Watch out for complacency.
65. Promptly admit when you are wrong.	84. Maintain a spiritual condition.
66. Make regular use of prayer.	85. Carry the message of AA.
67. Meditate.	86. Have faith.
68. Seek God's will for you, and the power to carry it out.	87. Count your blessings.
69. Practice these principles in all your affairs.	88. Try not to dwell on the faults of others.
70. Laugh.	89. Accept life as it comes.
71. Avoid getting too hungry.	90. Admit and correct your errors today.
72. Listen.	91. Believe that you are not alone.
73. Share your pain.	92. Avoid using the truth to injure others.
74. Choose positive thinking.	93. When you are shaky work with another alcoholic.
75. Be available for service.	94. Avoid gossip.
76. Look for similarities rather than differences.	95. Work to eliminate self-deception.
77. Beware of phony pride.	96. See adversity as opportunity.
78. Try to replace guilt with gratitude.	97. Develop self-restraint.
79. Avoid self-righteousness.	98. Don't fear needed change.
80. Practice rigorous honesty.	99. Let go and let God.
81. Keep it simple.	100. Take life a day, even a minute, at a time.

RESULTS AND DISCUSSION

A tool-by-tool similarity matrix* divided the 100 tools of the free sort into four clusters. The first cluster consisted of six tools which, upon analysis, were most often "tools not used." These included Tools 22, 23, 30, 33, 36, and 37.

The three remaining major clusters in the free sorting task were labeled Working the Steps, Self-change, and Sobriety. It is interesting to note that although the Twelve Steps of Alcoholics Anonymous (see Table 2) were not singled out from the other tools during presentation, they nonetheless formed a coherent subset within Cluster 2. The AA aphorisms (Tools 4, 12, 17, 81, 99) also formed a coherent subset within Cluster 4.

---

* The cluster analyses and Table 3 made use of a computer program written by Richard Degerman, University of California, Irvine.

TABLE 2.   TWELVE SUGGESTED STEPS OF ALCOHOLICS ANONYMOUS

1. We admitted we were powerless over alcohol—that our lives had become unmanageable.
2. Came to believe that a Power greater than ourselves could restore us to sanity.
3. Make a decision to turn our will and our lives over to the care of God *as we understood him*.
4. Make a searching and fearless moral inventory of ourselves.
5. Admitted to God, to ourselves, and to another human being the exact nature of our wrongs.
6. Were entirely ready to have God remove all these defects of character.
7. Humbly asked Him to remove our shortcomings.
8. Made a list of all persons we had harmed, and became willing to make amends to them all.
9. Made direct amends to such people wherever possible, except when to do so would injure them or others.
10. Continued to take personal inventory and when we were wrong promptly admitted it.
11. Sought through prayer and meditation to improve our conscious contact with God *as we understood Him*, praying only for knowledge of His will for us and the power to carry that out.
12. Having had a spiritual awakening as the result of these steps, we tried to carry this message to alcoholics, and to practice these principles in all our affairs.

Working the Steps, Cluster 2.   This cluster broke down into three subclusters: "Guidelines to the Program," "Surrender, Analysis, and Change," and "Working with Others." In "Guidelines to the Program," four of the tools increase direct involvement in the AA program (Tools 5, 6, 10, 29).

The second subcluster, "Surrender, Analysis, and Change," included the 12 Steps. "Surrender" was divided into powerlessness, Steps 1 and 2, and dependence on a Higher Power, Step 3 and part of Step 11. "Analysis and Change" contained the remaining steps divided into meditation (Step 11), inventory maintenance (Step 10), inventory sharing (Step 5), making a list of amends and making amends (Steps 8 and 9), seeking God's will (Step 11), taking an inventory (Step 4), and practicing the principles of AA (Step 12).

The third subcluster, "Working with Others," was divided into two kinds of service. Service to improve oneself was characterized by "practicing rigorous honesty," "carrying the AA message," and "admitting and correcting errors." Service to help others involved "being available for service" and "respecting the anonymity of others."

Self-Change, Cluster 3.   The third major cluster subdivided into "Responsibility for Self-change" and "Methods of Self-change." Tools in the "Responsibility for Self-change" cluster included service, sharing, responsibility, courage, and gratitude.

"Methods of Self-change" contained 28 tools and was the largest subcluster in the free sort. It broke down into tools proposing a "now orientation" and "readjustment." "Keeping an open mind" and "fending off loneliness" were examples of developing a "now orientation."

"Readjustment" divided into "attitude and thinking adjustment" and "raising morale." "Thinking adjustment" broke down into dealing with shortcomings such as self-pity and judgment, and eliminating "stinking thinking," which included the avoidance of nostalgia, anger, resentments, phony pride, complacency, and criticism of self and others. "Raising morale" came through accepting life as it comes and being good to yourself.

Sobriety, Cluster 4.   Cluster 4 was divided into "Motivation" and "Ways to Cope with a Drinking Problem." "Motivation" was increased through "being willing," "laughing," "listening," and "having faith."

"Ways to Cope with a Drinking Problem" broke down into "awareness of the problem" and "specific prescriptions for not drinking." "Awareness of the problem" was increased by remembering the last drunk and looking at the whole drinking record. Such tools as "Being wary of drinking occasions" and "Staying sober for yourself" clustered with remembering that alcoholism is incurable, progressive, and fatal, and seemed to support the disease concept of alcoholism in AA.

"Specific prescriptions" included getting comfortable by following directions, and not getting too hungry, too lonely, or too tired. Avoiding the first drink clustered with going to meetings, reading the AA message, living one day at a time, and using the telephone.

Distribution of Free Sort Clusters over Time Phases.   Table 3 indicates the way the tools within the free sort clusters were distributed in applicability over the time phases of sobriety. As Cluster 1 of the free sort contained mainly tools not used, it is not included in Table 3.

It is interesting to note that the major emphasis in Stage I, one day to one week of sobriety, is on the cluster labeled *Sobriety*. From Cluster 2, *Working the Steps* or the *Program* in Table 3, only one tool, "Admit you are powerless over alcohol," was applied. The only suggestion for self-change was "Believe that you are not alone."

In Stage V (over one year of sobriety), there is a gradual shift in emphasis from tools to maintain sobriety to tools for promoting self-change. In this time phase, the only tool suggested for sobriety is the maintenance of a spiritual condition.

TABLE 3.   TOOLS FOR RECOVERY

	Sobriety	Program	Self-change
Stage I One Day to One Week	Stay away from the first drink. Avoid getting too hungry. Go to AA meetings. Come with me to a meeting. Use the 24-hour plan. Eat or drink something—usually sweet. Make use of telephone therapy. Take life a day, even a minute, at a time. Avoid all chemical mood-changers. Listen. Get plenty of rest. Read the AA message. Be willing. Be wary of drinking occasions. Stay sober for yourself. Look for similarities rather than differences. Remember your last drunk.	Admit you are powerless over alcohol.	Believe that you are not alone.

Stage II *One Week to 60 Days*	Laugh. Keep it simple. Have faith. Remember that alcoholism is incurable, progressive, and fatal. Avoid major decisions in early sobriety. Easy does it. Be wary of drinking occasions. Remember that alcoholism is cunning and baffling. Try not to place conditions on your sobriety. Do first things first. When all else fails follow directions. Let go and let God. Share your happiness.	Find a sponsor. Try to turn your life and will over to a Higher Power. Share your pain. Use the Serenity Prayer. Come to believe in a power greater than yourself. Get active. Respect the anonymity of others. Make regular use of prayer.	Salute the daily progress you make. Keep an open mind. Fend off loneliness. Replace old habits with new, sober habits. Steer clear of emotional entanglements. Try not to test your willpower. Get out of the "if" trap.
Stage III *60 Days to Six Months*	Live and let live. Look at your whole drinking record. Let go and let God. Share your happiness. Count your blessings.	Try the Twelve Steps. Be available for service.	Eliminate self-pity. Change old routines. Look out for overelation. Let go of old ideas. Accept life as it comes. Avoid nostalgic sadness. Live in the now. Choose positive thinking. Be good to yourself. Try to replace guilt with gratitude.

(continued)

TABLE 3. (*continued*)

	Sobriety	Program	Self-change
Stage IV *Six Months to* *One Year*	Be grateful. Share your happiness. Count your blessings. Cherish your recovery.	Take a searching and fearless moral inventory. Share your inventory with someone else. Carry the message of AA. When you are shaky work with another alcoholic. Seek God's will for you and the power to carry it out.	Accept responsibility. Work to eliminate self-deception. Watch out for anger and resentments. Let go of old ideas. Accept life as it comes. Get out of the "if" trap. Develop the habit of gratitude. Try to heal yourself by helping others. Share your experience, strength, hope. Find the courage to change yourself. Avoid using the truth to injure others. Avoid gossip.

Stage V
Over one year

Maintain a spiritual condition.

Continue to take a personal inventory.	Watch out for complacency.
Promptly admit when you are wrong.	Avoid self-righteousness.
Meditate.	Find your own way.
Make a list of those you have harmed.	Try not to dwell on the faults of others.
Make amends to them when possible.	See adversity as opportunity.
Practice these principles in all your affairs.	Don't fear needed change.
Practice rigorous honesty.	Try to do a good mental housecleaning.
Admit and correct your errors today.	Try to become a part of the world you have rejected.
Seek God's will for you and the power to carry it out.	Develop self-restraint.
	Suspend judgment of yourself and others.
	Find the courage to change yourself.
	Find the serenity to accept others.
	Beware of phony pride.
	Avoid using the truth to injure others.
	Be good to yourself.
	Cherish your recovery.

The 100 tools elicited in this study can be viewed as activities engaged in by members of Alcoholics Anonymous. Results of the sorting tasks indicate the organization of tools and the semantic rules that govern how the activities are applied, thus leading to a new understanding of the "mystery" of the AA process. The intuitive, implicit knowledge of the AA sponsor can thus be rendered explicit, illuminating the structure of the recovery process.

AA activities were found to be semantically organized and to vary systematically over the time phases of the newcomers' sobriety. The advice given to the newcomer with two months or less of sobriety is both qualitatively and quantitatively different from the advice given at later stages of sobriety. Most pertinent to the newcomer is surrender and powerlessness, participation in the fellowship, and specific prescriptions for sobriety. As length of sobriety increases, there is a shift from specific advice and morale-building to self-change, spirituality, and the action steps. The newcomer progresses from the awareness of powerlessness to reliance on a Higher Power, a reliance that enables him to cope with that powerlessness and from achieving sobriety to maintaining a sobriety contingent on self-inventory and his spiritual condition.

It is important to note that many terms used by AA members have a specialized meaning within the subculture. "Surrender," for example, involves giving up the prolonged attempt to control both the consumption of alcohol and the course of life itself. It does not, however, imply subjugation. Similarly, "acceptance" is viewed as a positive action without reference to resignation.

Another term, "spirituality," often associated with religion, has no such connotation in AA, wherein its use deals with principles of conscious life as distinguished from the practice of sacred rituals. AA is not a religious organization. It is a spiritual fellowship offering sobriety to those who seek it. The experience of enlightenment accompanies this sobriety, sometimes quickly, sometimes slowly.

IMPLICATIONS

A hospital treatment program based on AA principles would feature specific behavioral prescriptions for achieving sobriety together with developing awareness of the drinking problem. It would not include therapy oriented toward self-change during the inpatient phase. Participation in the outpatient phase would be considered integral to the treatment program, as it is only at this time that principles for the maintenance of sobriety can be evolved.

Such a hospital program would also emphasize working with other alcoholics after one week of sobriety as a treatment modality in itself. According to members of AA, someone with a week or more of sobriety can be of great help to an alcoholic in the first few days of sobriety. The alcoholic with a week of sobriety, having such current experience with the trauma of the freshly sober alcoholic, can be most genuinely effective in the areas of trust and identification. He is, in turn, more enthusiastic about his own sobriety.

The method of tool elicitation and analysis employed in this study could be productively applied to the investigation of differences between the AA member as sponsor and the AA member as professional counselor. Recovering alcoholics who function in both capacities may select different tools for each setting. There may also be differences between the recovering alcoholic who works as an alcoholism counselor and the nonalcoholic counselor that could be investigated in this way.

The question of individual differences in sponsors (or folk therapists) is an important one. A further investigation could determine how types of sponsors match with types of protégés. It is common knowledge in AA, for example, that some sponsors require strict adherence to their instructions, while others are more lenient.

Elements of the AA recovery process as determined by this study could be compared with the recovery process of some other treatment program with a well-defined set of tools. The tools used by persons achieving sobriety through a specific inpatient–outpatient program, for example, could be elicited and sorted in a similar way.

By AA's own admission, at least half the newcomers relapse into drinking during the first year of sobriety. The current method could be adapted to analyze the considerable wisdom of AA sponsors about the conditions under which newcomers suffer relapse. With somewhat greater effort, one could also directly study differences between AA successes and AA failures during the first year of sobriety.

An investigation of the "spiritual experience" as described by AA members, and its relation to sobriety, could also be made using the methods of the present study. Some members describe "sudden illumination," while others experience a slow enlightenment.

An important implication of this study is the vast source of information about recovery from alcoholism available from those who are recovering. It is fair to say that most studies employ alcoholics who are in detoxification programs, but have little capacity to maintain sobriety. Further investigation of those who have found a new way of life in sobriety, of those who are emotionally and physically healthy, could be invaluable in improving alcoholism treatment, as well as unfolding the alcoholism process itself.

REFERENCES

The AA grapevine. New York: The Alcoholics Anonymous Grapevine, Inc., January, 1963.

The AA way of life, a reader by Bill. New York: Alcoholics Anonymous World Services, 1967.

Alcoholics Anonymous, the story of how many thousands of men and women have recovered from alcoholism. New and revised edition. New York: Alcoholics Anonymous World Services, 1955.

Bateson, G. The cybernetics of self: A theory of alcoholism. *Steps to an ecology of mind.* New York: Ballantine Books, 1976.

Living sober. New York: Alcoholics Anonymous World Services, 1975.

Madsen, W. *The American alcoholic.* Springfield, Ill.: Charles C Thomas, 1974.

A member's-eye view of Alcoholics Anonymous. New York: Alcoholics Anonymous World Services, 1970.

Questions and answers on sponsorship. New York: Alcoholics Anonymous World Services, 1958.

III

TREATMENT OF SPECIFIC POPULATIONS OF ALCOHOLICS

Chapter 14

The Psychotherapy of Alcoholic Women

John S. Tamerin

Introduction

The population of female alcoholics in the United States is large and possibly increasing. It is estimated that a minimum of 20% of the alcoholics in this country or one million of the estimated five million American alcoholics are women (Beckman, 1975). The number may be even higher, as the ratio of female to male alcoholics appears to be largely a function of the subsample from which it is drawn. Hence, this ratio may vary from 1 female to 11 males in prison populations (Jones, 1971) to a 1-to-1 male–female ratio in private hospital or private practice settings (Lindbeck, 1972; Tamerin, Tolor, and Harrington, 1976).

While the number of female alcoholics is obviously considerable, we must still ask whether it is meaningful to speak of alcoholic women as a separate clinical subgroup from the point of view of their psychotherapy. In order to answer this question, we must first consider whether there are special characteristics of female alcoholics and, second, if these distinguishing characteristics do exist, whether they suggest different approaches to the evaluation and treatment of alcoholic women.

JOHN S. TAMERIN • Clinical Associate Professor of Psychiatry, Cornell University College of Medicine, New York, New York.

Characteristics of Women Alcoholics

The issue of defining the special characteristics of alcoholic women has been addressed in a number of papers (Curlee, 1967, 1970; Schuckit, 1972) and more recently in a book edited by Greenblatt and Schuckit (1976), which includes seven chapters specifically devoted to alcohol problems in women. In an overview article in that book, Schuckit and Morrissey (1976) point out that the average female alcoholic drinks at home, alone. In view of the solitary aspect of their drinking, women as a group are inclined to conceal and deny their drinking. Their drinking is rarely done in bars. They are frequently protected by their husbands from facing the consequences of their drinking. They tend to be 40 to 50 years of age at the time of hospitalization. Between 20% and 50% are married, depending on the socioeconomic status of the participants in the study. The characteristic sexual pattern of alcoholic women also appears to vary according to the socioeconomic status of the particular group being studied. Hence, promiscuity is cited in lower-class felons and sexual inhibition in upper-middle-class patients studied in private hospital settings.

Studies (Tamerin *et al.*, 1976; Curlee, 1967) that specifically compared male and female alcoholics and controlled for the factor of socioeconomic status produced the following findings: (1) women are less likely than men to have school and antisocial problems before becoming alcoholic; (2) women are less likely to have alcohol-related legal difficulties; (3) women are less likely to have alcohol-related automobile accidents; (4) women are less likely to have experienced a job loss secondary to drinking. The drinking histories of women suggest that they are more likely than men to telescope the stages of their alcoholism into a briefer time span and that women are less likely to be hospitalized from the medical complications of alcoholism.

The major difference between male and female alcoholics from the point of view of treatment strategy, however, is the repeated observation that a higher degree of psychiatric dysfunction has been observed in female than in male alcoholics (Curlee, 1970). The primary difference lies in the area of affective disorder. Female alcoholics have repeatedly been found to have a higher rate of depression and a higher incidence of suicide attempts (Schuckit, 1972). In some cases, such as those observed and documented by Schuckit, Pitts, Reich, King, and Winokur (1969), depression that conforms to clinically definable criteria precedes the development of the drinking problem and, in such cases, the designation of primary affective disorder and secondary alcoholism has been suggested to indicate that we may be dealing with a different clinical condition than in the case of primary alcoholism.

Tamerin *et al.* (1976), in a study of male and female alcoholics' spouses and self-perceptions, found that females were more often characterized as guilty or depressed. Consequently, alcohol was likely to be experienced by women as a stimulant or antidepressant, temporarily helping them to feel livelier and more "full of pep." The study also revealed that female alcoholics and their husbands described the women in identical terms regarding their feelings and behavior for the sober state. In describing the female alcoholic when intoxicated, however, their husbands characterized them in far more negative terms than did the women themselves. The husbands saw a great deal more psychopathology emerging with intoxication. These differences were related to areas of anxiety (i.e., "restless," "jittery"), friendliness (i.e., "refuses to speak" and less "pleasant," "kind" and "warmhearted"), and affect, where spouses saw more unhappiness and weariness. In general, female alcoholics as a group characterized themselves when intoxicated as relaxed, friendly, warmhearted, and kind. Their spouses, on the other hand, perceived them as irritable, depressed, and unhappy. Only one of ten spouses characterized his wife as happy when intoxicated. Male alcoholics, in contrast, tended to be characterized by their wives as having a character disorder. This was exemplified by such traits as "inconsiderate," "uncooperative," "stubborn," "generally acts helpless," "thinks only of self," "often exhibits childish behavior," "contrary in actions," "deliberately upsets routine," and "needs a lot of attention."

Another area that has received scientific attention is related to the physiological and psychological experience of being a women and an alcoholic. Several authors (Belfer, Shader, Carroll, and Harmantz, 1971; Podolsky, 1963) have cited sex-related hormonal factors as significantly related to the drinking experience of the female alcoholic. Drinking has been associated with the stress of the menses or with the menopause and problems of the midlife identity crisis (Curlee, 1969).

Also under investigation is the sense of sexual identity in female alcoholics. McClelland, Davis, Kalin, and Wanner (1972) suggested that the male alcoholic drinks as a means of increasing his sense of power. The dependency theory of drinking (Blane, 1968) also focused primarily on male alcoholics and conceptualized their drinking as a means of gratifying passive, oral dependency needs in a setting that permitted these men to maintain an independent, assertive facade. Certainly the grandiose denial of the male alcoholic described and therapeutically elaborated by Tiebout (1949, 1954) in his discussions of the need for reducing the alcoholic's "ego" through the process of "surrender" appears central to the dynamics of the male alcoholic. But is this also true of the female alcoholic? Do women alcoholics drink for the same reasons? Are they drinking to increase their feelings of power? Are they drinking to act out while consciously denying underlying dependency needs? Wilsnack (1973a, 1973b, 1976) has examined this issue in several papers and concluded, both from her review of the literature and from her own independent study, that female alcoholics drink for different reasons than men. Wilsnack noted that female alcoholics value their traditional roles as wives and mothers. They have characteristically feminine interests, attitudes, and values. Despite these conscious feminine interests, however, it was demonstrated that the female alcoholic has an unconscious masculine identification. Wilsnack then went on to conduct other experiments which demonstrated that in a population of nonalcoholic women, alcohol increased feelings of femininity. While her leap from these findings to a theory of female alcoholism may be premature, her formulations are challenging and heuristically useful since she has evolved the following hypotheses to explain the progression of drinking in the female alcoholic: Drinking is seen as an attempt by the female alcoholic to gain an artificial feeling of womanliness. In this context, it may serve a reparative function for the woman with chronic doubts about her femininity. Unconscious sexual-role conflicts may create symptoms when life stress threatens the woman's sense of feminine adequacy. Wilsnack indicated that stressful events frequently occurred in her sample of alcoholic women as precipitants of drinking and as exacerbating factors relevant to the progression of the disease. Such life stress events cited were divorce, separation or death of a spouse, marital problems, children growing older and leaving home, and obstetrical–gynecological disorders. Furthermore, Wilsnack found that in her sample of female alcoholics 77% reported a specific obstetrical disorder that might have had impact on the feminine identity of these women. These problems included difficulties in conception, repeated miscarriages, infertility, and disappointments about an inability to have children. These alcoholic women did not consciously reject their femininity. Under stress, however, they turned to alcohol to increase and reinforce feelings of femininity.

Wilsnack also cited other relevant literature. Miller and Ely (1971) observed a modal personality of the alcoholic female—"hyperfeminine" and consciously denying masculine traits. Jones' (1971) study similarly concluded that the female alcoholic was consciously feminine but stylistically masculine. Also cited was Busch, Kormendy, and Feuerlein's (1973) study of the husbands of alcoholic women, which revealed that these men tended to characterize their wives as assertive and masculine. These spouses rated their wives as the dominant partner during the first two years of marriage. Self-ratings of these men, in contrast, revealed that they were less masculine than were the husbands of control subjects.

Another issue cited in the literature on the female alcoholic is the relationship between discernible life stress and the onset of problem drinking (Beckman, 1975; Schuckit and Morrissey, 1976). This connection is more characteristic of female than male alcoholics.

An additional feature highlighted in examining the female alcoholic is the family environment during childhood. The typical constellation cited has been a cold, distant mother and a warm, affectionate father with whom the girl typically identifies (Schuckit and Morrissey, 1976). This dynamic creates an inability to develop a strong feminine identification. It is also of considerable clinical interest that there is a much higher prevalence of alcoholism in the fathers of alcoholic women than in their mothers. Alcoholism in fathers of female alcoholics may be as high as $33\frac{1}{3}\%$ compared to 7%–8% in mothers (Schuckit, 1972). A survey by Curlee (1970) found alcoholism in 25% of fathers and only 4% of mothers of alcoholic women.

The literature is limited regarding the husbands of alcoholic women. Curlee (1967) has commented on the tendency of husbands to stay with these women until treatment is sought and then leave them, in contrast to the wives of male alcoholics, who for socioeconomic and cultural reasons tend more frequently to stay with their alcoholic husbands.

The variety and number of observed differences between male and female alcoholics would suggest the legitimacy of considering gender as a meaningful differential factor in conceptualizing and formulating different psychotherapeutic approaches to the female alcoholic. An attempt will be made in approaching this task to relate clinical techniques and formulations to those qualities found to characterize the female alcoholic. It should be pointed out that, although many articles have been written on the psychotherapy of the alcoholic in general, many of which have been cited by Zimberg in Chapter 1 of this book, no single reference currently exists dealing specifically with the psychotherapy of the female alcoholic. However, single case reports do exist (Noble, 1949).

EVALUATION OF ALCOHOLIC WOMEN

When one takes a history from the female alcoholic, it is not unusual for the patient to cite specific events associated with the onset and progression of problem drinking. This is in marked contrast to most male alcoholics, who report specific causal or precipitating factors far less frequently. It is not unusual for female alcoholics to cite times, events, situations, and even feelings which parallel the progression of the drinking problem.

Female alcoholics, in contrast to males, more frequently perceive themselves as psychiatric patients who are suffering and need help. In fact it is not unusual for female alcoholics to enter psychotherapy for other psychiatric problems, with the drinking problem emerging subsequently.

This suggests the importance of considering the possibility of alcoholism in a female psychiatric patient who may be providing only vague clues suggesting the use of alcohol as a means of coping with interpersonal conflict or dysphoria. In fact, cases that begin as symptomatic drinking can progress to alcoholism unless the clinician is alert to this possibility. One such case seen by the author involved a woman in her mid-30s who began to use alcohol as a means of medicating an anxiety neurosis with varied phobic and psychophysiologic accompaniment. In alcohol she discovered an effective "treatment" which she could employ with predictable results. She had entered analytic psychotherapy with a previous therapist and, although she derived some benefit from the treatment, her symptoms persisted—as did her attempts to medicate them. Eventually she became "anxious" and tremulous in the mornings on a regular basis. Her therapist treated the symptom as a neurotic manifestation suitable for interpretation. When this patient was seen in consultation by the author, she had become increasingly concerned about her drinking. It was obvious that she had become addicted to alcohol and that her morning anxiety was evidence of a withdrawal syndrome, rather than a neurotic symptom.

It is important in dealing with the female psychiatric patient who drinks to keep in mind the possibility that she may be an alcoholic, lest we miss diagnosing this important and treatable disease. The diagnosis of alcoholism generally mandates abstinence. When such a patient continues to drink while in treatment, the seriousness of her drinking is either minimized or ignored and the treatment is rarely of much benefit. It has been my frequent experience that when such patients eventually face their alcoholism, they have extremely negative feelings about therapists whom they have "fooled." Usually their response is an admixture of resentment for not having been confronted earlier and contempt for the therapist whom they deceived.

The converse of this problem, however, should also be pointed out. The fact that a woman may use alcohol as a means of periodically expressing her despair and frustration at her husband, whom she feels unable to cope with in any other way, does not necessarily mean that she is an alcoholic. One such case involved a woman in her early 50s, married for almost 30 years to a man whom she was finding progressively more withholding. She had a large family and found no other alternative for coping with this rejecting husband than periodic "explosions" in which drinking played a significant role. Her husband had no interest in changing or in conjoint therapy, which he contemptuously viewed as "handholding." His attitude at the initial consultation was "can't you teach her to stop complaining about me and realize how much better off she is than the people in India?" His attitude was "See how lucky you are," which was communicated as "be grateful and don't complain." The patient, who had raised ten children essentially by herself, was a competent and warm mother. However, periodically, when she could stand the situation no longer, she would get drunk and verbally attack her husband while threatening suicide. When she was seen in initial consultation, it was obvious that although she was sullen and resentful, she was neither clinically depressed nor alcoholic. Subsequent clinical experience reinforced this initial impression. The patient never became clinically depressed, nor did she experience a loss of control of her drinking except on rare occasions, always associated with angry outbursts at her husband. She regularly had one or two drinks in the evening, never more. Nor was there a desire for more. She never drank at any other time of the day. In short, although both "depression" and "alcoholism" were cited by her referring internist, neither was the significant issue, and insistence on abstinence, a most appropriate treatment for alcoholism, would have been a most inappropriate treatment for this woman.

In taking the drinking history of a female with a presumed drinking problem, certain points should be kept in mind. The duration of the drinking problem is often likely to be shorter than would be expected in the case of the male alcoholic. This is particularly true in outpatient treatment. This is not to suggest that one does not encounter women with 20-year histories of a drinking problem. However, it is not unusual to obtain a history of a drinking problem which may not exceed a year or two. This history is frequently confirmed by the spouse. In such instances, one should focus on specific life events and their particular meaning for the patient (e.g., a recent loss, a change in status, a geographical move, a change in the marital relationship, the death of a spouse, children leaving home, etc.). Furthermore, there is often an awareness in female alcoholics of using alcohol to medicate mounting anxiety, despair, loneliness, depression, or rage. This is in marked contrast to the history taken from male alcoholics, with whom the search for causal or precipitating factors often is experienced by the therapist as most unrewarding. This suggests a difference in treatment strategy in treating the female alcoholic. It is not only fruitful but necessary to establish connections between life events, affects, and drinking behavior. In contrast, the treatment of most male alcoholics must focus on their omnipotent denial and grandiosity.

PSYCHOTHERAPY OF ALCOHOLIC WOMEN

A corollary of the awareness of connections between psychological phenomena and drinking on the part of the female alcoholic is that the therapist may reasonably expect to obtain an adequate psychiatric history from the female alcoholic patient. This is in marked contrast to the majority of male alcoholics, in whose cases one must interview the spouse before any treatment can occur. The fundamental difference is that the female alcoholic is more often drinking to medicate a symptom of psychic distress, whereas the male alcoholic tends to express his character pathology when intoxicated, with limited awareness or recall, when he sobers up, of what has transpired. Consequently, sessions with male alcoholics alone can often consist of meaningless renditions of business events or attempts to turn therapy into a conversation between the therapist and patient, thus subverting the purpose of treatment. This is less likely to occur with the majority of female alcoholics, who are more comfortable in accepting the role of patient and thus willing to discuss their feelings and problems.

The female alcoholic tends to drink alone. The determinants of her drinking are therefore less likely to be social factors in the immediate environment. In contrast, the male alcoholic often drinks heavily in the company of friends or associates or within the context of business. The female who drinks alone must contemplate dealing with her future loneliness without alcohol. She must deal with self-monitoring of her drinking when no one else is around to observe her. She must deal with her shame at not having controlled herself in the past and fear of not being able to control herself in the future. She must examine how she will be able to cope with her complex feelings about her husband and about herself in the absence of alcohol. For these reasons an initial period of disulfiram (Antabuse) is often recommended. In addition, AA often helps to fill the psychological void experienced at home. Furthermore, actual changes in life style (including a new job or, at least, increased social or community involvement) are often necessary for many alcoholic women to maintain sobriety. This is in contrast to the majority of male alcoholics seen as outpatients, who will continue in the same vocational pattern.

In exploring the family background and history of a female alcoholic, the frequently observed constellation of the warm, overidealized father and a cold, competent perfectionistic mother should be kept in mind. In the author's clinical experience, the patient's mother is seen frequently as "perfectly organized," and "extremely controlling." The mother is perceived as running everything—particularly the patient. The patient measures herself in terms of her mother and feels inadequate. There is usually intense jealousy, which often is not conscious initially. What is conscious is the feeling of chronic inadequacy and unworthiness and rage at a cold, critical, demanding mother. There is less awareness of the internalization by the patient of the same demand system that has plagued her throughout her life, creating chronic feelings of self-disparagement. The exalted ego ideal together with a harsh, unforgiving superego leaves many female alcoholics chronically depressed and dissatisfied with themselves. The majority of female alcoholics encountered by the author in private practice are anxious, insecure, and constantly striving for the acceptance from others that they are rarely able to give to themselves.

The situation is made more complex because of the rage most of these women feel, not only toward their actual mothers, but toward the internalized demanding, perfectionistic, and controlling maternal introject within themselves. The result is a periodic oscillation between perfectionistic strivings with a compulsive submission to the maternal introject and resentful, rebellious, defiant, negativism—which is usually associated with drinking. The result of the drinking bout, which represents more an escape from the superego introject than an escape from actual reality, is ultimately feelings of guilt, shame, and failure. These feelings again set the stage for repentant submission to the demanding introject. The swing between perfectionism, compulsiveness, and order on one hand and resistance, resentment, and defiance on the other, between being overcontrolled or out of control, is the central issue in the psychotherapy of most female alcoholics.

The transference implications of this dynamic lie in the tendency to project the superego demands onto the therapist. There is an initial pattern of submitting to and overidealizing the therapist. This is followed by rage and disappointment with the therapist when all the pain does not disappear, followed by a desire to rebel and a fear of punishment. Often the battleground relatively early in therapy is the issue of minor tranquilizers, which the patient feels she needs in order to cope with the same dysphoria previously medicated with alcohol. I am not referring to the discomfort associated with withdrawal, but rather to the anxiety that may emerge within the first few weeks or months of treatment following abstention. It is essential that the therapist adopt a position somewhere between gratifying the need (i.e., functioning as the warm, permissive father) and rigidly refusing the request (i.e., acting like the cold, rejecting mother). The patient's request for tranquilizers from her new therapist must be seen as both a test and as evidence of some emerging trust. Since poly drug abuse is a major problem in female alcoholics, such patients frequently have already established sources for obtaining medications. A blanket refusal from the therapist will only push the problem underground and diminish the possibility for the development of honesty in the relationship. In fact, if the patient starts to use tranquilizers obtained elsewhere and does not report them in treatment, this is as destructive to the treatment as continued abusive drinking. A proper strategy is to explore the situational context of the dysphoria, to examine carefully all of the feelings and fears, to respect the patient's pain and her fear of losing control, and to work with her to establish a compromise regarding the use of tranquilizers. This might consist of prescribing a limited number of sleeping pills, preferably flurazepam (Dalmane), 15–30 mg to deal with mounting insomnia, which, if not addressed, could easily destroy all gains in treatment by resulting in drinking. Similarly, limited use of diazepam (Valium), that is, 10–20 5-mg pills used over a week or two of particular tension, may not only reduce the anxiety that might drive the patient back to drinking but also conveys to the patient a compassion for her pain, combined with an emphasis on control and/or limit setting and with a serious concern for the potential of habituation and addiction to such agents if they are used frequently and over long periods of time.

Alcoholic women often tend to idealize their fathers while blaming their mothers for all of the problems at home. This is particularly evident where the father has had a drinking problem, which can be expected in at least 25% of cases. Although the alcoholic woman demands that she perform like her mother in order to be acceptable, she frequently identifies with her father, whom she sees as poorly organized, dependent, and often out of control. Frequently she attacks herself as she has observed her mother attacking her father. The therapeutic implications of the perceived overidealized, weak, poorly organized father are feelings of reassurance at the therapist's organization and strength, together with rage at the absence of these qualities, which these patients would have welcomed, in their fathers, particularly in order to protect them against the demands and control of their mothers.

When the father of the female alcoholic was himself an alcoholic, additional dynamics must be kept in mind. Often the female alcoholic has observed a violent interaction between her parents, particularly if her father was drinking. Drinking, therefore, becomes associated with the expression of rage. Drinking may also be associated with love and sexuality. An alcoholic woman will frequently report that her father was warmer to her and, possibly, even overtly sexual when drinking. It is not rare to obtain a history of actual sexual experience during childhood with either the father or an older male relative, when that individual was drinking. Sometimes the alcoholic father will take his young daughter out to bars with him. In such settings either the father or other men may sexually stimulate the young girl. The implications of these experiences are enormous in creating conflict associated with sexuality, the sense of feminine identity, and ambivalent feelings about drinking.

The adolescence of the female alcoholic is often stormy. One frequently obtains a history of submissive compliance alternating with angry rebelliousness. Drinking generally plays a significant role in the latter, and guilt, conscious or unconscious, is pervasive and almost continuous. Such patients are often shy and inhibited when sober and sexually uninhibited when drinking.

In the marriages of female alcoholics, themes relating to dependency and rage are often prominent. Ambivalence toward the maternal figure is frequently reexperienced with the husband, who is often perceived as demanding, ungiving, and perfectionistic. There is often considerable rage, which may be conscious but is usually expressed only when the patient has been drinking. The fear of expressing these feelings when sober is based on the guilt associated with their intensity and anticipation of rejection. Consequently, such feelings can be expressed only in an altered state of consciousness (i.e., while intoxicated) and then partial'y or totally forgotten. Often the anxiety which these women experience late in the day, prior to the arrival home of their husbands, or the fears they experience when their husbands travel or work late at the office are symptomatic manifestations of their rage. Such feelings need to be made conscious and discussed in therapy. Often conscious or unconscious shame at being so needy prevents these women from honestly facing the basis for their rage. In therapy it is essential to help these women differentiate between the reasonable expression of their needs and blind, unexpressable rage, which they feel they must suppress.

Case Histories

Two case histories will now be presented to illustrate some of the psychodynamic issues discussed. These dynamics will be related to the onset and progression of each patient's drinking problem, and a therapeutic approach to these issues will be suggested.

Case 1.   The first case is that of a 45-year-old widow who entered treatment because of excessive drinking several months following the death of her husband. The treatment initially focused on her drinking and its physical and behavioral consequences. The patient was aware that she had lost control of her drinking. She intellectually accepted the reality of her alcoholism and the necessity for abstinence. She accepted the need for Antabuse and the value of AA, but she felt completely lost. She was confused, helpless, and depressed following the death of her husband. The necessity of having to cope with the ensuing financial and emotional problems of running a home and caring for two teenage sons by herself added to her problems. Her rage at her husband for leaving her in this predicament was not conscious in the early stage of her treatment. The only feelings the patient was aware of were anxiety and depression. In her words, she was using alcohol "to relax" and "to settle her nerves."

After the initial phase in treatment, the patient became aware of the parallel between her current palliative use of alcohol and the factors associated with the development and progression of her drinking problem. She reported that, although she had not sought treatment for her drinking problem during her husband's lifetime, she had had a drinking problem for a number of years.

She indicated the experience of anxiety in rather concrete and somatic terms and the effects of alcohol were similarly experienced: "I felt as tight as a knot and when I would drink, the drinking seemed to dissolve this knot." Her drinking began in the late afternoon and early evening prior to her husband's arrival home. She never thought about it very much, although she was aware that she was becoming more tense and nervous as she anticipated his return. Her tension embarrassed her, expecially since she felt that she was expected to be calm and under control, and there was no ostensible reason for her anxiety. So she discovered the soothing effects of alcohol, which produced a surface calm and momentary inner peace. Behind this anxious and tense exterior, the patient learned in treatment that she was "boiling with resentment." But neither during her husband's lifetime nor at the beginning of treatment was she aware of this rage. She was aware only of "trying to do everything that her husband wanted" and feeling that nothing that she did seemed to be enough. She was consciously aware that her husband was difficult and demanding. But her response was simply "to try harder" while feeling more inadequate. She was aware of feeling unappreciated and unloved, but she tried not to think about it. She believed that whatever dissatisfaction she felt with her husband must be her fault since he was "successful" and so capable.

As the patient's anxiety and "unhappiness" mounted so did her drinking. As the drinking progressed, her husband became aware of it. His attitude and behavior were both critical and controlling. The problem was seen, not as a manifestation of possible alcoholism nor as an attempt to cope with otherwise unmanageable feelings, but rather as his wife's lack of self-control. Her response was quite characteristic. The problem went underground and she began sneaking drinks. It is of interest and by no means unusual in such cases that the patient's husband, who resented her drinking "for relaxation," in fact encouraged her to drink before going to bed with him in order to "loosen up" so that she might be more amorous and receptive to his sexual advances.

When her husband died quite suddenly one might have expected the patient's drinking problem to disappear. No longer subject to the controls, criticisms, and demands that she never seemed to be able to fulfill, she was at last free to pursue her own life. With the cinder removed, one might assume that the vision would now be clear. Exactly the opposite occurred. The patient's drinking increased dramatically. The reasons for her increased and continuous drinking following her husband's death shed some additional light on the interesting and not infrequently observed syndrome of the alcoholic widow. Following her husband's death the patient was initially consumed with feelings of guilt. She stated repeatedly, "I should have done more. If I had done more, maybe he wouldn't have had the problems he did at work. I should have pushed him to see another doctor." The real basis for her guilt emerged only later in the treatment. It became apparent to the patient after a number of months of twice-per-week individual psychotherapy that she had wished her husband dead. Her guilt was not for what she had *not* done to save her husband, but for unconsciously hating him and for her unconscious feelings of relief at his death. In fact her initial obsessive preoccupation with her financial dilemma screened her unconscious relief at her husband's death.

The patient first needed to work through her feelings of self-pity and rage before she was able to deal with her feelings of guilt and depression and with her compulsive drinking. She recognized that she had been suppressing these feelings of rage and self-pity during her husband's lifetime and had attempted to cope with them via her medicinal use of alcohol. She began to recognize that the real cause of her despair was not her husband's death, but the loneliness that she had felt for years. Eventually she was able to complain bitterly and openly, really for the first time in her life. "He loved life so much but he never loved me. He just looked at me as a good breeder of children. He never cared about how I felt. He was more interested in how I would look on his arm. Everyone else saw how great he was. I saw the other side." Because of profound feelings of guilt and self-hatred, such women characteristically blame themselves when they are angry, dissatisfied, or needy. The problem is often compounded by the arrogant certainty of the husband, who projects all of the blame onto his already guilt-ridden wife. A polarization then occurs in the minds of such women. Although they may be furious at their husbands, and this rage may even be conscious during sobriety and frequently expressed when intoxicated, there is a deep underlying sense that they are "wrong." They see their husband as the successful, healthy, normal achiever, whereas they see themselves as the sick, unsuccessful, abnormal alcoholic. This polarization obviously fuels further self-destructive drinking. Ultimately, the only way such women can cope with their self-hatred, resentment, and jealousy of their husbands is by unconsciously attempting to "drag him down to (their) level" by the excessive use of alcohol as an unconscious means of inflicting pain while establishing a pathological control over their husbands. In effect, if they cannot control their own lives, at least they can attempt unconsciously to control their husbands'. Of course this unconscious desire to destroy their husbands increases the guilt of alcoholic women and thus further intensifies their drinking problem.

Although this interpersonal dynamic may be strikingly apparent to the clinician, it is important to realize that the patient may never have consciously recognized the interpersonal implication of her drinking and it may come as a startling and highly therapeutic insight to her, provided it is presented when the patient is ready to hear it (i.e., not at the beginning of treatment.) In the early stages of treatment, all the patient generally is able to recognize is the existence of a drinking problem and the palliative use of alcohol to remove pain (i.e., her tension, nervousness, unhappiness, fatigue, or boredom). Only later in the treatment is the patient ready to recognize the deeper dynamics of her drinking (i.e., her rage and ultimately her masochism) and the role these dynamics play in perpetuating her drinking problem. Although a strong conscious desire to stop excessive drinking may exist for many years, until these patients deal with their unconscious rage and masochism, the unconscious need to drink in a destructive manner will continue. This is why AA alone is insufficient treatment for such patients.

In the case of this alcoholic widow, the dynamics of a female alcoholic who drinks in response to a live interpersonal conflict with a live husband are complicated by the husband's death. A link exists, however. The patient's drinking following her husband's death was still in response to him. She drank following his death, not because of what he was doing to her, but because of what he had done in the past and because of what she had tolerated. Although she drank presumably "to forget," her drinking in fact kept the marriage alive in a most pathological form. It provided an unconscious means of "getting back" at her husband (i.e., "see what you have done to me") while actually punishing and degrading herself. While the superficial reasons for her drinking were reported early in treatment, only later did she come to grips with the less conscious reasons for her drinking problem. It may be paradoxical that before she could start a new life—free from her husband by whom she felt oppressed—she had to give him up. It was not enough merely for him to die. The neurotic link continued. Only when this was analyzed and worked through could the patient give up the self-destructive drinking, which was a link to the past. Once these issues were worked through, the patient had no further slips and no further desire to drink. She had accepted her alcoholism as she finally accepted her right to start a new life. She was then able to symbolically as well as actually remove the wedding band she had worn for many months following the death of her husband.

Conjoint Marital Therapy.   The second case is presented to illustrate the importance of the role of conjoint marital therapy in the treatment of the female alcoholic. Marital therapy has a rather different role in the treatment of male and female alcoholic patients. This difference is attributable to the fact that in the male alcoholic the marital discord is generally the consequence of the drinking, whereas for the female it is often a major cause. The drinking problem tends to be the primary issue for the male alcoholic and marital discord ensues as his wife attempts to cope with the behavioral aberrations associated with his drinking. These most often take the form of verbal and occasionally physical outbursts of anger directed toward his wife and less frequently toward his children. The situation is very different for the woman with a drinking problem. It has been the author's experience that many women with drinking problems are drinking in an effort to cope with marital problems that they find frustrating and at times insoluble. Their drinking represents a desperate attempt to deal with their frustration, helplessness, and despair while expressing the rage which they have tended to suppress when sober, but which finally explodes when they are intoxicated. Recurrent drinking episodes in women are generated by this mounting rage at their husbands. The rage is suppressed during sobriety because of profound feelings of guilt at least partially related to prior drinking episodes and because of projected fears of retaliation. This rage can be expressed only during intoxication and thus becomes the precipitant of their drinking.

With male alcoholics, since marital discord is usually the consequence of drinking, it has been the author's experience that when the drinking is terminated, the marital problem is often markedly diminished. However, the approach and expectation in the treatment of the female with a drinking problem must be different. Although the drinking may have reached the stage of alcoholism, clearly indicating the necessity of abstinence as a treatment goal, the drinking must still be considered the symptom and not the cause or the primary problem. As a result, the therapist cannot assume that cessation of drinking will represent an adequate treatment goal for the female alcoholic. In such cases, unless the underlying marital confict is confronted and worked through, any improvement in the clinical picture will be fleeting and relapse can be expected. Focus on the marital conflict is essential and conjoint marital therapy is the treatment of choice.

Case 2. The patient was a woman in her late 40s who was seen initially in outpatient consultation following a brief stay in a general hospital where she had been placed by her internist to "dry out" following a protracted binge. She indicated in the first interview that she had been "feeling rotten, down in the dumps, bored, and trapped." She reported that she had "no interest in anything" and that she "felt lonesome." She indicated that all of her friends were in another community from which she "had been moved" by her husband and "his company." In brief, she felt lost and discovered that the only thing that predictably "picked her up" was alcohol. She remarked, "when everything seems so worthless, drinking permits you to go on—to do the wash and the ironing. For a while you don't even feel so unhappy about it. Alcohol gives me the energy to push the vacuum and then after a few drinks I feel so good I'll stop working and go and watch T.V."

This had been the patient's third hospitalization for excessive drinking and obviously she felt depressed. The patient rejected the use of Antabuse and AA attendance. Antidepressant medication was considered but not used. It is important for the clinician to evaluate, not merely what the patient says regarding her mood, but how she appears. Although this patient expressed feelings of depression, in fact her predominant affect was rage. The focus of her rage was also obvious and unambiguous—her husband. She found him "boring," "passive," and uncommunicative. She reported that she and her husband talked very little in the evenings and that he generally fell asleep after dinner. She described him as a "nice, easy-going guy whom everyone else thinks is the salt of the earth." She, on the other hand, was furious at him for his detachment and for his passivity and fear of confronting her or dealing with any of their teenage children, which left the total responsibility and burden of providing discipline for the children to her.

The predominance of rage rather than depression in this patient and the very clear focus of this rage suggested that her husband's participation in meetings might produce a rapid shift in her mood. This is precisely what occurred. It is important to note that the patient's husband had played no part in any of her previous hospitalizations or outpatient treatments. Since the marital conflict was the major precipitant of her drinking, it is not surprising that her drinking problem persisted despite a more than adequate medical approach to the problem in the past, a reasonable orientation to the disease concept of alcoholism, and an appropriate introduction to AA. This time, however, her husband's willingness to participate in the treatment produced a rapid and dramatic change in the clinical picture.

In the experience of the author, rapid improvement in the clinical picture is more characteristic in conjoint marital treatment than in the individual treatment of the female with a drinking problem. The reason for this is that the sharing of responsibility by the spouse and the willingness to make the effort to regularly attend conjoint therapy sessions does a great deal to rapidly diminish the patient's guilt and rage while opening channels for constructive communication, the development of mutual respect, and individual growth. In this particular case the spouse was willing to accept his share of responsibility for the problem. In fact, even in his first visit, he was able to acknowledge his fear of confrontations and his tendency to avoid them. He revealed that throughout his marriage he had tended to avoid any expression of feeling, believing, or at least rationalizing, that this might further upset his wife. The patient would often become enraged at him when she would drink. His characteristic response was to distance himself (i.e., by ignoring her or by working late hours at the office rather than dealing with any of her feelings or with any of the issues that she raised when she was intoxicated). Instead, he preferred to withdraw and attribute all of her feelings to the drinking.

By the third conjoint session the patient's mood had lifted dramatically, although no antidepressant medication had been prescribed. Furthermore, she was experiencing no need or even desire to drink.

The patient reported that she "was feeling great" and that her husband "was doing a lot of thinking" . . . "and trying to express himself with the kids rather than leaving it all to me." He commented that he "was struck by the fact that the therapist was saying many of the same things his wife had said to him, but now he found that he was listening." The same comments that he had, in the past, considered "irrational because his wife was totally irrational (drunk) when she said them" now were being heard for the first time rather than "tuned out." This tendency to "tune his wife out" had left her frustrated and furious and had driven her to further drinking, ultimately resulting in her severe drinking problem.

Within five or six sessions the patient was beginning to realize and accept the connection between her frustration, her anger at her husband, and her chronic "depression." Her depression cleared entirely within a month following the initiation of treatment. It became apparent that despite this patient's obvious anger, this affect surprisingly had not been apparent to her in the past. She had experienced herself as depressed but not as angry. Only once she had begun to express this anger could she acknowledge that for years she had been angry at her husband. Furthermore, she was able for the first time to see the dynamic connection between this anger at her husband and her drinking episodes. Her husband traveled frequently and she was able to observe that her drinking while he was away was actually her way of "getting even" and "making him remember me." While she was beginning to face her chronic rage and its relation to her drinking, her husband began to realize how he had been hiding rather than communicating with his wife and that he had been afraid to express himself most of his life. He commented that his fear of offending his own alcoholic mother ("the queen bee") had led to his tendency to avoid any confrontation with his wife and his children. Once he received and accepted reassurance from the therapist that it was proper, and in fact desirable, for him to express his feelings, and particularly his anger, he was able to express himself toward both his wife and his children in an appropriate manner, much to his wife's delight.

Just as the therapy legitimized his anger, it also gave his wife the right to accept her resentment and anger without the guilt that she felt and that many female alcoholics feel about expressing their needs. She was aware of her jealousy of her husband's devotion to his job, which traditionally far surpassed his interest in her. But she had always felt that it was wrong to complain and therefore had expressed her feelings and complained only when she had been drinking. As she became more in touch with the reasons for her rage and more accepting of her right to be angry she remarked, "I always thought a wife went along and did what her husband wanted and did not open up her mouth. When the company said jump, I always thought you had to jump. He was always so busy pleasing the company. He never said 'no.' I guess I also felt too guilty to say no."

Rapid improvement in therapy continued and the treatment was concluded after three months of meetings, which were initially twice a week, then once a week, and then once every two weeks. This clinical improvement was in marked contrast to all prior attempts at treatment, which had not included the husband.

CONCLUSION

Certain generalizations have been presented in an attempt to highlight differences between male and female alcoholics and to delineate an orientation and approach specific to the treatment of alcoholic women. Obviously, all of the dynamics presented are not unique to alcoholic women. Furthermore, the clinician must always be sensitive to specific differences among women. This chapter has tended to highlight differences between groups (i.e., alcoholic men versus alcoholic women); however, there are obviously considerable intragroup differences. At the most obvious level, one female alcoholic may drink to medicate delusions of a paranoid psychosis and must be treated with a phenothiazine and supportive therapy, while another may drink primarily when in the manic phase of a manic–depressive illness and should be treated with lithium carbonate. Both patients, however, may need Antabuse and referral to AA. More frequently one female alcoholic may be drinking in a desperate attempt to cope with a rejecting husband and will need to be treated in marital therapy; while another with intrapsychic conflicts should be treated in long-term, individual, dynamically oriented psychotherapy, which will facilitate the development of the necessary transference distortions that will ultimately enable the patient to recognize the difference between her projections and reality.

The observations presented in this chapter are based primarily on work with upper-middle-class patients treated by the author in a setting of private practice in a suburb of New York City. The majority of these patients were referred by their family physicians and, in contrast to many other groups of female alcoholics who have been studied, the majority of these women were married to men who did not leave them during the course of treatment. This obviously is a specialized subsample of the total female alcoholic population. Whether the observations presented can be generalized to the treatment of other groups of alcoholic women will depend on the findings of other clinicians and researchers working with more varied populations. It is hoped that this preliminary attempt to formulate some of the significant issues in the treatment of female alcoholics will stimulate further interest on the part of other workers in the field.

REFERENCES

Beckman, L. J. Women alcoholics: A review of social and psychological studies. *Journal of Studies on Alcohol*, 1975, *36*, 797-824.

Belfer, M. L., Shader, R. I., Carroll, M., and Harmantz, J. S. Alcoholism in women. *Archives of General Psychiatry*, 1971, *25*, 540-544.

Blane, H. T. *The personality of the alcoholic: Guises of dependency*. New York: Harper and Row, 1968.

Busch, H., Kormendy, E., and Feuerlein, W. Partners of female alcoholics. *British Journal of Addictions*, 1973, *68*, 179-184.

Curlee, J. Alcoholic women: Some considerations for further research. *Bulletin of the Menninger Clinic*, 1967, *31*, 154-163.

Curlee, J. Alcoholism and the "empty nest." *Bulletin of the Menninger Clinic*, 1969, *33*, 165-171.

Curlee, J. A comparison of male and female patients at an alcoholism treatment center. *Journal of Psychology*, 1970, *74*, 239-247.

Greenblatt, M., and Schuckit, M. A. (Eds.). *Alcoholism problems in women and children*. New York: Grune and Stratton, 1976.

Jones, M. C. Personality antecedents and correlates of drinking patterns in women. *Journal of Consulting and Clinical Psychology*, 1971, *36*, 61-69.

Lindbeck, V. L. The woman alcoholic: A review of the literature. *International Journal of Addictions*, 1972, *7*, 567-580.

McClelland, D. C., Davis, W. N., Kalin, R., and Wanner, E. *The drinking man*. New York: Free Press, 1972.

Miller, R. T., and Ely, N. E. Hyperfemininity in the female alcoholic. Seattle Alcoholism Treatment Clinic (unpublished manuscript), 1971.

Noble, D. Psychodynamics of alcoholism in a woman. *Psychiatry*, 1949, *12*, 413-425.

Podolsky, E. The woman alcoholic and premenstrual tension. *Journal of the Woman's American Medical Association*, 1963, *18*, 816-818.

Schuckit, M. A. The alcoholic woman: A literature review. *Psychiatry in Medicine*, 1972, *3*, 37-43.

Schuckit, M. A., and Morrissey, E. R. Alcoholism in women: Some clinical and social perspectives with an emphasis on possible subtypes. In M. Greenblatt and M. A. Schuckit (Eds.), *Alcoholism problems in women and children*. New York: Grune and Stratton, 1976.

Schuckit, M. A., Pitts, F. N., Reich, T., King, L. J.,and Winokur, G. Alcoholism I. Two types of alcoholism in women. *Archives of General Psychiatry*, 1969, *20*, 301-306.

Tamerin, J. S., Tolor, A., and Harrington, B. Sex differences in alcoholics: A comparison of male and female alcoholics' self and spouse perceptions. *American Journal of Drug and Alcohol Abuse*, 1976, *3*(3), 457-472.

Tiebout, H. N. The act of surrender in the therapeutic process. *Quarterly Journal of Studies on Alcohol*, 1949, *10*, 48-58.

Tiebout, H. N. The ego factors in surrender in alcoholism. *Quarterly Journal of Studies on Alcohol*, 1954, *15*, 610–621.

Wilsnack, S. C. The needs of the female drinker: Dependency, power, or what? *Proceedings of the Second Annual Alcoholism Conference of the National Institute on Alcohol Abuse and Alcoholism*, 1973a.

Wilsnack, S. C. Sex role identity in female alcoholism. *Journal of Abnormal Psychology*, 1973b, *82*, 253–261.

Wilsnack, S. C. The impact of sex roles and women's alcohol use and abuse. In M. Greenblatt and M. A. Schuckit (Eds.), *Alcoholism problems in women and children*. New York: Grune and Stratton, 1976.

15

Treatment of Socioeconomically Deprived Alcoholics

Sheldon Zimberg

Introduction

This chapter will discuss the problem of alcoholism among socioeconomically deprived alcoholics living in urban areas. The experience in treatment approaches is based on extensive work with Black alcoholics in Harlem and Puerto Rican alcoholics in East Harlem.

It has been noted that there is a high prevalence of alcoholism among the urban poor. The Harlem and East Harlem areas of New York City have higher death rates due to cirrhosis of the liver than any other area of New York City.

A household survey conducted in the Washington Heights area of Manhattan indicated that the prevalence of alcoholism was inversely related to socioeconomic factors such as income and education (Bailey, Haberman, and Alksne, 1965). A national survey of drinking practices among men showed that men of lower socioeconomic status had a higher proportion of drinking problems (Cahalan, Cisin, and Crossley, 1974).

A study conducted in St. Louis used interviews of Black men in a sample obtained from public-school records (King, Murphy, Robins, and Darvish, 1969). In addition to the interviews, a record search in

---

Sheldon Zimberg • Director of Psychiatry, Joint Diseases, North General Hospital, New York, New York; Associate Professor of Psychiatry, Mount Sinai School of Medicine, New York, New York.

various medical, police, welfare, and other agencies was undertaken to determine the respondent's alcohol-related problems. The authors concluded that increasing use of alcohol was related to an increasing number of social problems and seemed to be a crucial factor in many of the social problems of these men.

A study of the prevalence of alcoholism in New York City service agencies indicated that alcoholism existed in 26% of individuals on parole, 17% on public assistance with most in the home relief category, and 8% of individuals in the family court (Staff and Peterson, 1975).

A prevalence study conducted on the medical wards of Harlem Hospital Center indicated that 60% of the male medical inpatients and 34% of the female medical inpatients had diagnosable levels of alcohol abuse (McCusker, Cherubin, and Zimberg, 1971). About 18% of the admissions to the medical service during the period of the study were directly due to the medical consequences of alcoholism. A study conducted in the emergency room of the Joint Diseases, North General Hospital, which serves the East Harlem area, using the same questionnaire as in the Harlem Hospital study noted that one-third of the patients who came to the emergency room of the hospital were alcoholic (Zimberg, 1979).

Data about the prevalence of alcoholism among Puerto Ricans are scarce. In a paper on alcoholism in Puerto Rico, Aviles-Roig (1973) indicated that with a steadily rising per capita consumption rate there had been increasing amounts of alcoholism. He noted that for 1970 the death rate for liver cirrhosis was 23.0 per 100,000 population, with a rate of 34.5 for men compared to 12.0 for women. The rate for Puerto Ricans living in New York City for this same period of time was 26.7 per 100,000 (New York City Health Department, 1970). The sex-adjusted rates were 44.4 for men and 10.8 for women. Thus, Puerto Ricans living in New York experienced a substantially higher death rate from cirrhosis of the liver among men and a lower rate for women compared to people living in Puerto Rico. Apparently the impact on men living in a dominant culture with a different language and cultural attitudes contributed to a higher rate of alcoholism.

It should be noted that there is a much higher rate of alcoholism among Black women, as noted in the Washington Heights study, compared to White women: 20 per 1000 for Black women compared to 5 per 1000 for White women. The ratio 3.6 male alcoholics to 1 woman alcoholic was noted for the population as a whole compared to a ratio of 1.9 Black male alcoholics to 1 Black woman alcoholic. Among Puerto Rican women 75% reported in a survey in New York City that they do not drink at all, thus accounting for a much lower rate of alcoholism among Puerto Rican women in New York City compared to male Puerto Ricans (Haberman, 1970). These sex differences in alcoholism rates among men and women are interesting and may suggest some answers to the problems in treatment approaches among Black patients and Puerto Rican patients to be discussed below.

At this point it should be explained that the urban groups of socioeconomically deprived alcoholics under discussion in this chapter must be distinguished from the skid-row homeless and disaffiliated alcoholics. The alcoholics described in this chapter are living in poverty in urban ghettos. They have a residence and some family ties and are either employed or maintained on public assistance. Their poverty preceded their alcoholism and may have been a significant contributing factor in their alcoholism. The skid-row alcoholics' alcoholism caused, in many cases, a severe physical and social deterioration, leading such individuals to lose contact with their families and friends and to drift into the skid-row area. These people are homeless and are therefore not eligible for public assistance cash grants. They live in the street and are given chits for flophouse sleeping and meals. They are at the bottom of the barrel socially. The prognosis for recovery with appropriately designed programs is much better for socioeconomically deprived alcoholics than it is for skid-row alcoholics, and therefore these distinct alcoholic subpopulations should not be confused with one another.

The enormously devastating impact that poverty, racial discrimination, and limited opportunities for upward mobility have had on individuals' ability to cope are apparent to anyone who has worked in urban ghetto areas. Alcohol is a readily available source of relief from the pain such stress causes and is also a source of immediate pleasure and gratification. Among Blacks the historical pattern of drinking during slavery, which was permitted on holidays and other festive events and used as a reward for hard work, has had an influence (Bourne, 1976). Among Puerto Ricans heavy drinking is considered part of the concept of "machismo" (Aviles-Roig, 1973). Therefore certain cultural and historical factors combined with severe social stresses associated with poverty, discrimination, and limited hope for advancement have contributed to the high prevalence of alcoholism among these groups. These social and cultural conditions in the socioeconomically deprived must be considered as major contributory factors in the causation of alcoholism, and appropriate treatment interventions must be directed toward these factors.

TREATMENT APPROACHES: BLACK ALCOHOLICS; PUERTO RICAN ALCOHOLICS

In spite of the magnitude of the alcoholism problem among the poor, there have been few treatment programs established in the areas where they live. An investigation of social class as a determinant of diagnosis, prognosis, and therapy of alcoholism indicated that the lowest-social-class alcoholics were more likely to receive a diagnosis of psychosis or chronic brain syndrome, were given less intensive treatment, and had a poor or poorer prognosis than higher-social-class alcoholics (Schmidt, Smart, and Moss, 1968). An analysis of outcome in treatment in eight alcoholism clinics conducted by Gerard and Saenger (1966) suggested that poorer alcoholics do less well in treatment. Work by Kissin, Rosenblatt, and Machover (1968) and Mindlin (1959) on prognostic factors in the treatment of alcoholism suggests that alcoholic patients with few social or economic resources tend to do poorly in treatment.

A study by Pattison, Coe, and Rhodes (1969) suggests that it is necessary to develop more specific treatment approaches for particular alcoholism subpopulations, since alcoholics do not represent a homogeneous population with similar requirements. The following discussion will focus on treatment approaches that have proved effective with socioeconomically deprived alcoholics with particular reference to urban-ghetto dwellers in the Black and Puerto Rican ethnic groups.

Treatment Approaches for Black Socioeconomically Deprived Alcoholics. A pilot treatment program was established at Harlem Hospital in 1966 to provide an effective treatment for socioeconomically deprived alcoholics (Zimberg, Lipscomb, and Davis, 1971). This model was expanded in an alcoholism clinic established in 1972 at the Joint Diseases, North General Hospital, which serves East Harlem. The populations that were being treated were characterized by marked social and psychological maladaptations and chronic and acute physical disorders. Many of the patients were too sick to use community and social services effectively but were considered not acutely sick enough to require institutionalization. They frequented hospital emergency rooms, but never received adequate treatment. Many were estranged from their families, living in single rooms with no meaningful relationships. They had relatively little education and poor work histories. Many were maintained on public assistance or disability benefits. They often drank heavily and at times engaged in violent quarrels.

Clearly a traditional approach to establishing a clinic with an appointment system and a regular schedule of attendance for specific services could not effectively meet the multiple needs of these patients. A psychosocial model of treatment was developed. This model established day care as the core treatment approach and the modality designed to engage patients initially in treatment.

The day-care program provided a 9-to-5 structured treatment program in an alcohol-free environment. The staff of the day-care program consisted of recovered alcoholics who were residents of the area and who served as alcoholism counselors. They were under the professional supervision of social workers and a psychiatrist. The alcoholism clinic also provided medical examinations and treatment, psychiatric evaluations and treatment, individual and group therapy, and disulfiram (Antabuse). Patients graduated from the day-care program to the more intensive treatments that were available. The day-care program permitted many patients to be effectively detoxified from alcohol on an ambulatory basis through their daily attendance and close supervision. The ambulatory detoxification regimen provided daily doses of vitamins and decreasing doses of chlordiazepoxide (Librium). Patients were given daily doses by the nurses and a two-day supply for weekends.

The day program provided large group discussions and alcoholism-education lectures. There were recreational activities and outings and a great deal of socialization. Patients were encouraged to develop patient governments and make an increasing number of decisions on their own.

Because they understood the patients' situation in relation to drinking as well as their socioeconomic circumstances, the recovered alcoholism counselors served as effective role models for the patients. The patients could easily identify with the counselors and were thus encouraged in their own efforts at recovery.

When patients had achieved a significant period of sobriety, at least 90 days, they were provided with vocational counseling. Since most patients had little education, poor work histories, and no marketable skills, the emphasis on the vocational counselor was to increase their education and have patients learn skills rather than try to place them in menial, low-paying jobs without a future. Many vocational-training programs were utilized and over 160 patients became involved in training during one year.

The patients' involvement in day care and the rehabilitation process has been observed to occur in five fairly distinct and predictable stages. These stages represent progressive levels of social, psychological, and functional improvement.

The first stage occurs when the patient appears at the alcoholism clinic for evaluation and lasts one to three weeks. Initially all patients receive a complete psychosocial evaluation, a psychiatric evaluation, and a medical history and examination. Patients are detoxified on an ambulatory basis or hospitalized if too sick medically or unable to stop drinking on an ambulatory basis. The availability of a small number of hospital detoxification beds enables the sicker patients to enter treatment during the beginning stage. This stage is characterized by the patients' almost obsequious acceptance of the program and abstinence from alcohol.

The first stage then fades away and the patient may start drinking or act out in other ways. This stage represents a testing by the patient of his acceptance by the group and the counselor. It tends to last two to six weeks and may clear up through the directive counseling of the staff or require the use of disulfiram. The patient who has not established a positive transference at this time may drop out of treatment. Patients who cannot become engaged in treatment in an outpatient setting will require more intensive, structured treatment in a halfway house. A halfway-house program has become available in recent years and can be useful for the recovery of such patients.

The third stage is reached when the patient has become abstinent and has become a regular participant in the day-care program. The patient has established a positive transference and is engaged in treatment. The patient has developed close attachments to the staff and other patients and becomes concerned about the welfare of his fellow patients, who are now his friends. At this point more intensive treatment including individual counseling, small-group therapy, family therapy (if a family member is available), and the beginning of vocational counseling can be made available to the patient. This stage lasts from three to six months.

The fourth stage involves the beginning of independent functioning of the patient. The patient has by this point achieved at least six months of sobriety and is ready to move out of the day-care program into employment, training, or education. This stage produces severe anxiety in some patients and may result in a return to drinking. If it is dealt with therapeutically by the staff and if a good vocational or educational opportunity can be found for the patient, he leaves the day-care program and enters stage 5.

Stage 5 is of indeterminate length, since it is recognized that alcoholism is a chronic disease with a high potential for relapse. This stage involves some achievement of success in the patient's employment or training situation. The patient is followed in a once-a-week evening or weekend clinic group therapy with or without disulfiram depending on the degree of internalized control over the impulse to drink. He is encouraged to attend AA meetings regularly. The availability of evening and Saturday clinics is important for the working patients and those who graduate to this status as well as for providing accessible treatment for a crisis situation. Weekend clinics are particularly helpful in providing socialization and recreational opportunities during a crucial period when drinking frequently occurs. There is emphasis during this last stage on reintegration of the patient into his family if one exists, and family therapy is intensified at this time. The patient may visit the day-care program or return for brief day-care treatment whenever this is indicated.

A particular problem with this population has been involving the family in treatment. Often by the time the patient has reached treatment, he is estranged from his family and reintegration is not possible. Another problem has been engaging female Black alcoholics in the day-care program, although the prevalence is high for this group. Some recent efforts at establishing all-female groups have increased attendance of the female patients.

The psychosocial process of treatment described can be an effective modality in the treatment of socioeconomically deprived alcoholics. The crucial elements of this psychosocial approach include the use of a structured day-care program staffed by recovered alcoholism counselors; the provision of alcoholism education; socialization, recreation, occupational therapy, and patient government activities; the availability of multidisciplinary services including psychiatric, medical, social case work, and vocational counseling; and the phasing in of more intensive treatment and rehabilitative modalities as the patient becomes engaged in the treatment process.

Treatment Approaches for Puerto Rican Socioeconomically Deprived Alcoholics. Many of the concepts regarding the treatment of socioeconomically deprived alcoholics apply to the treatment of Puerto Rican alcoholics in urban areas on the mainland. The use of day care as the primary method of engaging patients in the psychosocial rehabilitation process has validity for this group of alcoholics. In addition, the use of recovered alcoholics as effective therapeutic agents and role models is also useful.

However, there are somewhat different emphases and requirements that apply to the Puerto Rican alcoholic. First, it is necessary to recognize and understand Puerto Rican culture and heritage and the way alcohol is used and viewed. The rum industry is a major contributor to the Puerto Rican economy, and the use of rum is widely accepted and, according to Dr. Aviles-Roig (1973), "associated with sex, happiness, social status and Puerto Rican identity." The man who drinks to excess and becomes intoxicated is a "whole man" and part of the cult of "machismo." Therefore positive social status and acceptance are associated with getting drunk. Women are supposed to drink soft drinks and be primarily concerned with the home and raising children.

It is therefore necessary to have staff involved in the treatment of Puerto Rican alcoholics who have extensive knowledge of Puerto Rican culture and are bilingual. Since drinking is such a cultural attribute among men and social stigma among women, being comfortable with treatment in terms of being able to communicate effectively one's feelings and to feel that one is accepted and understood is essential in the treatment process.

Another aspect of the treatment of the Puerto Rican alcoholic that differs from that of the Black alcoholic is the fact that most of the Puerto Rican patients are accompanied by their families during their initial visit to the treatment program. This involvement of the family should be capitalized on through the development of family-therapy approaches. Such approaches have included joint therapy of married couples and couples' therapy groups. The impact of the family on the therapeutic process has been noted to be extremely effective and should be utilized early in the treatment process.

The use of Alcoholics Anonymous among Puerto Rican alcoholics has been noted to be much less than among Black alcoholics. There are about 20 AA groups in Central Harlem, which is largely Black, but very few in East Harlem, which is largely Puerto Rican. The reason for this seems related to the fact that the leadership of the few Hispanic AA groups are people who have come from South and Central America as opposed to Puerto Rico and the hostility felt between these groups of people has interfered with the development of a significant number of AA groups among Puerto Ricans. This observation points out the cultural differences and antagonism that may exist among the various cultural groups that make up the Hispanic peoples.

Treatment efforts have been less effective among Puerto Rican women alcoholics than Black women alcoholics. These results seem based on the much greater stigma associated with a Puerto Rican woman becoming an alcoholic and failing in her womanly duties. There is much greater denial of the drinking problem and less willingness to talk about it and take effective steps toward treatment.

The acceptance of disulfiram has also been noted to be significantly different among Puerto Rican alcoholics than Black alcoholics. Many fewer Puerto Rican alcoholics are willing to continue to use disulfiram due to an apparently higher incidence of side effects, particularly those relating to loss of libido and impotence. Possibly smaller doses of disulfiram at the level of 125 mg would be better tolerated than the standard 250 mg dose.

Treatment approaches for Puerto Rican alcoholics require that the day-care approach be conducted in a bilingual and bicultural setting. There should be more emphasis on family therapy. The use of AA and disulfiram seems less accepted among this population. Puerto Rican women alcoholics seem even harder to reach than other women alcoholics and will require even more specialized treatment approaches.

The treatment approaches described have been successful in increasing the percentage of Puerto Rican alcoholics in treatment at the Joint Diseases, North General Hospital from 15% to 30% over a three-year period.

EVALUATION OF TREATMENT OUTCOME IN SOCIOECONOMICALLY DEPRIVED ALCOHOLICS

An evaluation study was carried out in the Harlem Hospital Alcoholism Program (Zimberg, 1974). This study compared the outcome of a group of patients receiving a comprehensive array of ambulatory treatment services including day care provided by a multidisciplinary staff and a group of patients receiving medication and supportive psychotherapy from an internist. Among the patients assigned to day care, 55% achieved a stage 4 level of involvement, the beginnings of independent functioning. However, many were frustrated at this stage because of the lack of vocational training and job opportunities. It was noted further that there were no significant differences in outcome between the two groups studied. The patients who achieved a significant period of abstinence in both groups were married, not on public assistance, and not living in social isolation; were in a higher social class, working more often, and less impaired in vocational functioning; and had developed an alcohol problem at a later age (35 to 44 versus 15 to 24). Therefore the patients who improved to the greatest extent regardless of the intensity of treatment were those who had the greatest amount of social stability and socioeconomic status at the time they entered treatment and who had developed an alcohol problem at a later age. This result confirmed earlier studies showing that, even among alcoholics with socioeconomic deprivation, those with the greatest amount of social, vocational, and familial resources had the best prognosis for improvement.

It is clear that most deprived individuals with alcoholism do not experience treatment as enough of an incentive to give up alcohol. By contrast, working-class and middle-class alcoholics who, because of drinking, have experienced the reality, or the threat of, severe social, vocational, or family losses have a strong incentive to retain or regain through abstinence what they might lose through continued drinking. Among individuals who began drinking heavily early in life and have little to lose by continued drinking, no such incentive is operative. Treatment is necessary for such socioeconomically deprived alcoholics, but is not sufficient.

In recent years the alcoholism program at Joint Diseases, North General Hospital, has steadily increased its capability of securing vocational training and rehabilitation for its alcoholic patients. In 1976, 160 patients became involved in such activities. Recently developed data showed that these socioeconomic incentives have increased the recovery rate for the population served by this program. Changes in policy of the State Office of Vocational Rehabilitation regarding greater willingness to accept alcoholics for their services and the development of the Employment Program for Recovering Alcoholics (EPRA) have greatly increased training and employment opportunities for alcoholics. A specific contract between the Federation Employment Guidance Service and the hospital's alcoholism program has provided many patients with these opportunities and has resulted in patients earning high school equivalency diplomas, entering and graduating from college, learning specific marketable job skills, and obtaining well-paying jobs with a future. The hospital itself, as an employer, has hired recovering alcoholics who turned out to be excellent employees.

Looking at outcome of treatment for chronic alcoholics among the socioeconomically deprived should be broader than simply the individual alcoholic's attainment of sobriety, or even his or her involvement in a productive work situation. The economic and social costs to the community of the enormous consequences of alcoholism include medical and surgical complications requiring hospitalization, public assistance costs, broken marriages, child abuse and impaired child development, criminal activities, and home and automobile accidents. Any one or several of these can serve as bases for the evaluation of the cost-effectiveness of alcoholism programs among the socioeconomically deprived.

An example of such an approach was an economic analysis of the treatment of chronic alcoholics in a hostel-type alcoholic rehabilitation program compared to the involvement of the patients with the criminal justice system through arrests for public intoxication. This study was carried out by graduate students in Monroe County, New York (Sample and Mairs, 1971). The study determined that the alcoholism rehabilitation program generated a benefit of $147,556 greater than the cost of the program through the patients' increased productivity, work program operation, jail-costs savings, reduced judicial case loads, and increased public services. Additional studies of this type are needed in relation to alcoholism treatment for the socioeconomically deprived. The last chapter of this book describes some of the techniques involved in clinical evaluation of alcoholism treatment. Adding variables related to the social, health, welfare, and criminal-justice system costs of no treatment can demonstrate that alcoholism treatment for the poor can have major economic impact for society beyond the help for the particular patient in treatment.

The importance of this viewpoint relates to the fact that in the current era of cost-containment efforts, unless programs can demonstrate cost-effectiveness they will not be continued to be funded. Effective treatment approaches are not enough to justify continuation of programs for the socioeconomically deprived.

DISCUSSION

Evidence has been presented that alcoholism is a major public health problem among the urban poor. Many hospital admissions are related to the consequences of alcoholism. Significant amounts of public assistance costs, many family disruptions, accidents, unemployment, and law-enforcement costs are related to the consequences of alcoholism. Therefore it is important to try to develop effective treatment approaches for the socioeconomically deprived.

It is important to distinguish between the primary socioeconomically deprived alcoholic and the skid-row homeless alcoholic who can be seen in any urban area of this country. The primary socioeconomically deprived alcoholic has been poor prior to developing alcoholism, has begun drinking early in life, and is trapped in the cycle of poverty with little chance of upward mobility. These people have, in general, maintained some family relationships and community contacts, have a residence, are able to utilize community agencies with some help, and can be maintained on public assistance. The communities of the urban poor are indeed communities with strong kinship bonds, well-established community organizations, and often articulate political representation. The approaches necessary to effectively treat the primary socioeconomically deprived alcoholic are therefore quite different from those for the homeless skid-row alcoholic population.

The treatment approaches for the primary socioeconomically deprived alcoholic should utilize a model of social and psychiatric interventions that is based on an understanding of the social and psychological factors that have contributed to the development of alcoholism in this population and its resistance to traditional treatment approaches. The core treatment modality is the day-care program, which serves as the entrance point into treatment and as the method of engaging patients in treatment. The day-care program should be staffed with recovered alcoholics who have had life experiences similar to the patients'. Initially, all patients should have a thorough psychiatric and medical examination because psychiatric and medical disorders often coexist with the alcoholism. In addition, initial efforts at assisting the patients with housing, public assistance, and legal problems will be required.

The day-care program should be a large group program with a variety of activities. The emphasis should be on socialization and identification with the recovered-alcoholic counselors, who serve as role models. Patient government, occupational and recreational therapy, alcoholism education, and discussion groups should be provided. As patients achieve some sobriety and become engaged in the treatment process, more intensive treatment approaches such as individual therapy, small-group therapy (eight to ten in number), and family therapy should be utilized. At a later stage of recovery, vocational counseling that can lead to vocational rehabilitation should be available. In addition, educational services that could lead to obtaining a high school equivalency diploma should be available. These vocational and educational services are essential components of the rehabilitation process. It has been proven that many poor alcoholics can achieve sobriety but will not maintain it unless there is a chance of improving their socioeconomic status. Such patients have little to lose by maintaining their drinking, which is often established to blot out their lack of opportunity in life. Unless some tangible socioeconomic incentives can be built into the program, only the patients with the greater amounts of socioeconomic resources will recover.

In looking at the outcome of the treatment of such alcoholics, it can be expected that 30%–40% will recover if the sociopsychiatric approaches described are utilized. Higher rates of recovery can be anticipated if a well-developed program of educational and vocational rehabilitation services is readily available for these patients.

Since funding agencies require evaluation of program effectiveness, variables other than drinking status should be utilized. Improvement in functional status as well as drinking status should be looked at. In addition, the impact of treatment on the consequences of alcoholism such as hospital usage, public-assistance costs, law-enforcement costs, and changes in vocational status should be evaluated as important factors that may be significantly altered by effective alcoholism treatment for this population.

Somewhat different approaches are required for Puerto Rican alcoholics compared to Black alcoholics, although the day-care model is also appropriate for this population. However, programs serving both patient populations should take into account that some antagonism might exist between these groups and among various Hispanic groups, and counselors must be tactful in the establishment of the somewhat differing services for these patient populations. These services can be provided at the same location with the scheduling of the more specialized services at appropriate times.

As is generally applicable to the treatment of alcoholism, specific treatment approaches must be tailored to specific alcoholic subpopulations. This chapter has presented effective treatment approaches for primary socioeconomically deprived alcoholics among the Black and Puerto Rican urban populations. The techniques of psychosocial day care with socioeconomic incentives built in, which are culturally and linguistically syntonic with the patient population served, and staffed with recovered alcoholic counselors of the same ethnic group as the population can be effective for other minority groups such as native Americans and those living in rural areas.

SUMMARY

Significant amounts of evidence have been accumulated that alcoholism is a major public health problem among the urban poor. Past treatment efforts have been largely ineffective for this population. The primary socioeconomically deprived alcoholics are distinguished from skid-row alcoholic population, which is a disaffiliated, homeless population. Treatment approaches for the poor urban alcoholic population should be based on a sociopsychiatric intervention model that utilizes a structured large-group setting as a socializing and ego-enhancing experience in an alcohol-free environment. More intensive treatment, as well as educational and vocational rehabilitation, should be part of the program to provide socioeconomic incentives to patients who will achieve sobriety but will require the hope of upward mobility in order to maintain the sobriety. Somewhat different approaches, particularly a greater emphasis on family intervention, will be required by Puerto Rican patients.

Outcome of treatment of the socioeconomically disadvantaged alcoholic should look at variables including drinking status and health, social, vocational, housing, economic, and family status. In addition, impact of treatment on hospital costs, public-assistance costs, law-enforcement costs, and benefits to society from increased vocational productivity should be a major aspect of review in terms of the cost-effectiveness of these treatment programs.

REFERENCES

Aviles-Roig, C. A. Socio-cultural components of the alcoholism problem in Puerto Rico. Presented at the National Institute on Alcohol Abuse and Alcoholism Area II Interstate Conference on Alcoholism, New York City, December 5, 1973.

Bailey, M. B., Haberman, P. W., and Alksne, H. The epidemiology of alcoholism in an urban residential area. *Quarterly Journal of Studies on Alcohol*, 1965, *26*, 19–40.

Bourne, P. Alcoholism in the urban black population. In F. D. Harper (Ed.), *Alcohol abuse and black America*. Alexandria, Va.: Douglas Publishers, 1976.

Cahalan, D., Cisin, I. H., and Crossley, H. M. *American drinking practices: A national survey of drinking behavior and attitudes*. New Brunswick, N.J.: Rutgers Center of Alcohol Studies, 1974.

Gerard, D. L., and Saenger, G. *Outpatient treatment of alcoholism*. Toronto: University of Toronto Press, 1966.

Haberman, P. W. Denial of drinking in a household survey. *Quarterly Journal of Studies on Alcohol*, 1970, *31*, 710–717.

King, L. J., Murphy, G. E., Robins, L. N., and Darvish, H. Alcohol abuse: A crucial factor in the social problems of Negro men. *American Journal of Psychiatry*, 1969, *125*, 1682–1690.

Kissin, B., Rosenblatt, S. M., and Machover, S. Prognostic factors in alcoholism. In J. O. Cole (Ed.), *Clinical research in alcoholism, psychiatric research report 24*. Washington: American Psychiatric Association, 1968.

McCusker, J., Cherubin, C. F., and Zimberg, S. Prevalence of alcoholism in general municipal hospital population. *New York State Journal of Medicine*, 1971, *71*, 751–754.

Mindlin, D. F. The characteristics of alcoholism as related to prediction of outcome. *Quarterly Journal of Studies on Alcohol*, 1959, *20*, 604–609.

New York City Health Department, Vital Statistics, 1970.

Pattison, E. M., Coe, R., and Rhodes, R. J. Evaluation of alcoholism treatment: A comparison of three facilities. *Archives of General Psychiatry*, 1969, *20*, 478–488.

Sample, R. W., and Mairs, L. S. Chronic alcoholics' rehabilitation: An economic analysis. Unpublished report presented to Gordon A. Howe, Manager, Monroe County, New York, May, 1971.

Schmidt, W., Smart, R. G., and Moss, M. K. *Social class and the treatment of alcoholism*. Toronto: University Press, 1966.

Staff, C., and Peterson, B. *Prevalence of alcoholism among clients in three government service systems: Family court, parole and welfare*. Unpublished report to Manhattan Borough President's Advisory Committee on Alcoholism, 1975.

Zimberg, S. Evaluation of alcoholism treatment in Harlem. *Quarterly Journal of Studies on Alcohol*, 1974, *35*, 550–557.

Zimberg, S. Alcoholism prevalence in general hospital emergency rooms and walk-in clinics. *New York State Journal of Medicine*, 1979, *79*, 1533–1536.

Zimberg, S., Lipscomb, H., and Davis, E. B. Socio-psychiatric treatment of alcoholism in an urban ghetto. *American Journal of Psychiatry*, 1971, *127*, 1670–1674.

Psychotherapy of Adolescent Alcohol Abusers

JAY FISCHER

INTRODUCTION

Teenagers are a highly visible segment of our population. They are a reflection of our own behavior and morals—the carriers of our societal structure. For these reasons we are increasingly concerned about the problem of teenage alcohol abuse. Despite this, we are as yet unclear about the meaning of abuse; nor have we arrived at a satisfactory definition that holds implications for treatment.

Traditionally, teenage problem drinking has been defined in terms of quantity and frequency of alcohol consumption, as well as the presence of alcoholism-related symptomatology (Rachal, 1976). Since adolescent drinking is often characterized by frequent use of limited quantities, any attempt to define problem drinking using quantity and frequency data may lead to false diagnosis or overestimation of the problem. Moreover, such a definition does not allow for the possibility that problem drinking measured in terms of symptomatology associated with years of heavy drinking might not be applicable to adolescent abuse. Alternatively, studies which attempt to assess the extent of adolescent alcoholism, using survey methodology, often produce unrealistically low prevalence rates that are uniquely dependent on how adolescent alcohol abuse is operationally defined (Robertson, 1982). Additionally,

JAY FISCHER • Assistant Director for Management and Administration, The Door-Center of Alternatives, New York, New York.

we are unclear about the extent to which young persons who are diagnosed as alcoholic, or alcohol abusing, cease doing so as a function of maturation (Mandell, 1983). Given this, it would seem that conceptualizing adolescent alcohol abuse in terms of epidemiological concerns (i.e., quantity, frequency, and prevalence) has little direct relationship to treatment considerations. In order to obviate these difficulties, Strauss (1976) has suggested that teenage problem drinking be defined as occurring when "an individual drinks . . . 'too much' as defined by its effect on health, interpersonal relations or ability to fulfill social expectations and meet responsibilities."

Alcohol abuse defined in terms of interference with individual goals would allow us to include those individuals who are abusing alcohol but have yet to experience the physical sequelae of alcoholism. Such a definition also allows us to include teenagers whose abuse is a transitory or temporary phenomenon and who are not likely, therefore, to develop chronic alcoholism. Most important, Strauss' definition holds implications for treatment. By equating drinking with impeding the attainment of goals, it affords a circumscribed area upon which early treatment can be based.

Much of our early work has focused on prevalence, to the detriment of delineating techniques necessary to treat the adolescent abuser. In an attempt to bridge our knowledge gap, this chapter will review some of the characteristics of teenage alcohol abusers. The review is not exhaustive, but focuses on those characteristics and dynamics which are most likely to bring about adolescent alcohol abuse. It is these that must first be considered when planning for the treatment of the teenage abuser. We will then proceed to delineate those strategies and techniques which follow from the characteristics and dynamics of the population.

CHARACTERISTICS OF TEENAGE ALCOHOL ABUSERS: SOME IMPLICATIONS FOR TREATMENT

O'Leary, O'Leary, and Donovan (1976) noted that teenage alcohol abusers tended to choose friends and role models who were heavy drinkers. The importance of the sociocultural environment as a determinant of alcohol abuse is supported by Schuster (1976), who indicated that, within our inner-city ghettos, substance-abusing adolescents are exposed to very high levels of environmental and peer support for their substance abuse.

The alcohol- and drug-abuse peer culture, according to Kamback, Bosma, and D'Lugoff (1977), provides a structure with definite social roles and obligations that compensates for a vague and inconsistent family environment. The abuser's family is often characterized by intense conflicts, familial instability, inconsistent behavior, unclear expectations, and substance abuse, so the adolescent abuser often experiences considerable role and identity confusion, along with arrested emotional development. Although chaotic to the outsider, the substance-abusing peer culture provides a milieu with clear obligations and roles—a setting where the adolescent can establish an identity, albeit dysfunctional. In short, the peer culture serves as a surrogate family.

The dysfunctional family environment often leads to the adolescent's developing marked feelings of depression. These may be masked by aggression or bravura behavior. However, the aggression and bravura may become inadequate coping mechanisms and give rise to alcohol and other substance abuse. During the course of treatment, therefore, efforts should be directed toward helping the adolescent work through any underlying depression and aggression.

Another important factor is parental attitudes toward alcohol. Because parents serve as adult role models, they are instrumental in helping to shape children's attitudes and behavior regarding drinking. It has been my experience that alcohol-abusing teenagers often come from households where parents or parental figures hold overly restrictive or overly permissive attitudes regarding teenage drinking. It is not surprising, therefore, that parental attitudes and drinking practices are important issues in the adolescent's treatment.

It would seem that sociocultural factors (including environmental considerations) are of primary importance in helping to shape *initial* patterns of adolescent abuse. The vast majority of teenagers who drink too much, in terms of alcohol interfering with attainment of goals and responsibilities, do so in order to meet their perceived expectations of social situations (Strauss, 1976). The exact nature of the social situation involved will vary. For inner-city ghetto youth, the need to conform to the drinking and social norms of the "street scene" is of primary importance. For more middle-class adolescents, it may be the need to compete in dating situations, or the desire to gain acceptance in social organizations, such as large peer groups, fraternities, or sororities, for which drinking is often an entry requirement.

In other words, initially, adolescents generally are not physically or psychologically dependent on alcohol, but often manifest anxiety if they are not doing what is thought to be appropriate to gain peer approval or acceptance into desirable social situations. Thus, it is the sociocultural demands that begin to shape initial patterns of abuse. Psychological or even physical factors may then serve to reinforce and maintain deviant alcohol consumption.

From an alcoholism–treatment perspective, the above findings suggest the need for intervention to help the young person develop coping mechanisms for handling existing sociocultural demands without having to resort to alcohol abuse. In terms of a treatment goal, this does not necessarily mean abstinence. A youngster who is just beginning to abuse alcohol in response to sociocultural demands may be able to return to moderate drinking if helped to deal more effectively with existing environmental pressures. This possibility is contraindicated when there is evidence of physiological dependence or a history of other drug abuse. Sometimes, even when there are no obvious contraindications, it may not be possible for the young person to drink socially within his or her existing environment. For example, an inner-city youth for whom daily alcohol and drug consumption is seen as a rite of passage into the "street scene" may find it difficult to alter drinking patterns. A major treatment goal in this case is to help foster the development of alternative social networks. Offering opportunities for patient socialization as part of the treatment program seems an ideal way to accomplish this.

The issue of variable treatment goals with respect to drinking is a complex one, needing additional clarification. The need for variable goals rests on the assumption that there are at least two main types of adolescent and young-adult abusers. These can be labeled the "early" and "advanced" alcohol abuser (Coyle and Fischer, 1977). The "early" abuser is characterized by a short history of alcohol abuse (perhaps not greater than one or two years). His drinking is in response to a particular emotional problem or crisis, with a direct relationship between the precipitating problem and the drinking, a previous history indicating an ability to drink without abusing alcohol, a general absence of symptoms indicating a physiological dependence upon alcohol, and a mild to moderate amount of alcohol-related behavioral problems such as fights, family arguments, or deterioration in school or work functioning. The "advanced" abuser, on the other hand, can be characterized by a pervasive pattern of abuse, no clear relationship between drinking and stressful situations, a prolonged history of alcohol abuse, the presence of alcohol abuse from the onset of drinking, loss-of-control drinking, and marked alcohol-related behavioral problems.

Given the marked contrast of these two groups, it would seem that some variation in treatment goals is in order. Clinical experience (Coyle and Fischer, 1977) suggests that the goal of moderate drinking is best suited to the early-stage abuser. To insist on abstinence for these patients places an unnecessary burden on them and discourages them from continuing treatment (Fischer and Coyle, 1976). The advanced abuser, on the other hand, has already demonstrated an inability to drink moderately, so abstinence would appear to be the necessary treatment objective (Coyle and Fischer, 1977). Staff might question the wisdom of treating patients with such divergent goals within the same program and perhaps even within the same therapy group. One may fear that under such circumstances the likelihood of patient rivalry in terms of hostility between those patients whose goal is abstinence and those whose goal is moderate drinking is increased. Another fear is that all patients would want moderate drinking and be incapable of accepting the need for abstinence. Clinical experience with older adolescents and young adults has shown that these potential problems have not materialized to any great extent, given that patients are adequately prepared for treatment (Coyle and Fischer, 1977).

There are patients who are on the boundary between early and advanced abuse. In these instances, the decision about an appropriate treatment goal becomes more difficult. It may be necessary to allow such patients to experiment with moderate drinking, with an understanding that the goal might have to be amended to abstinence, depending on performance and progress in treatment.

At times, the issue of varying goals becomes a tactical maneuver rather than a preferred goal. Occasionally, patients who should be abstinent may not be ready or willing to accept this. Moderate drinking can then be posited as a tentative goal. The patient may then be more willing to accept abstinence when confronted by peers and staff about his or her inability to sustain moderate drinking.

The possibility of varying treatment goals with respect to drinking is one of the few things that separates adolescent and young-adult treatment from that of the older patient. Since most older patients have a prolonged history of alcohol abuse before they seek treatment (Fischer and Coyle, 1977), as well as more limited ego strengths and coping mechanisms, the option of moderate drinking is less viable.

Differentiation, among alcohol abusing young persons, may also be made according to the individual's overall personality type (character structure) or, phrased alternatively, the characteristic way in which the individual interacts toward others in his or her environment. Mandell (1983) has indicated that youthful alcohol abusers can be classed into three subgroups. The first is the *depressed* individual. The second is the *shy-anxious* young person, while the last is the adolescent chronically exhibiting *low self-esteem*. As in the previous classification scheme, each subgroup has different treatment goals and tasks.

With respect to the depressed young person, the initial goal of treatment is to provide structured tasks to enable the young person to manage better the depressive episodes that underlie the alcohol abuse. For the shy-anxious individual, we must provide a climate in which social skills can be learned in comfort. Last, for the young person with chronic low self-esteem, we must facilitate the restructuring of the young person's interpersonal environment and interactions in such a manner as to allow the client to internalize the right to succeed. As in the previous classification scheme, treatment goals and tasks cannot be separated from the unique characteristics of the population under consideration. Therefore, it would be more difficult for agencies who do not have intensive adolescent treatment experience to develop successful treatment programs. Turanski (1982) provides various cogent arguments for why adolescent alcoholism treatment (in the social service agency context) should best be undertaken by an agency already providing such comprehensive services as alternative education, career counseling legal services, life skills workshops, and so forth. Given the resistances that impinge on the young person's willingness to seek treatment (discussed in the next section), the program or agency that can provide a range of services—seen by the adolescent as not necessarily alcohol related—may have an important mechanism through which an on-going treatment relationship can be established and maintained.

Parallels exist for the private practitioner. Persons treating alcohol-abusing adolescents within a private practice setting should be well-versed in both adolescent and alcoholism treatment. Moreover, they must be prepared, if necessary, to intervene in a variety of systems (e.g., legal, education, health, etc.) that are often seen as being outside the context of traditional therapeutic neutrality.

PROBLEMS ENCOUNTERED IN THE TREATMENT OF ADOLESCENT ALCOHOL ABUSE

Treatment strategies, whether broad or specific, must remain flexible to allow for issues, dynamics, and problems that emerge during the course of treatment. It is therefore useful to consider some problems likely to be encountered by the practitioner, along with their implications for the therapeutic intervention.

Denial. Denial is often the first problem encountered. Since most adolescents begin to abuse alcohol in response to sociocultural peer pressures, it may be difficult for the adolescent to perceive his or her level of consumption as a problem, particularly since peer group members are often consuming the same or greater amounts of alcohol. The therapist should be mindful that any attempt to meet the denial head-on may exacerbate the problem and discourage the youth from seeking treatment. Using the terms *alcoholic, problem drinker, alcohol abuser*, stressing the amount of alcohol consumed, or trying to persuade the adolescent to initially accept the existence of a drinking problem can increase defensiveness and therefore be counterproductive.

A more fruitful approach might be for the therapist, during the course of the initial interview, to help the patient delineate those areas of social functioning felt to be important. Depending on the patient's age (less appropriate for younger adolescents), the inquiry can be broadened to include personal or life goals. Once these have been explored, the therapist may then turn the discussion toward examining how current levels of alcohol consumption interfere with social functioning or attaining personal goals.

An example can be seen in the following case history: James, age 17, was referred by his family doctor because of repeated family fights about James' drinking. James, however, did not see his drinking as a problem and indicated that he did not drink much at all. I sensed James' defensiveness about drinking, but did not verbalize this. Instead I said that since he did come to see me, I wondered if there was anything he would like to talk about, stressing that he could use the time in any way he wanted. He indicated considerable difficulty in making friends, as well as being lonely. Upon further questioning, it became apparent that James saw himself as unlikable and unattractive. He also felt that he could not ask a girl out for a date unless he had a few drinks. I sensed that James' drinking was a way of soothing the hurt from anticipated rejection. Further questioning revealed that he coped with anticipatory rejection by staying in his room or going drinking alone. I commented that sitting at home or drinking alone was not the best way to make friends. Perhaps, I said, we might be able to help him develop social skills and increased self-confidence, thereby making it easier to make friends.

James was able to see that his drinking, which was not labeled excessive or alcoholic, interfered with his goal of making friends. Within this frame of reference, he was able to accept the offer of treatment.

Accepting the Need for Treatment. Helping the patient to see the dysfunctional aspects of current alcohol consumption does not necessarily engage the client in treatment. Adolescents, even if they are aware of a problem, often see treatment as stigmatizing—a sign of weakness, or an indication of their inability to achieve adult status. Moreover, they are fearful that being in treatment precludes socializing with peers who still drink. The adolescent often associates treatment with abstinence, which may, in turn, be equated with social isolation. During the course of the first or second interview, it is therefore a good idea for the therapist to inquire about such beliefs (along with other patient expectations) and, if they exist, to point out that seeking treatment is a sign of health and maturity rather than weakness or immaturity. It should be stressed that being in treatment and associating with peers who drink are not necessarily mutually exclusive, but will depend on the adolescent's ability to handle social and peer pressure without resorting to dysfunctional levels of alcohol consumption.

If, after the first few interviews, the therapist suspects that a change in peer group may be indicated, this suggestion should be withheld until a firm treatment relationship has been established. It is extremely anxiety-provoking for adolescents to contemplate breaking old ties, particularly if they lack self-confidence. A suggestion made prematurely might therefore result in the adolescent's terminating treatment.

Resistance of Family Members or Significant Others. Family members often contribute to the adolescent's resisting treatment. This may be due, in part, to the fear that treatment may disturb the existing social or psychodynamic equilibrium within the family. Parents may also view the need for treatment as indicating that they have not adequately fulfilled their parental role or obligation.

Parental resistances that may sabotage treatment must be actively dealt with. This is often done by requiring the parents or other family members to be in concurrent treatment. Simultaneous treatment of family members is also indicated when familial attitudes toward drinking, drinking practices, and/or family dynamics are related to the adolescent's excessive consumption of alcohol. It is necessary to recognize the adolescent's need for independence by obtaining consent before involving parents or other family members in the treatment process.

The adolescent's peers may also try to dissuade the patient from entering treatment. Many factors contribute to this, such as the fear that their own level of drinking might be called into question or that treatment may lead to the dissolution of the peer group. Friends may react by encouraging the adolescent to drink even more, rather than seek treatment. Recognizing the potential influence of peer group members in determining the level of alcohol consumed has led several treatment programs to establish significant other services for adolescents. The therapist should at all times be mindful of adverse peer pressure and therefore give considerable support to the young person seeking help.

Peer counseling can be effective for motivating the young person to seek treatment. Any suggestion as to the need for, or benefit from, treatment may be more likely to be accepted if made by a peer, than by an adult (Turanski, 1982). Additionally, peer counselors serve as a potent role model and a viable indication to the conflicted adolescent that change is indeed possible and beneficial. Moreover, peer counseling allows young people an opportunity to test out potential career choices. In developing a peer counseling program, be it individual or group counseling, care must be taken to insure that young persons are clear about their limitations as counselors and are not functioning in such a way as to primarily meet their own treatment needs.

Persons to Be Excluded from Treatment

Fortunately, very few youngsters need to be excluded from our treatment programs. Outpatient settings, except where there is the provision for prescription of medication or the backup of institutional facilities, would seem inappropriate for the psychotic or violently acting-out youth. It is also unwise to accept into an outpatient setting those individuals who exhibit chronic medical ailments necessitating frequent absence, since this is disruptive to treatment. The above patients are often best treated within inpatient or day-hospital programs.

Let us now consider the problems posed by the unmotivated adolescent. Should such persons be summarily excluded from treatment? We have already discussed the resistance of most adolescents to begin treatment. Indeed, this resistance or ambivalence is an age-appropriate response. Many adolescents make sporadic contact with agency staff over several months before accepting the offer of ongoing treatment. During this time they are constantly testing out and "sizing up" adult staff. Whether or not their behavior is accepted will be an important determinant in the adolescent's decision to make a treatment commitment. The fact that the patient returns for a second, third, fourth, or even tenth contact—however irregular—should be taken as the beginning of a positive relationship between patient and program, as well as the first sign of a budding interest in treatment. Therefore, the adolescent who maintains a sporadic contact with an agency should not be seen as unsuited for treatment. Recognizing this, it is important for the therapist to use any technique that will serve to strengthen this beginning relationship. Needless to say, the choice of techniques such as warmth, support, confrontation, pressure, and praise should be dictated by the patient's particular history and dynamics.

Treatment of Choice

Let us assume that the adolescent has now made an initial commitment to treatment. We must proceed to develop a long-term treatment plan that provides maximal opportunity for the patient's emotional and interpersonal growth and development. Should such a plan include individual therapy, group therapy, or both?

In general, group therapy is seen to be preferable to individual treatment. The group setting offers increased opportunity to bring into operation such curative factors as positive peer pressure, identification with the experiences of other group members, an opportunity to see that one is not alone in one's problems, and reduced dependency on the therapist. Within the group the adolescent also has the opportunity to observe positive emotional growth and behavioral change in other members. This offers the skeptical adolescent a sense of hope and reinforces both the importance and usefulness of therapy. Moreover, the interpersonal relationship among group members may offer an important opportunity for developing a mutual support system within the group. This human network of caring and concern may bring about important therapeutic changes. I have known several instances in which older-adolescent and young-adult group members have driven long distances or staged week-long telephone vigils in order to dissuade a depressed member from resuming drinking. The recipient of the group's concern has subsequently indicated this to be a positive turning point in treatment. Finally, the group format offers an opportunity for an increased variety of intervention techniques, such as multiple role-playing, psychodrama, and leaderless meetings.

Before placing an adolescent in the therapy group, some preparation is in order, particularly when there has been no prior exposure to group treatment. The therapist should briefly explain the nature of group therapy and the kinds of behavior required for successful participation in the group. At this time, material from previous individual sessions should be reviewed and tentative—but mutually agreed on—treatment objectives should be set. This includes the question of whether the adolescent should abstain from drinking. The factors pointing to the advisability of abstinence as opposed to a change in drinking behavior or a reduction in consumption have already been noted.

There are times, however, when individual treatment is clearly more appropriate. Some adolescents in the initial stages of treatment may be too intimidated by a group. They may be unable to reveal shortcomings and concerns among their peers. This is particularly the case with inner-city adolescents, who often view sharing any weakness, be it emotional or physical, as threatening to their existence in the "street scene." Last, there are those adolescents who are so deprived of attention or who are otherwise so narcissistic that they are unable to tolerate sharing the therapist's concern with other group members. In all these instances, individual therapy is more appropriate. Once the individual has gained sufficient ego strength, individual therapy can be reduced or eliminated.

An example of this can be seen from the following case history. Lucy, age 16, was referred to treatment because of declining scholastic performance, repeated absences, latenesses, and an otherwise lackadaisical attitude. These behaviors became evident six months prior to referral. Prior to that, Lucy was a superior student, but one who was characterized by teachers as "quiet, shy, and somewhat a loner." When I first met Lucy, I was struck by an aura of denial that pervaded her entire conversation. She did not see herself as having any problems, indicated that she drank only occasionally, could not understand why she was "referred" and was resistant to persuing any line of inquiry. I said to her that as long as she was here, was there anything she needed help with? She responded by saying she heard that people can come to the program to learn about jobs. More careful questioning revealed that she was unsure about what she wanted to do, felt that she could not do anything and was frightened about losing her "friends" when she finished high school. I indicated that finishing high school did not necessarily mean losing one's friends, and perhaps she might get some idea about jobs and/or careers from the vocational counselor. I felt that given Lucy's marked low sense of self-esteem and fear of interpersonal relationships, group treatment, at least at the inception, might not be indicated. Lucy, I felt, had to learn how to feel good about herself, along with developing a preliminary vocational-like, work plan. Poor school performance and drinking could be seen as manifestation of conflicts in these important areas. Perhaps if Lucy were able to see some viable options vis-à-vis vocational choices, she would then feel more likely to accept treatment for other areas including her drinking. In short, successful referral to vocational counseling with satisfactory outcome allowed Lucy to acquire enough self-worth to see the value of treatment and to accept the interest of those around her.

Occasionally adolescents who are willing and able to participate in a therapy group may require short-term individual therapy to supplement their group treatment. This need may be indicated by an acute emotional crisis, a sudden decision to drop out of the group, or the need to work through important concerns that cannot, in the opinion of the adolescent, be shared with the group and which, if not resolved, will jeopardize the individual's treatment progress or that of other group members. During these crisis periods I have also found it helpful to suggest that patients attend AA meetings. This gives added support and serves as an additional deterrent to alcohol abuse.

The decision to supplement group treatment with individual interviews is not without risk. Such an action may precipitate patient rivalries or encourage competition within the group for the therapist's attention. Should these behaviors develop, it is imperative that they be worked through during the course of the group meetings. To do otherwise robs patients of an invaluable opportunity to learn about their behavior and also jeopardizes the continuance of the group.

GROUP TREATMENT TECHNIQUES

Given the importance of the group as the treatment of choice, let us now consider some treatment techniques required during each stage of development. For the purposes of discussion, the group will be divided into the beginning and advanced stages. It should be remembered that this division is entirely arbitrary.

The Beginning Stage. Adolescents may anticipate the first meeting with considerable fear. Because they are normally highly concerned about how their peers—other group members—may view them, adolescents are often anxious about beginning "group therapy." The therapist should anticipate this and start the first meeting by sharing his or her feelings about commencing a new group. This often breaks the ice and allows the leader to act as a role model for appropriate and productive group behavior. Moreover, by sharing anxieties, the therapist enables the adolescent to see that feelings of initial apprehension are an appropriate response. It is hoped that this may in turn enable members to discuss their apprehensions, which can be explored during the beginning phase of the group. In instances when the group is unduly anxious, it may be helpful to spend the first few meetings discussing nonthreatening topics of mutual interest. Appropriate areas for conversation may be sports, movies, and the pop-music scene. These informal discussions will give members an opportunity to get to know one another and thereby lessen anxiety. The discussions will also provide the therapist with an excellent opportunity to observe the natural interaction patterns within the group.

The task of the beginning stage is to delineate the way in which members' alcohol and other substance abuse interferes with the attainment of personal goals and social responsibilities. Members should therefore be encouraged to discuss drinking and other drug-taking behavior as well as their personal goals and social responsibilities. This fosters a commonality among members, a factor necessary to insure continued commitment to treatment.

The direction of discussion must be carefully maintained by the therapist; otherwise there is a tendency for members to play the game of "one better" when sharing material relating to substance abuse. The purpose of "one better" is to avoid self-examination (which is a deviation from the group's task) and acquire a high status among the group members by emphasizing the bravura aspects of substance abuse. It must be repeatedly reiterated that the group's purpose is to discuss the dysfunctional aspects of substance abuse, rather than to foster the development of progressively more flamboyant "stories."

Material from these discussions can be used to further the development of the group's cohesiveness and purpose. It should be noted that although underlying problems may vary, each member has chosen to abuse alcohol, and perhaps other substances, in response to sociocultural and intrapsychic pressure. The therapist can then point to the more general purpose of the group, which is to provide an environment in which members can learn to cope with sociocultural pressures and other psychodynamics without having to resort to a level of drinking that impedes the fulfillment of personal goals and social responsibilities.

This often leads to the question of whether one must remain abstinent. In all probability the question will be directed to the therapist, who may be advised to respond by indicating that no absolute prescription can be given. Rather, the advisability of drinking should be determined by the individual's particular response to alcohol consumption.

For some individuals one drink may repeatedly interfere with personal and social responsibilities; in such cases abstinence is the most appropriate goal. For others with a higher tolerance for alcohol and a greater ability to cope with pressure, abstinence may be counterproductive. This whole matter usually sparks quite a heated debate, during which the adolescent may try to challenge the therapist's expertise and authority. It is advisable to allow ample opportunity for discussion, but remind the group that the whole question has already been discussed with each member prior to entering the group. It is advantageous to point out that although goals have been formulated, this does not preclude the possibility of modification or even reversal, based on subsequent performance and progress in treatment. The adolescent should, however, during the early stages of the group, be encouraged to accept the therapist's professional judgment. This should be possible if initial group cohesiveness and commitment to treatment have been established.

During this phase problems with family, school, employment, and legal authorities may emerge. In order to cement the initial treatment relationship, the therapist must be prepared to assume an advocacy role in helping the adolescent successfully negotiate difficulties within each of these systems. Needless to say, the type of advocacy will vary, based on a thorough exploration of the adolescent's problem. Some typical examples may be telephone calls, letter writing, or collateral contacts.

An example can be seen in the following case history: In the fifth meeting of the group, Steve, age 16, indicated that he was in danger of being fired from his part-time job because of repeated lateness. He did not want to lose the job since it was his main source of spending money. After discussing the circumstances surrounding his lateness, I suggested that the group help Steve develop a strategy for convincing his boss not to fire him. Several suggestions were made and we explored each one, using role-playing, until Steve found a strategy he was comfortable with. During the course of the sixth meeting Steve reported that the plan did not work and his boss had decided to fire him. We discussed Steve's anger and depression, and I suggested exploring how Steve might handle the situation. Sue wondered whether a letter from me might help to get Steve his job back. I indicated that I would be prepared to write the letter, provided this was acceptable to Steve and provided the group thought it was a good idea. About three months later Steve commented that his immediate reaction to being fired had been to drop out of the group, but he had decided against this because of my intervention and concern.

The Advanced Stage. While drinking continues to be a major theme during this stage, the group moves slowly to consider alternative coping mechanisms by which stressful situations—both sociocultural and intrapsychic—can be faced without resorting to alcohol and other substance abuse. The transition may develop spontaneously, but is more likely to be brought about by the therapist's intervention. For example: During the course of the tenth meeting, Peter, age 15, mentioned that his drinking was again causing him difficulty in school. Peter had already discussed this at two previous meetings. In response to Peter's discussion, John shared that he was beginning to cut classes in order to drink with friends. The group then launched into a rambling discussion about school problems and drinking. After a short time I noted the common concerns shared by the group and wondered whether members may be looking for some help. I suggested that it might be useful to talk about the need to drink during school hours.

During the 11th and 12th meetings, the discussion shifted to the conscious reasons for drinking. Some members discussed fears of being rejected if they did not drink with friends during school hours. Others said that drinking relieved the boredom of school, while one member felt that drinking would enhance his social desirability among girls.

At the beginning of the 13th session I posed the following question: How might you decline an offer to drink during school and still remain "cool" with friends? The members made several suggestions which were then "tried out" within the safety of the group, using role-playing and sociodrama.

By now the group should have begun to develop a definite sense of cohesiveness and commitment. If this is the case, the focus will gradually shift from discussing sociocultural reasons for drinking, e.g., peer pressure, dates, the street scene, to reasons that involve more personal concerns, such as loneliness, alienation, rage, and sexual identity. Moreover, there is an additional shift toward helping the members work through the pain associated with these newly expressed concerns. As before, the therapist is also concerned with helping the group develop alternatives to alcohol abuse.

An example of an advanced-stage group can be seen in the following case history: At the beginning of the 25th meeting, Sam, age 17, indicated that he had drunk heavily the previous week. Larry asked why, since Sam had been able to drink socially for the last two months. It seemed that at the time Sam resumed heavy drinking, he had been thinking about his father who had died four years before. Sam appeared to be in considerable pain—perhaps on the verge of tears. The group responded by questioning Sam in a gentle and supportive manner. Sam related that his father died from cirrhosis of the liver brought about by heavy drinking. We asked Sam to describe his father, at which time he became silent. With further probing and support, Sam was able to vent pent-up rage. He hated his father for repeatedly assaulting his mother and siblings. He also hated the fact that his father spent the family's money on drinking, which meant his mother had to go to work. Over the next several sessions it became apparent that Sam harbored considerable guilt in relation to these feelings and felt responsible for his father's death. The group helped Sam accept that, under the circumstances, his feelings of hate were to be expected and that, in reality, they did not cause the death of his father. Sam was gradually able to accept this, and his need to abuse alcohol (which was used to block out these painful feelings) diminished. The working-through was a slow process, but by the end of the 40th session Sam had become totally abstinent. He was able to maintain sobriety by continuing to attend the group, as well as local AA meetings.

This case is an illustration of the fluidity of goals concerning drinking. The initial goal for Sam was that of moderate drinking. One may question the soundness of this prescription since Sam is a child of an alcoholic father and therefore at increased risk of developing alcoholism. Yet his history did not reveal any incidence of prolonged alcohol abuse or other aspects characteristic of the advanced abuser. His drinking was a response to feelings of panic, which revolved around what he would do after finishing high school. In almost all respects, Sam could be considered an early-stage abuser. Therefore, moderate drinking was seen to be the goal of choice. As the group helped him to deal with plans following high school, along with deeper emotional problems, his need for drinking lessened. The decision to choose abstinence was Sam's, not the therapist's. He felt that although he could drink moderately, he had to be more mindful about monitoring his consumption, so drinking made him less rather than more spontaneous. His decision was respected by both the group and the therapist. Before he left the group, Sam indicated that it was important for him to have arrived voluntarily at the decision of abstinence. Had he been "urged," he said, he would have resisted. Too often we assume that the question of modified treatment goals is the province of the therapist and not the patient.

Treatment of the adolescent (and perhaps the young adult as well) differs in two main respects from that of the older patient. The first, as previously noted, is the issue of differential goals with respect to drinking. The second difference involves the degree of therapist activity needed to treat the adolescent abuser. As an illustration, let us consider the patient who must appear in court. If an older patient is facing legal difficulties, I might write a letter. With an adolescent, however, I might be more inclined to accompany him or her to court and make my intervention in person. In short, treating the adolescent requires much more activity on the therapist's part.

Another aspect of activity is the degree to which the therapist is required to "get down" to the level of the patient. With adolescents and young adults, I am more involved, show more of my own feelings, and share more technical dilemmas as they arise within treatment; I am also more prone to use humor, more inclined to share and explore existential uncertainties, more inclined to be silly or frivolous, and more accepting of social chatter involving sports, movies, or the pop scene. More frequently I provide reasonable answers to reasonable questions and am less concerned with the underlying motivation for a particular question. Last, I am more inclined to interact with patients outside the formal treatment setting, provided there is a potential therapeutic gain that can be realized from such interactions. An example of this occurred in Scotland, where a young-adult treatment group met in a pub, following alternate group-therapy sessions (Coyle and Fischer, 1977). Patients whose goal was abstinence had to learn how to buy drinks for others while ordering nonalcoholic beverages for themselves. Patients whose treatment goal was moderate drinking were able to learn to pace their consumption. This practice reflects a basic postulate of treatment discussed earlier: to help the young person cope with sociocultural pressures without resorting to alcohol abuse. From the above discussion it can be seen that the therapist who is a blank screen or a detached professional does not have a place in adolescent treatment.

Problems Arising within the Group

Let us now briefly consider those problems the therapist may encounter during the running of a group. The first problem is that of disruption. In a beginning group, members are often afraid to confront the disruptive member lest they be the target of future confrontation. If this is the case, the therapist might ask why members are reluctant to discuss the disruption. In extreme cases it may be necessary to ask the disruptive member to leave. In a more advanced group, however, members are willing to deal with disruption, which then becomes an important topic for discussion.

The second problem is posed by the nonverbal patient. In the beginning group, the therapist should take an active role. Such questions as "I wonder what is on your mind?" or "I wonder why you have not said anything?" may help to stimulate material. Often the nonverbal patient is extremely frightened about being in the group. Because the fear is not verbalized, the therapist must rely on nonverbal indicators, such as tics, shifting about, and tension in the arms and legs. Often, upon gentle probing or questioning, the patient will verbalize and then explore the anxiety. It is also possible that the nonverbal patient uses silence to become the focus of the group's attention. This should be pointed out and discussed with the group. In the case of the advanced group, the members can usually encourage the nonverbal patient to speak. In fact, interventions by experienced group members are often more effective than those of the therapist.

The last problem is that posed by the intoxicated patient. As part of the preparation for group treatment, I always tell patients that they will not be allowed to attend the group if intoxicated. The presence of intoxicated individuals usually causes a great deal of disruption; limits need be set to ensure the smooth running of the group. Although patients readily accept this, there is a periodic need to challenge either the therapist or the group. Perhaps it is a way of communicating anger. In general, patients who arrive intoxicated are asked to leave and return for the next group meeting, when their intoxication can reasonably become material for group discussion.

SUMMARY

This chapter has reviewed some of the characteristics of teenage alcohol abusers which have served to bring about and then maintain the abusive drinking pattern. It would appear that most adolescents begin to abuse alcohol in response to sociocultural pressures. Intrapersonal problems may serve to maintain abuse. The task of treatment, therefore, is to provide an environment in which the individual can learn to cope with sociocultural and emotional stress without resorting to alcohol abuse.

The problems encountered in beginning treatment were reviewed. The three main problems are denial, the adolescent's resistance, and the resistance of family members and peers. Several ways to overcome these problems were suggested.

In planning ongoing treatment it would appear that group therapy is generally superior to individual sessions. Reasons for this were discussed, as were the instances when group therapy is contraindicated. The therapy group undergoes a series of developmental changes. The beginning-stage group is characterized by considerable member anxiety and lack of clarity. The therapist must work actively to lessen anxiety and build group cohesiveness and treatment commitment. The task of the beginning group is to explore the relationship between drinking and interference with personal goals or responsibilities.

Once initial cohesiveness and commitment have been established, the group moves into the advanced stage. In the beginning of this stage, discussion is characterized by exploration of drinking behavior. As the group develops, however, the focus shifts to exploring and then "trying out" alternative coping mechanisms for dealing with sociocultural pressure. In the latter part of the advanced stage, the focus shifts from exploring external causes for drinking toward considering the intrapersonal factors involved. Members are helped to work through the pain associated with these and are helped to develop more adequate coping mechanisms. Problems encountered during the course of the group's development are also considered.

References

Coyle, B., and Fischer, J. A young problem drinker's programme as a means of establishing and maintaining treatment contact. In J. H. Madden, R. Walker, and W. H. Kenyon (Eds.), *Alcoholism and drug dependence—a multi-disciplinary approach*. New York: Plenum Press, 1977.

Fischer, J., and Coyle, B. Treating young problem drinkers. *Focus*, 1976, *49*, 12–14.

Fischer, J., and Coyle, B. A specialized treatment service for young problem drinkers (16–30 years): Treatment results obtained during the first six months of the treatment programme. *British Journal of Addiction*, 1977, *72*, 317–319.

Kamback, M. C., Bosma, W. G., and D'Lugoff, B. C. Family surrogates. The drug culture or the methadone maintenance program. *British Journal of Addiction*, 1977, *72*, 171–176.

Mandell, W., *Personal communication*, 1983.

O'Leary, D. E., O'Leary, M. R., and Donovan, D. M. Social skill acquisition and psychosocial development of alcoholics: A review. *Addictive Behavior*, 1976, *1*, 111–120.

Rachel, J. V. Defining adolescent alcohol abuse: Measurements used and results from a national study of junior and senior high school students. In P. S. O'Gorman, S. Stringfield, and I. Smith (Eds.), *Defining adolescent alcohol use: Implications toward a definition of adolescent alcoholism*. New York: The National Council on Alcoholism, 1976.

Robertson, J. Problem assessment for adolescents with alcohol problems. In D. Leslie (Ed.), *New perspectives for youth treatment: Book of readings*. Rockville: National Institute on Alcohol Abuse and Alcoholism, 1982.

Schuster, R. Trust: Its implication in the etiology and treatment of psychopathic youths. *International Journal of Offender Therapy*. 1976, *3*, 128–133.

Strauss, R. Conceptualizing alcoholism and problem drinking. In P. S. O'Gorman, S. Stringfield, and I. Smith (Eds.), *Defining adolescent alcohol use: Implications toward a definition of adolescent alcoholism*. New York: The National Council on Alcoholism, 1976.

Turanski, J. A treatment approach to youth with alcohol related problems. In D. Leslie (Ed.), *New perspectives for youth treatment: Book of readings*. Rockville: National Institute on Alcohol Abuse and Alcoholism, 1982.

17

Management of Children of Alcoholics

Joseph C. Kern

Introduction

There are large numbers of children of alcoholics in the United States, but there have been only two attempts to arrive at scientifically derived estimates of prevalence in recent years. One is provided by Booz-Allen and Hamilton, Inc. (1974); a more recent one by Woodside (1982).

In 1974, Booz-Allen and Hamilton, Inc. reported that there were 28 million children of alcoholics (COA) in the United States. Woodside, in 1982, reviewed the methodology employed by them and concluded that this was an overestimation. Instead, she found that, based on corrected methodology, there are 6,988,103 children under age 20, of alcoholics in the United States, or 9.6% of that age group.

An equally important statistic is the number of adult children, over age 20, of alcoholics. Although it is commonly reported that adult COA are found in abundance in alcoholism treatment facilities (Woodside, 1982), a sound, scientifically based prevalence estimate is lacking. Those that are available have used adult patient populations currently enrolled in treatment programs. There is a clear trend that points to a link between being a child of an alcoholic and developing adult alcoholism. As early as 1933, Pohlisch reported that 47% of fathers of alcoholics he studied were also alcoholics and, as recently as 1982, Woodside reported that 58% of alcoholics enrolled in the New York State operated alco-

Joseph C. Kern • Nassau County Department of Drug and Alcohol Addiction, Hempstead, New York; Lehman College, City University of New York, Bronx, New York.

holism treatment rehabilitation units had at least one alcoholic parent. This range of statistics has been repeatedly reported both in the literature and by clinical and program directors.

We do not know the prevalence of adult COA. COA carry their childhood problems into adulthood. As will be explained in more detail later, these problems take many forms and include addictions (i.e., alcoholism, food, work, gambling, etc.), compulsive and rigid behavior patterning and medical, psychological, and interpersonal problems.

Personality Characteristics of COA

Children who live with chronic stress and crisis develop a variety of problems. Children living with a disabled parent develop an array of psychological, social, and interpersonal problems. As the children adjust to the chronic nature of the parental illness, they learn to avoid the honest and spontaneous expression of feelings since this might worsen the condition of the ill parent. They also learn to limit their demands for emotional and social support and finally lose touch with both their feelings and needs. The chronic nature of the parent's illness takes center stage and they tend to limit and withhold their needs in favor of the ill parent. This results in raising children who are out of touch with their needs and who assume that adults are not consistent sources of support and gratification. Additional information on family dysfunction and distinctive roles of children in alcoholic families can be seen in Chapter 8 in this book on family therapy.

COA share many of the problems of children living with other disabilities, but clinicians report that COA have these special difficulties: (1) The scope and depth of the child's problems persist long after the chronic drinking has ended and, in fact, does persist down through the generations with or without active alcoholism.

Long after the alcoholic parent is sober, removed from the home by separation, divorce, or death, the child still persists with destructive attitudinal and behavioral problems. They continue into adolescence and adulthood and color the entire complexion of relationships and child-bearing practices. (2) The process by which the child's problems develop and persist are marked by greater compulsion, rigidity, and delusional quality of beliefs and values.

Compulsion. COA develop various survival strategies (discussed later) in order to exist from day-to-day. These survival strategies are reinforced very frequently and because they work—the child has survived another day. The irony and tragedy is that various coping mechanisms that sustain survival in childhood are very destructive in adolescence and adulthood. For example, one survival strategy of COA, the "family hero", is to try and rescue the family from alcoholism by their good deeds. The child tries to control the alcoholism and rescue the family from disaster by being perfect and hence, a source of pride to the family. This behavior is reinforced very frequently by the alcoholic family ("At least I can depend on my Michael to be responsible around here" says the sober parent). Schools and teachers reinforce this behavior through awards of excellence and high grades and a visibly responsible role in the community. Hence, this mechanism is "stamped into" the child as *the* single best way to cope with feelings and gain approval. The child does not experience a variety and range of ways of coping with stress (e.g., express anger through talking it out), but has learned only one way to get along in life—by being a perfectionist.

For COA, the compulsive nature of this coping mechanism results in being trapped with a rigid personality in adolescence or young adulthood. All attempts at problem-solving are approached in the same inflexible manner. The repetition of the same stress reducing mechanisms in adolescence and adulthood produces the opposite of healthy relationships because the children cannot choose from a variety of anxiety-reducing and problem-solving mechanisms. Instead, they are driven to use the only one they learned in the alcoholic home. Errors in judgment enter as the growing child is unable to match a coping strategy with a reality problem and instead applies the same problem-solving strategy to all new situations, regardless of its appropriateness.

The child's response to anxiety, stress, and reality problems is determined while living with alcoholism. The preferred survival strategy (PSS) becomes the only way the child knows to adapt to new situations and problems. The strategy takes on strong anxiety-reducing properties and hence, becomes what Allport (1961) describes as "functionally autonomous."

The compulsive nature of the child's response to stress can be altered through appropriate intervention, preferably in an alcoholism specific treatment agency or, if one is not available, in a mental health clinic with alcoholism specific trained staff. Also, participation in the Al-Anon groups Alateen and Adult Children of Alcoholics is essential.

Rigidity. The compulsive nature of the child's response to chronic stress in the alcoholic home is matched with a rigid insistence that it works. Life calls for a variety of responses based on an assessment of the reality of a situation and evaluation of possible alternate responses by the individual. A critical part of the maturing process is to learn by trial and error which response fits various situations.

COA experience very few mature adult role models for stress reduction. The range of responses by the alcoholic family is limited and stereotyped. Rather than responding to the stress of alcoholism with a variety of appropriate responses, alcoholic families rigidily fixate on a single set of strategies. Although these are effective in the short-term by promoting physical survival, in the long run they are ineffective.

For example, a 16-year-old family "scapegoat" may rigidly continue his acting-out behavior despite the fact that his alcoholic father is in recovery and his mother in Al-Anon. His teenage misbehavior served the purpose of drawing attention away from the alcoholism. Now that the family secret is public, he no longer needs to misbehave. Yet, the rigidity of his response to family alcoholism (learned over the course of 12 to 15 years) is such that he simply does not know how else to cope with life and to get attention from the family. The child needs to learn how to obtain acceptance from the family in an age appropriate manner; at the same time, the entire family must alter their distorted perceptions and expectations of him.

Rigid means fixed and unbending. COA do not see the changing realities of life, even during sobriety, and fixate on time honored stress reducing coping mechanisms. Their loyalty to them, persisting long after they have served their purpose, speaks to their addiction to destructive attitudes and behaviors that accompany the physical addiction of the alcoholic.

Delusional Quality of Beliefs and Values. The alcoholic home is the training ground for the teaching of a belief system that is encapsulated within the household and bears minimal resemblance to the real world. The child believes that the alcoholic family's values and beliefs are facts. Rather than "checking them out" with the real world, they become self-deluded into generalizing from their unique and very private experience to the rest of reality outside the home. They are unable to accept the pain of corrective feedback from the environment and continue in their distorted views. The COA personality rigidly reinforces the false set of beliefs. The inability to learn from reality and experience leads to continual conflict and need deprivation. These false beliefs are based on the denial of the alcoholism as the major problem in the family.

What are some of these false beliefs? Wegscheider (1981) has outlined the "rules" of the alcoholic home developed and learned over the years of active alcoholism and continued into adulthood. These rules form the core of the alcoholic family's delusional belief system that, in turn, children of alcoholics come to accept as representative of reality. The manifestation of these rules in the form of destructive attitudes and behavior has been graphically summarized by Al-Anon Adult Children of Alcoholics (1979). Their list of 14 "characteristics of adults who grew up in alcoholic households" has been derived by wide experience with adult children of alcoholics. Table 1 compares the rules learned in childhood in the alcoholic home with their adult manifestations.

The first 3 rules lead to the children not being able to identify problems within themselves as the source of their unhappiness. Problems in the family are externalized and projected onto the environment. Although the children internalize guilt and responsibility, in accepting responsibility for the family chaos, they learn that the route to change is someone else's responsibility. The result is children who are unable to focus on themselves.

Rules 4 and 5 deal with taking risks. For children to learn and grow they must be able to "try out" new behaviors in the world within the protection of a family that provides freedom for exploration as well as setting limits.

Children living in alcoholic homes do not have this luxury. These rules teach the child to accept the minimum that life has to offer. They learn not to ask for anything (physically or emotionally) since this might precipitate another explosion in the household. They watch and wait and slowly give up the expectation that adults can be responsive individuals.

A critical issue here is that of abandonment. The ultimate rejection is to be physically abandoned. Children will do anything to avoid this terror. The implicit threat of abandonment is everpresent in the alcoholic home. It may not be articulated, but being egocentric by their very nature, COA will assume that the chronic chaos in the household will result in their abandonment. The question for the child is how to avoid it. The answer is not to ask for anything. The ultimate realization of this process is that the children believe that they alone can satisfy their own needs without outside connections or help. Largely, children of alcoholics find it difficult to develop warm, open relationships with others. This requires a perception of need and that the children understand they need other people in order to be complete and fulfilled. They need experiences with adults they can trust and whose behavior is predictable. Therefore, they are deluded in the belief that they can be "encapsulated" as self-sufficient individuals. Obviously, this false belief results in tremendous problems for COA, especially in the areas of social isolation and fears of abandonment.

School counselors and therapists report that COA are resistant to intervention and change. One of the reasons is that they are taught to keep the "family secret" and not to ask for help. They see their parents struggle with the alcoholism, however unsuccessfully, without self-help or therapeutic intervention. Modeling their parents, they assume that outside intervention is not necessary and that "the family can solve its own problems." Hence, it is not surprising that COA are resistant to interventions from outside agencies and helpers. Ways of overcoming this block to help will be discussed later in this chapter.

Rules 6 and 7 flow directly from the earlier ones. Here the child learns three self-delusional beliefs: (1) together with the earlier rules, that alcoholism is not the problem; (2) that loyalty to the family is essential—talking to outsiders is a sign of disloyalty, and (3) that one's mature expression of feelings is forbidden.

Prior to intervention and treatment, the alcoholic family believes

TABLE 1. COMPARISON OF CHILDHOOD "RULES" OF ALCOHOLIC HOME[a] AND THEIR ADULT MANIFESTATION[b,c]

Rules of alcoholic home learned during childhood	Adult manifestation
1. The alcoholic's use of alcohol is *the* most important thing in the family's life.	We became approval seekers and lost our identity in the process.
	We have an overdeveloped sense of responsibility and it is easier for us to be concerned with others rather than ourselves as this enables us not to look too closely at our faults.
	We confuse love and pity and tend to "love" people we can "pity" and "rescue."
2. Alcohol is not the cause of the family's problems.	We judge ourselves harshly and have a very low sense of self-esteem.
	Para-alcoholics are reactors rather than actors.
3. Someone or something else caused the alcoholic's dependency; he is not responsible.	We get guilt feelings when we stand up for ourselves instead of giving in to others.
	We became addicted to excitement.
4. The status quo must be maintained at all costs.	We either become alcoholics, marry them—or both—or find another compulsive personality such as a workaholic to fulfill our sick abandonment needs.
	We live life from the viewpoint of victims and are attracted by that weakness in our love and friendship relationships.
	We are dependent personalities who are terrified of abandonment and will do anything to hold on to a relationship in order not to experience painful abandonment feelings which we received from living with sick people who were never there emotionally for us.

continued

TABLE 1.   (*continued*)

Rules of alcoholic home learned during childhood	Adult manifestation
5. Everyone in the family must be an "enabler."	Alcoholism is a family disease and we became paraalcoholics and took on the characteristics of that disease even though we did not pick up a drink.
6. No one may discuss what is really going on in the family, either with one another or with outsiders.	We became isolated and afraid of authority figures.
7. No one may say what he is really feeling.	We are frightened by angry people and any personal criticism. We have stuffed our feelings from our traumatic childhoods and have lost the ability to feel or express our feelings because it hurts so much [denial].

[a] From Wegscheider (1981).
[b] As developed by Al-Anon COA, 1979.
[c] As adapted by Kern, 1983.
  Note: The relationships above do not suggest a discrete cause–effect but, rather, suggestive ways in which "rules" act as the basis for adult COA attitudes/behaviors.

the societal myth that alcoholism is a moral issue. They accept this stigmatization and will define the problem as anything except alcoholism. In an attempt to define the family's problem, COA will assume that their behavior is the cause of the family's problems. As will be discussed later, intervention steps with COA should begin with this in mind and gradually move toward helping the child identify with a disease model of alcoholism.

COA remain loyal to their alcoholic parent. This is puzzling to counselors who only see the child as being victimized by the alcoholic's behavior. The loyalty is based on the shared family secret (i.e., alcoholism) which all have implicitly denied. The shared secret is one of the few bonds of intimacy that hold the family together. For the child, talking to outsiders is breaking the bond and a sign of family disloyalty.

There is an additional factor that reinforces the child's loyalty to the alcoholic. Skinner (1969) has shown how human behavior is shaped by various schedules of reinforcement. If a child is rewarded for desired behavior every time, he will continue that behavior until such time as the positive reinforcements cease. The behavior will completely drop out of his repertoire once reinforcement is withdrawn. This is what is called a *continuous reinforcement schedule*. The other option is what Skinner called a *partial reinforcement* schedule. Here the child is reinforced on a random basis for desired behavior. When reinforcements cease, the child will still perform the desired behavior for long periods of time. The expectation of reward drives the child to perform the desired behavior because he never knows if and when reinforcement will occur.

COA are on a partial reinforcement schedule. The alcoholic can be punishing, surly, and physically abusive while intoxicated; yet cordial, effusive, and responsible when sober. The child will attempt to initiate behavior that is designed to control the alcoholic's behavior. The child is never able to accomplish a "match" between his controlling behavior and the outcome as displayed in the alcoholic's behavior. Some of the child's behavior seems to "work" in being reinforced by the alcoholic in a positive way at one time; while at another, when the alcoholic is intoxicated, the child's behavior "fails" in the sense that the child is punished. Hence, the child's behavior is "partially" reinforced.

Skinner has shown that children on such a partial schedule of reinforcement will persist in such behavior long after reinforcement ceases. The overwhelming desire of the child is to be accepted and loved by the alcoholic parent. For years, the child will persist in yearning for and shaping his behavior to elicit acceptance from the alcoholic parent. This fantasy of the child will persist for years in the expectation that there is something he can do to "win over" the alcoholic parent.

It is easier for children to reject a parent who is continuously negative and punishing; which is the healthy response for them, but the children living in an alcoholic home, despite anger and rage, live in the delusion that they can make the alcoholic well. Hence, they never let go of the yearning for acceptance by the alcoholic parent.

Children also see human behavior in simplistic cause–effect terms. They see alcohol being consumed by the alcoholic and followed by his bizarre behavior. This is a primitive, but understandable, explanation of the alcoholic's immediate behavior. On the other hand, they generally do not see the sober parent drinking and hence, cannot understand the difficult behavior of the sober parent. For them, the sober parent has little reason to be nonsupportive of them. Unlike the ingestions of alcohol, they cannot see their silent suffering and despair and the subtle loss of energy and hopelessness. The children are more often critical of the sober parent since they cannot see any visible reason for their lack of energy and involvement with them.

Finally, children of alcoholics learn very early to deny their feelings and not to take the risk of honest, spontaneous expression. They function at a primitive level of need gratification—survival—and rarely move to higher order needs. As Maslow (1968) has indicated, individuals have to have "lower order needs" (i.e., physical safety) met before they are capable of asking for and having "higher level needs" (i.e., love, recognition) met. COA often remain at that safety level and give up the expectation of having higher order needs met.

This situation is especially evident in the handling of anger. They do not see the healthy expression of anger and resolution of conflict in the alcoholic home. The honest expression of anger is too great a risk to take; the child might be rejected again and possibly abandoned. Hence, they will tolerate tremendous abuse and neglect without a proportional emotional response to their treatment. As anger is suppressed, the related feelings of joy and intimacy are also lost. Having years of practice of not expressing feelings in a spontaneous manner, they eventually lose touch with what they are feeling. The end result of this process is children who cannot identify their emotional needs, much less ask them to be met.

In terms of the delusional quality of children of alcoholics, the above process results in children who believe that they do not have the right to feelings (especially anger); that they can only expect minimal needs of a survival nature being met; and that they should not ask for what they need. This results in adult children of alcoholics who are terrified of abandonment and change and will "put up" with disasterous marriages and interpersonal relationships; who are fearful of authority figures and who ask for very few things physically or emotionally; they are physical and emotional "door mats" who do not put themselves first in family or interpersonal relationships.

ROLES PLAYED BY COA IN ALCOHOLIC FAMILIES

Beyond the compulsion, rigidity, and delusional quality characteristic of COA, what specific problems do they exhibit? Two problem areas warrant special attention because of their critical importance in developing an appropriate treatment plan: The first deals with stereotyped roles of COA developed in their families and the other with their developmental problems.

Wegscheider (1981) has described the roles COA develop in the alcoholic household. The roles are developed largely on the basis of birth order and take on significance because the children confuse the roles they play with their real selves and these roles become fixed and provide very poor need gratification. Table 2 summarizes the roles, feeling states, and outcomes and will be discussed briefly below.

TABLE 2. ROLE STRUCTURE FOR CHILDREN OF ALCOHOLICS[a]

Role	Visible characteristics	True feelings	Value to family	Without help	With help
Family hero	Achievement Happy—"smiling" Good—pleases people	Failure Guilt Low self-esteem Humiliated	Pride Takes focus off of the alcoholism	Workaholic Escapes intimacy Frenetic life style Emotionally blocked	Good executives Able to be open and vulnerable Accept failure Slower pace in life
Scapegoat	Angry Defiant/acts out	Failure Rage Guilt Low self-esteem	Takes the focus off of the alcoholism; often the identified patient	Legal problems Defiant of authority Drug/alcohol problems	Sensitive Abandons rage Good counselor potential
Lost Child	Withdrawn Isolated	Powerless Unemotional	Relief	Emotionally shallow Withdrawn Passive Drug/alcohol problems	Assertive Creative and imaginative Artistic
Mascot	Clowning "Life of the party"	Terror Hysterical	Comic relief	Fragile/poor stress tolerance Compulsive clown Drug/alcohol problems	Appropriate humor Ability to handle stress

[a] Adapted from Wegscheider (1981).

Family Hero. This is usually the oldest child in the family who quickly asserts their alliance with the sober spouse. They are the "good child" who become the stable source of dependability in a chaotic family. They have an excellent reputation in the school and community, achieving good marks, excelling in sports and club activities, and going out of their way to be helpful. Their role in the family is to "fix it"—to rescue the family from disaster. However, their good deeds of rescue are to no avail; no matter how well they do, their parent still continues to drink and the family slides into disaster. Family heroes do not see themselves as successful. Their attempts to rescue the family have met with failure and they harbor a deep sense of guilt about their alleged failure and a crushing sense of low self-esteem. Behind the smile is a child who is constantly self-critical and humiliated by the alcoholism. This is an important role for a child to play in an alcoholic family since the parents can point to their oldest child as proof that they are "good parents." Untreated, this child will become addicted to work or some other form of compulsive behavior. Unable to tolerate the pain of failure, or intimacy, they move into high energy professions which are demanding and take them away from the opportunity for warm intimate relationships. Since they have to understand that they were trapped in a survival role as a child and now have the chance to change, it is critical that the family hero enter treatment in an alcoholism specific treatment agency, even though they may not present a primary alcoholism problem.

Scapegoat. This child, who usually is second in birth order, realizes that their older sibling has a corner on being "good;" being older, they are more skilled and well-liked in the family and the community. The scapegoat develops a strategy for getting the family's attention by developing defiant, angry behavior. Although negative and disapproving, it is better than no attention at all. They develop a surly, arrogant, defiant posture which belies their feelings of failure and guilt. Like the family hero, they are trying to create change in the family by acting-out, but they feel failure in that their bad deeds have not netted any improvement. Every alcoholic family believes unconsciously that they should have a scapegoat! They become the identified problem so that the alcoholism can be hidden and the family's problems misdiagnosed as having an acting-out child. Although the hero is family oriented, the scapegoat is peer oriented and will often turn to drugs and alcohol as acts of defiance. This is the child who is most likely to be referred for treatment. It is critical that the counselor see this child as part of a dysfunctional alcoholic family and not as the identified patient. Alcoholic families cannot tolerate this child getting well; that takes the focus off of the child's behavior and runs the risk of exposing the alcohlism. Hence, it is preferable that the whole family be engaged in treatment. If this is not possible, it is critical that at least one parent also be in treatment, preferably in their own modality and, as appropriate, with the scapegoated child.

Lost Child. This is commonly the third child in the birth order and who is quickly overwhelmed by their older siblings (who are expending tremendous energy in their respective roles). Unable to find an opening in the family system, this child simply gives up. Characterized as withdrawn and a follower, the lost children isolate themselves both emotionally and physically from the center of activity. Neither excelling nor failing, they limit their demands on the family and slide into a powerless role and an extended fantasy life. Unlike their older siblings, they have very few living skills. They need long-term individual treatment since they have had little practice in developing in-depth relationships and in being independent and assertive. Being high risk for drug/alcohol problems, this child can also exhibit sexual identity problems and is often the victim of incest. During treatment, their fantasy life can be unraveled in a productive manner by encouraging artistic expression.

Mascot. Frequently the youngest in the alcoholic family, the family mascot present themselves as carefree, fun-loving children. Unable to compete with the older serious hero and the surly scapegoat siblings, they adopt a clowning strategy in attempting to gain parental attention and relieve family tension. Despite apparent conviviality, they feel a sense of hysterical terror. They are afraid of losing touch with reality. The alcoholism, by now, has progressed and the family is further deteriorating. They see the deterioration; hear the fights; see the drinking—yet are told there are no problems in the family. The hero is so invested in presenting a perfect family image, that they will tell the mascot what they see, feel and hear are not true. After awhile the mascot provides welcome comic relief; they always have a "wise crack" even in the midst of family chaos. Mascots are frequently hyperactive in school; have short attention spans and end up in classes for the learning or emotionally disabled. They cannot tolerate stress and are frequently anxious. Commonly misdiagnosed in school settings, they should be seeing the school's addiction specialist instead of being prescribed antihyperactive drugs unless there is well-documented evidence of attention-deficit disorder. Given appropriate alcoholism–specific treatment, the mascot can learn to manage stress, tolerate feelings, and exhibit humor in an appropriate manner.

These roles are a general characterization of a child's life in an alcoholic home. Each child individualizes their own, based not only on birth order, but also on sex of the alcoholic, the stage of progression of the alcoholism, sex of the child, number of siblings, and developmental level, to which we now turn.

DEVELOPMENTAL PROBLEMS OF COA

Ackerman (1983) had detailed the 8 stages of human development according to Erikson (1963). Table 3 is a summary of these stages with notes of the risk factors for children of alcoholics on each level. Each stage builds on the last one and is the basis for entering the next one in a stable, healthy manner. Without the completion of earlier stages, later ones become almost impossible to accomplish. COA do not have difficulty at all eight stages. However, development begins to be arrested when the alcoholism takes on chronic, debilitating features in the family. If the alcoholism became acute when a child is a late adolescent, he may escape with minimal effects, but for younger adolescents and children in the family, the damage can be devastating.

The clear implication is that COA will, of course, grow physically, but will stop growing developmentally. Hence, a COA therapist may be working with a seventeen-year-old family scapegoat who developmentally is a latency age child. Once growth restarts, the adolescent will need to accomplish development tasks of latency age before able to finish those of adolescence.

Erikson's (1963) 8 stages of development provide useful insights in understanding COA and developing working treatment plans. COA do respond well to intervention and treatment and generally are surprisingly resilient.

Table 4 shows a checklist of COA characteristics that has been discussed here and can be found in the literature. These characteristics should be looked for when interviewing COA and their families.

There is some evidence that COA may have a higher prevalence of hyperactivity, or as in DSM-III, attention-deficit disorder. Cantwell (1972) has studied this question and supports this observation. Therefore, it is necessary to do a differential diagnosis of COA who are hyperactive or who have had learning disabilities to determine if they meet the attention-deficit disorder criteria. If so, treatment for this condition should be provided along with treatment for psychological consequences that occur in children of alcoholics.

A small number of children born of alcoholic mothers may have a fetal alcohol syndrome due to the intrauterine effect of alcohol. This syndrome consists of prenatal and/or postnatal growth retardation, central nervous defects leading to mild to moderate mental retardation and

Table 3. Erikson's Developmental Stages as They Relate to Children of Alcoholics[a]

Stage	Age	Risk Factors for COA
Trust versus Mistrust	First year	Maternal deprivation by alcoholic mother; emotional unavailability due to drain of alcoholism; inconsistent nurturing.
Autonomy versus Shame/Doubt	Two to four	Limit setting either excessive, leading to self-doubt, or extremes in discipline resulting in timidity.
Initiative versus Guilt	Four to seven	Playful curiosity and testing of limits suppressed due to chronic tension in the alcoholic home; unpredictable inconsistent responses to child's curiosity lead to suppression of creative urge—all resulting in guilt. Role modeling of alcoholic parent occurs here.
Industry versus Inferiority	Seven to eleven	Parents lack of interest in school achievements, due to exhaustion of alcoholism, leads to child's feeling that successful task accomplishments are meaningless; a useless/failure feeling at home will generalize to school; homework and school assignments often ignored.
Learned Identity versus Identity Diffusion	Twelve to fourteen	Extreme negative identification with alcoholic household; family identity disorganized overshadows adolescent's ability to carve out an individual identity.
Intimacy versus Isolation	Fourteen to young adulthood	Legacy of partial failures at earlier stages leads to inability to share and be open, resulting in an inability to "establish primary relations with others."
Generativity versus Self-absorption	Adulthood	Deprivation in learning how to form primary relationships produces shallow relationships with their children; emotional impoverishment of parent breeds new generation of children affected by alcoholism.
Integrity versus Despair	Senior years	Blaming others for life's misfortunes leads to despair.

[a] As adapted from Ackerman (1983).

TABLE 4. BEHAVIORS CHILDREN OF ALCOHOLICS MAY EXHIBIT[a]

1. Inability to form primary relationships
2. Distorted sense of reality
3. Pseudomaturity
4. Depression
5. Delayed physical and emotional development
6. Night terrors; excessive fears
7. Apathy
8. Anxious to please others
9. Excessive use of fantasy
10. Oblivious to hazards
11. Lack of creativity and exploration
12. Gender role confusion
13. Low self-esteem
14. Isolated and lonely
15. Poor impulse control
16. Inability to function in peer group
17. Lack of knowledge about environment
18. Inability to accept responsibility for self at age-appropriate levels
19. Inability to trust their own feelings and judgments

[a] Order does not indicate priority rankings. COA do not exhibit all of these behaviors simultaneously; they appear depending on developmental level and other factors.

hyperactivity, and a characteristic facial dysmorphology that includes microcephaly, microopthalmia and/or short palpebral fissures, and poorly developed philtrum, thin upper lip and flattening of the maxillary area (Rosett, 1980). Such children are diagnosed by these abnormal features and the history of maternal alcoholism. These children can also have attention-deficit disorders and should be treated for this condition as well as being provided with special education for the mental retardation.

TREATMENT

Several principles have been developed in working with COA in an alcoholism clinic setting. The first principal involves education about alcoholism. Regardless of age, COA need to learn the basic facts about alcohol as a drug and alcoholism as disease. This is the entry point, the beginning, which then blends into group and individual treatment. Basic information is transmitted in an age appropriate manner, and rarely in a classroom type setting. An education series for latency age children will work as long as there is plenty of time for free exchange and sharing. For adolescents, who will not relate to a structured lecture series, information is integrated into the group as various issues arise.

Regardless of the format, there are a number of information components about alcoholism which are a must for all COA. Table 5 lists them in summary form.

The principles that follow are involved in the treatment of COA:

1. *Children should be seen and accepted as "primary" clients as well as members of an alcoholic family system.* The chaos resulting from the alcoholic's frequent drinking demands crisis intervention. The suffering of the alcoholic's spouse can at least be articulated by the adult; children generally do not talk about this. They are often seen as "collaterals" whose problems will evaporate as the parent recovers. The treatment agency and counselor can unintentionally become "professional enablers" by only responding to adult needs and agreeing with the adult's minimization of their children's problems. Many counselors were raised in alcoholic homes. Unresolved feelings around their childhood often find professional expression in conflicts over agency policy regarding serving COA, responding to community pressure, and from the criminal justice system in treating the alcoholic as the only primary client.

In order for the COA to be the "primary client," there must first be strong administrative support for services to COA. Without this support from the highest levels of administration, middle management and treatment staff will consume endless hours in fruitless discussions about the need for services to COA. A strong administrative policy must be communicated frequently to all staff in a clear and decisive manner and supported by appropriate training/orientation of all staff on the needs and problems of COA. Second, an appropriate staff member must be hired to work *only* with COA. Asking existing staff to include COA in their current caseloads does not work. A children's specialist must be hired and designated to work only with COA and their families. Later, we will outline the ideal staff qualifications of a children's specialist. In addition, separate and private space in the clinic must be reserved for children. The area should be children's space with age appropriate posters, drawings, toys, books and other materials to set it off from adult activities. This immediately dignifies the importance of children within the clinic and indicates to them the commitment of the agency to helping them. Finally, all staff, including custodial, security, and treatment personnel, should be aware of the names of the children who regularly attend the clinic and be especially warm and enthusiastic in their greetings. This "family lens" approach to treatment adds to the warmth of any clinical setting and helps provide a positive experience for all clients.

2. *Group is the treatment of choice.* This provides an arena to work on issues such as isolation, socialization, and trust. To be effective, group must be closely age matched. For example, groups for COA are usually

Table 5. Cognitive Information about Alcoholism Important for COA to Understand

Information	Value for COA in their recovery
Alcoholism is a blameless disease.	Depersonalizes responsibility for the drinking and family chaos; "It's not my fault"; reduces guilt.
Alcoholism is a progressive physical, emotional and spiritual disease.	Removes morality conception of alcoholism; helps child identify with disease process rather than guilt over alleged failures; identifies alcoholism as the problem; makes possible entry into addiction-specific treatment and self-help groups.
Blackouts of the alcoholic are a physical manifestation of alcoholism.	Explains memory lapses of alcoholic; his absence from treasured events (school, sports, etc.); explain discontinuity in alcoholic's behavior.
Alcohol is a mind and mood altering drug. It is not a "truth serum."	Depersonalizes alcoholics abuse while intoxicated; explains discontinuity between sober and intoxicated behaviors.
COA are trapped in rigid prescribed roles.	Explains COA being developmentally "stuck"; sees roles of other siblings and helps identification with disease model; reduces guilt.
Paraalcoholic acts and thinks like the alcoholic; is sick and needs help.	Explains emotional unavailability of codependent and mood swings.
COA have choices; they can choose to live.	Dispells the illusion that COA must "wait around" for alcoholic to get sober for them to live. Places responsibility on them for making choices; can no longer hide behind the alcoholism.
Alcoholics appear arrogant and hostile, but are really hurting and helpless.	Depersonalizes distance and abuse of alcoholic; helps see parent in broader perspective and as ill.
What COA see and feel is real.	Validates their experiences which are often discounted in the home and by others; "I'm not crazy."
You are not alone.	Fosters identification with self-help movement and "privilege" of becoming part of it.
Alcoholics do get well.	Hope that the family can recover; energizes.
COA need help.	Helps them focus on themselves; reduce denial of their own illness and facilitates entry into treatment.
COA must end their obsession with rescuing, controlling and managing the alcoholic.	Fosters focusing on themselves; can see route to change, despite decision of other family members, for health.
Feelings are neither "good" nor "bad"; they just are.	Relabel as "comfortable" and "uncomfortable"; gives permission to feel and to act responsibly.

Note: Order of presentation does not suggest greater or less importance.

grouped by developmental level: 6 to 9, 10 to 13; 14 to 16, and 17 to 19. This depends, of course, on the number of COA in treatment at any one time. Broader age groups can be arranged but it is particularly important to separate latency age from early adolescent and mid-adolescent COA. Grouping should also take into account the maturity level of each child; a mature 12-year-old might feel better in an older group than in one including only his own age peers.

Ideally, once a group of 6 to 10 COA is formed, it should be closed to new members. The prolonged interaction of the same small group creates the potential for trust building and learning the skills of establishing and maintaining relationships. New members often become the focus of "rescuing" attempts of more experienced group members and disturb the steady flow of communication so that the group regresses until the new member(s) are incorporated.

Groups, initially, can be structured to avoid premature intimacy (for which members are not ready) by the leader taking a dominant position and establishing an educational focus. COA need to have time and space to begin to open up and share. This process cannot be rushed. Beginning with a quasi-educational focus protects them from premature self-disclosure and insures a safe place for later, more intimate, sharing.

Despite the COA preference for individual therapy, the therapist should use a strong hand in encouraging the COA to accept group. This is not to rule out the importance of individual therapy, but this should be seen as adjunct to group. There are certain COA who are not ready for group or who find it very painful and threatening. For example, the lost child often finds group intimidating and overwhelming. They may require some individual sessions in order to prepare them for group as well as for additional individual sessions. Some COA may require individual treatment based on an assessment of the entire family.

It is important that only nonsubstance abusing COA be retained in COA focused groups. Some adolescents in a COA group will begin to show early stage symptoms of alcoholism or other drug dependencies. They should be carefully evaluated and switched to an adolescent alcoholism modality in order that they focus on their chemical abuse. Mixing them in a COA group will only serve to confuse issues for the group as well as for the alcohol-abusing youth.

Finally, group provides a family setting where members experience interaction and practice new behaviors and skills. They then try them out in their family of origin and report back to the group results which then become the focus of more planning and practice.

3. *Clinicians must be careful not to fall into the trap of seeing only one child (usually the family scapegoat) in the alcoholic family.* All available mem-

bers of the family should be assessed and provided with at least basic alcohol education.

Frequently, the family scapegoats are the "identified patients" by the family. Their misbehavior serves to take the focus off the alcoholism. Clinicians who accept them as the only members of the family requiring treatment only serve to reinforce the family's denial of alcoholism.

In order for the family to present themselves as intact, they will under report problems of their children. Especially vulnerable to being overlooked are the family hero and the lost child. Both will be presented as functioning adequately in the family and hence not requiring help. The hero, of course, especially brings pride to the family by his deeds of excellence. We have stressed the fact that all children of alcoholics are at high risk. Despite their outward behavior, they carry the family secret of guilt and responsibility for the family's failure as a unit. It is important that the intake worker involve all available members at intake and then designate treatment modalities as appropriate. Exposure for all children to a basic education series on alcoholism will serve to help them identify their roles in the alcoholic family. This motivates them for treatment, and to support the recovery of the alcoholic and other family members as they come to understand alcoholism as a family systems disorder and help the members of the family become self-generating individuals.

4. *At least one parent of a minor child must be involved in alcohol therapy in order for the child to be in treatment at an alcoholism clinic.* The child's growth and changes in treatment will have a "domino" effect on the rest of the alcoholic family system. Unless at least one adult is in alcoholism treatment, they will not support the child's growth and will withdraw the child from treatment in an attempt to reestablish the equilibrium of the closed system interaction of the family.

This is especially true in the treatment of the family scapegoat. This client is often referred to the clinic because of deviant behavior in school and the community, as well as an outward angry, surly, uncooperative attitude. As they improve their academic and interpersonal skills, the diseased alcoholic family system loses the excuse for family dysfunction. Since they are still denying alcoholism, the scapegoat's recovery will only serve to increase tension within the closed and rigid alcoholic family system; the system will have to find a new focus to scapegoat their problems. Often the family will not be able to tolerate the scapegoat's progress in treatment and will attempt to undermine it.

Likewise, as the family hero recovers, he may begin to misbehave by not being perfect and by pulling back from being quasi-adult. These changes, unless understood and supported by at least one parent, will be especially threatening as the family sees its hero change. Any change in behavior in the closed, rigid alcoholic family system will be perceived as a threat not only to the alcoholic, but to each family member. Clinical staff must be keenly aware of this and work creatively in supervision and case conferences to avoid premature termination.

5. *Intake procedures should involve at least one meeting with all available family members so that all receive identical information, particularly as it relates to issues of confidentiality and the need for continued family secret keeping.* The dysfunctional alcoholic family will, of course, distort the treatment contract to meet their own preconceived ideas. The treatment system must confront these distortions immediately, not only within therapy, but also in terms of the way the treatment contract is structured. The intake worker should make it clear that the clinic is there to help the entire family and that it does not "take sides" in the family's problems. The needs of absent family members can be at least partially met by addressing the needs of the typical dysfunctional alcoholic family.

Hence, the intake session is partly educational. Each member of the family is advised of their therapist and modality, which is often separate from other family members. For example, an 8-year-old boy might be placed in a latency age COA group which would be separate from his mother's significant other group. Guidelines of the clinic regarding confidentiality of therapist/patient relationship are then reviewed. It is made clear that, especially with children, information is not shared with the parent without the express consent of the child. It is common for parents to be threatened by their child being in a COA group. The parents' fantasy is that the child is criticizing them and sharing the family "secret." Their fantasies should be verbalized as early as possible and the parents made to feel that the agency is there to aid their parenting, not to compete with them for their child's affection and loyalty.

The procedures for involving the entire family in joint sessions should be made clear. One family member, for example, adult significant other/parent, may want to call their child's therapist to "see how he is doing." The guidelines for disclosing confidential information should be clearly specified at intake so that the child and parent feel structure and hence, protection. The question of the parent may lead to a joint family meeting structured around certain topics (e.g., homework). The family can then be taught mature ways of asking for information and help.

It is also common for the initially uninvolved and hostile parent to call the child's therapist and question his child's involvement. Reference can be made to the initial family meeting where confidentiality was discussed and the parent invited to come to the agency for more information. This initial complaint by the parent often is converted into an intake session for the previously uninvolved parent. Here again, it is important to involve the entire family, at least once, in a joint session in order to review ground rules. As children recover, they will, of course, upset the equilibrium of the alcoholic family. It is critical that available family members be prepared for this predictable occurence by suggesting various ways family members can cope with change.

Finally, it is critical that the intake worker have a family orientation to the disease of alcoholism. Their covert and overt behavior will transmit the philosophy of the agency and set the tone for as complete family involvement as possible. Experience shows that intake workers who have already taken sides (however unconsciously) only serve to reinforce the dysfunctional behavior of the family as well as enable the family's denial of a problem to continue.

6. *Although clinical supervision is, of course, important for all treatment staff, it is critically important for therapists working with children of alcoholics.* First the supervisors themselves should have a holistic family orientation to alcoholism in order to support the importance of children's services. They should be skilled in the dynamics of childhood development as well as the family dynamics of alcoholism. Hence, the supervisor's training and background should not only include alcoholism, but also knowledge and experience with generic mental health practice issues. Secondly, the supervisor should be particularly sensitive to the staff issues around treating children of alcoholics and how staff can act themselves as a dysfunctional alcoholic family system. Children trigger deep feelings in staff. Not only their own childhoods (often as adult children of an alcoholic) are touched but also their own adequacy as parents is threatened. The child specialist in a clinic is vulnerable to staff isolation and criticism. The supervisor must be aware of these family dynamics as they impact on professional practice and work through these issues in staff conferences and meetings.

This is best accomplished by encouraging staff to function as a healthy family system. For example, a therapist for the alcoholic may get caught in the family "dance" by becoming a partner with the alcoholic in being overly critical of his children. Likewise, the child specialist can covertly be opinionated about the recovering alcoholic's slow response to the needs of his children. A clinical supervisor must identify these issues and meet with staff to verbalize them and work through potential or actual conflict in a direct and mature manner. This serves to act as a role model for the family to emulate as they struggle to work through their own conflict in a mature manner. The recovering alcoholic and family members are acutely sensitive during the stage of early sobriety. They can and will detect subtle competition and conflict within an agency's staff. Rather than avoiding these issues, a clinician supervisor is best advised to confront them internally as part of an ongoing effort to have the agency and staff function as a healthy family system.

7. *Treatment for COA ranges from short-term education (8 to 10 weeks) up to three years.* Short-term educative treatment is sufficient for COA who live in a recovering family which is committed to appropriate self-help groups.

This does not include, however, the vast majority of COA. The majority require much more time, usually 1½ to 3 years in order to gain from the healing process because the child's changes will have a domino effect on the entire family's equilibrium which may result in some family members getting worse and others getting better. The child will need continual support to adjust to these changes and especially to commit themselves to self-growth, sometimes in the face of family disapproval. For example, a lost child may begin to assert himself, to ask for emotional support and time with the family. The co dependent parent, if not in treatment, will see this child's growth as a negative— another child demanding attention. The child will need to be encouraged to grow and ask questions despite rebuffs. A common misconception held by some counselors is that when the alcoholic attains sobriety, this alone is ground to believe that he will begin to re-parent and that the children's needs will begin to be met. For some COA, parental sobriety is as equally empty as were the active drinking years. Expecting to have a parent emotionally ready and able to help them, they are instead let down by finding a sober parent who is so committed to his program for recovery that he has little time or energy for them. The fantasy of instant recovery needs to be explained to children. Their parent needs their time and space, but the child does not have to wait around until the parent is emotionally available for them to recover. The slowness of children of alcoholics to open up to change, combined with the shifting family dynamics, call for a treatment process that is not hurried and gives due respect to the need for time to recover. In addition, many adolescent COA already have incorporated into their personalities patterns of adult children of alcoholics. These personality patterns will persist for a lifetime unless challenged and changed while the adolescent personality is still in the formative stage.

8. *COA are best treated in an alcoholism specific agency.* There are four reasons for this recommendation: (1) COA need to identify with a disease model rather than a morality view of the family's dysfunction. Many report overwhelming feelings of guilt and shame about their family. Identification with disease model depersonalizes responsibility for the

drinking of the alcoholic; helps the children identify their roles in the disease process; teaches them that they were trapped in rigid survival roles and that they can change. In addition, group involvement is tremendously rewarding as they meet other COA who provide ready identification and a support system. (2) Placement in an alcoholism agency will aid the process of self-diagnosis and reduce denial. This awareness is critical in charting the course to recovery. Without the understanding of alcoholism, the child will continue to be guilt ridden and bear responsibility for the family's chaos. (3) An alcoholism specific agency has the capability to treat other family members in appropriate modalities. For example, the child's father may eventually seek treatment and should be enrolled in the same agency but in his own early sobriety group. Other siblings can also be enrolled in age appropriate groups. In short, the entire family can enter modality specific treatment in the same agency, which enhances the recovery process for all. (4) The alcoholic family is reported to have special and unique characteristics unlike those of other patient groups. Just one uniqueness of the system is the enormous availability of self-help groups and the critical role they play in the recovery process. Other agencies understand little about these groups or the special character of the alcoholic family system. Hence this family recovers best in an alcoholism specific agency whose philosophy and staff are engrossed in and committed to the disease of alcoholism.

9. *COA are involuntary clients.* COA usually reach treatment through the mandate of a parent, school referral, or via the criminal justice system. Either explicitly or implicitly, the child is there at the wish and directive of another party. The implication of this is that they will be as resistant to treatment as is the alcoholic adult who is mandated to treatment by an employer or through a drinking driver arrest. The same time and patience is required to work through the initial resistance of the child as we assume is necessary with the alcoholic adult. Initially, the COA therapist has to accept distance and anger as two realities of the child and gradually work through them to a place where the child desires and wants change. Furthermore, the child views the COA therapist as an authority figure who initially seems similar to their parents. Obviously, it takes time to work on developing a trusting relationship. Agency staff should not be discouraged by the initial apparent lack of response of COA to treatment. As with their alcoholic parent, they should be viewed as mandated clients who initially present as angry and resistant, but who hold great promise for positive change.

10. *Treatment staff should structure rituals into the treatment program.* Family rituals (e.g., birthday parties, anniversaries, holiday parties, etc.)

are tremendously important for emotional bonding. For the child, they also provide continuity in generations of the family and a reaffirmation of a stable set of values and norms that the family is committed to. The alcoholic family often has few rituals. Those opportunities commonly available (e.g., religious holidays, etc.) are usually marked by chaotic outbursts ending in pain and disappointment. Hence, it is important for the children's specialist to plan regular rituals around any and all events that occur in the group and the community. Obvious ones include religious and country-wide celebrations, as well as birthdays and group anniversaries. Group members plan, execute, and enjoy the celebration as they develop routine rituals in their lifestyle.

11. *The treatment agency and staff should integrate knowledge of developmental tasks and stages into the treatment process.* Although alcohol specific in content, the structure of treatment should aid children in accomplishing developmental tasks appropriate to their age level. Latency age children require a therapist directed group and enjoy repetition of games of skill as they develop conceptual and physical competency. Adolescents respond better to a peer-oriented system where the therapist is more of a guide than a leader. Even here, though, we have found that many adolescent COA have not completed the developmental tasks of latency age children and some have problems with early bonding issues. Here the group may be more focused on "going back" to developmental tasks of those earlier years rather than going forward. The treatment staff should integrate what is known about the developmental tasks of childhood/adolescence into their specialized knowledge of alcoholism in designing treatment for this needy population.

THE COA THERAPIST

The personal qualities of the COA therapist are critical in facilitating the healing process. This is also true, of course, in working with alcoholic adults, but it is even more important with COA due to their vulnerable and dependent status. The therapist, in many ways, becomes a mature role model and consistent source of support and patience. Hence, it is critical that they possess not only appropriate education, but a variety of personality qualities which are listed below.

Educational background should include generic mental health training with a special emphasis in childhood/adolescent development stages and education/teaching skills; knowledge of alcoholism with special emphasis on the child's response to generational and current alcoholism both during active drinking and following sobriety and knowledge of family dynamics with special knowledge of the alcoholic family both during the active stages and later in sobriety. The most productive model is the therapist who is trained foremost in working with children—either in a school setting, or child guidance clinics—and then adds on the additional generic mental health and family dynamic skills. This is probably because of their total commitment to the child.

1. *Many COA therapist are themselves adult children of alcoholics and/or have children who have had addictive problems.* Therefore, they should avoid over-identifying with the client COA or forcing upon them their own way to recovery. The need for professional treatment for COA therapist who themselves are recovering from an addictive household is essential.

2. *The COA therapist should not personalize acting-out by COA during the treatment process and recognize that such acting-out is a treatment issue.* It is critical that the COA therapist be comfortable with honesty. Children are less defended than adults and will perceive feeling states in the therapist that they themselves may not be aware of. The COA therapist should be able to receive honest and accurate feedback from COA and also to be honest in their interactions with children.

3. *The COA therapist should be willing to use themselves as a therapeutic tool and be comfortable with appropriate levels of self-disclosure.* In the alcoholic home, there is very poor ability to develop conflict resolution skills. As treatment progresses, it is appropriate for the COA therapist to give examples of how to resolve conflict and teach a COA group how to resolve conflict within the group.

4. *COA therapist should be aware of their own counter-transference and avoid taking sides in the dysfunctional alcoholic family.* There is always a danger of the therapist becoming a "rescuer" and "pseudo-parent" for the COA. The COA therapist should resist the impulse to solve all the child's problems and to assume the good parent nurturing role. Although appearing to be helpful, overdoing this role will only serve to weaken the child's ability to solve their own problems.

5. *The COA therapist should be able to be tough and sensitive at the same time.* COA often blame their poor school performance on the chaotic nature of their household. The COA therapist will accept the reality of the impediments to completing homework assignments, but will quickly move to help the child define ways to meet school demands.

6. *The COA therapist must show patience and consistency in the treatment setting.* Whereas the alcoholic will often present at intake with anger and the codependent with martydom, the children will present with emotional distance. This is their particular form of denial; they appear not to care. This is simply a defense against the deep craving for acceptance and approval. The COA therapist must be patient in permitting the COA time to lay aside the defense of "not caring" as they begin to

trust the therapist and treatment process and open up to their own feelings and wishes.

7. *COA usually underreport the impact of alcoholism on their lives.* This denial should not be taken at face value. They minimize and discount the impact of such traumatic events as parental fighting, separation, child abuse, and criminal justice system problems. This defense against feelings can be incorrectly interpreted by the therapist as meaning that the child is coping well. The COA therapist should not be deluded into believing that children who can function well under such circumstances are not being negatively impacted by these experiences—they are! A common technique of COA therapist is to constantly ask the child to report how they feel about such events; to have other group members comment and themselves report how they might feel about such traumas.

8. *The COA therapist must be able to tolerate small increments of improvement in the child.* Unlike the alcoholic in whom dramatic changes can be measured in fairly brief periods of time, the child's growth is often subtle and private. The COA therapist is "planting a seed" of self-awareness and self-power of which they may only see a small portion.

9. *COA require a therapist who they can trust completely with their feelings and with sensitive information.* At intake, the agency rules regarding sharing of information among therapist and family members must be outlined and adhered to. Common confidentiality guidelines include the rule that the COA therapist will not speak to the parent without the child's permission and/or presence, that family meetings can be called by any family member to share concerns, that the child's disclosures to the COA therapist are private, and that these and similar rules may be broken in the event of an emergency (examples are provided as guidelines).

10. *The effective COA therapist should be able to understand the importance of play in the therapeutic process.* COA are often pseudo-adults who take on adult responsibilities long before maturational readiness. Part of the healing process is for them to learn again how to be children. Some COA therapists have adapted popular games and toys with alcohol specific questions and outcomes. This combines the best of playful activity with the importance of learning about alcoholism.

11. *Finally, the COA therapist should know the relevant local child abuse and neglect statutes, reporting mechanisms, and school and local laws as they pertain to children at risk.* The therapist should also act as an advocate and negotiate for the child and family with criminal justice, school, and other legal systems.

The task of being an effective COA therapist is a demanding one both professionally and personally. COA deserve the very best in professional talent; the rewards are the prevention of a new generation of alcoholics, substance abusers, and co-dependents. Three case histories follow of children seen in an alcoholism out-patient clinic with a child specialist within a family oriented program.

CASE HISTORIES

Susan

This case involves an 11-year-old girl referred to an alcoholism clinic by a school social worker. The presenting problem was school truancy, a chaotic family who were difficult to contact, and the "hunch" on the part of the school social worker that alcohol might be involved. This worker had considerable training in alcoholism.

The child was seen by the children's specialist and presented as a pleasant, physically mature but emotionally immature child who denied any problems at home and refused to comment on her truancy and runaway behavior. Father and mother were seen and although both agreed that Susan was a "bad" girl, disclosed little else. In further conversations with the school personnel, it was found that Susan was the youngest of six children, all of whom had been school problems. The family had been referred through the years to various mental health clinics and had never followed through on treatment.

The children's specialist observed Susan and one or both of her parents during several sessions of an alcoholism education series and felt strongly that this was a secret-keeping family. Possible sexual abuse was suspected and the children's specialist, trained in intervention, brought this issue to Susan and her parents. Several sessions, in addition to psychological testing on Susan, turned up no signs of sexual abuse or incest. The detective work continued with Susan's truancy while her periods of time away from home were increasing. Susan's one revealing statement was, "I don't like my father." Continued sessions with the parents revealed marital discord of some years' duration and was highlighted by the demand of the father to remove Susan and place her in a secure facility.

After two months of working with the family, the children's specialist was contacted by the mother and an immediate appointment was requested and scheduled. Mother and father appeared together and mother with trembling voice told the family secret of alcoholism. The father, a child of two alcoholic parents, had a long history of alcoholism and numerous alcohol related arrests. He had been abusing alcohol daily for the past 10 years. Mother, totally ignorant about alcoholism and its effect on the family, had not only kept the secret to protect her husband but had raised all the children never to reveal to anyone what happened when father drank.

The family is now beginning to learn through education and therapy who they are and how their lives have been focused almost totally on father, his drinking, and the resulting chaos. All need long-term treatment, particularly Susan's father, a deprived child himself, whose diagnosis is more complex than alcoholism addiction. Susan is being placed temporarily in a residential setting; the older siblings are receiving education on alcoholism and individual assessments and the father is being encouraged to enter an in-patient alcoholism rehabilitation facility. Prognosis for this family, with continued alcoholism specific treatment is good.

Jane

This case involves an eleven-year-old girl who was brought by her mother to an education series on alcoholism for latency COA. On initial questioning by the group leader, it became apparent that Jane had no idea that anyone in her family was alcoholic. She appeared shy, unable to carry on a relevant conversation with either the group leader or fellow group members, and presented herself as either very slow or retarded.

The group leader set up an appointment with Jane and her mother. The mother, with great reluctance, revealed that her husband, a prominent professional, had been drinking alcoholically for over 10 years. The mother described Jane as a slow child, learning disabled, and the apparent victim of considerable verbal abuse by the family. The family was involved in treatment; the mother in a spouse group, the father in an alcohol group and Jane in a latency-age group. Contact was made, with appropriate written consent, with Jane's school and a treatment plan was developed for the family. Engagement of Jane, frightened and ignorant of what was causing the chaos in her family, took several months. Jane continued to have great difficulty in following conversations, responding appropriately, and found group a painful experience.

The children's therapist, after ongoing conferences with the parents' therapists, asked for a family meeting. It became apparent that Jane's inability to communicate was the result of a lifetime spent with two adults who spoke in phrases, gutteral responses, and never communicated with each other. Jane's sense of self was damaged due to neglect and lack of any positive feedback.

This family had to deal with several setbacks, one due to the premature death of the alcoholic father. The morning following the death of the father, Jane called the agency to speak with her counselor. The counselor was unavailable but the receptionist called her at home to make her immediately aware of this traumatic event. The counselor immediately called Jane and followed-up by attending the funeral for her father. Jane had fantasized and wished the death of her father for many months; the guilt surrounding his eventual death became a major topic to work through in her group. The family has completed treatment and are leading productive lives.

Jane had been misdiagnosed as learning disabled and as treatment progressed was able to integrate into a regular classroom. This was a process that required ongoing conferences with school personnel. As Jane's self-esteem improved so did her abilities to communicate and her ability to express appropriately her needs and to gain gratification in life. She developed extraordinary leadership skills and has since received several citizenship awards as well as scholastic achievements.

Jane was in treatment for five years. She is now 18 years old and recently graduated from high school, spent a summer in Europe in an exchange program and is college bound, preparing for a career in teaching. Without appropriate intervention in an alcoholism clinic, life for Jane, in an alcoholic family could have been very different.

Betty

This is a 17-year-old girl who self-referred to an alcohol out-patient clinic when she was 15 complaining of anxiety and depression. Her alcoholic mother had been sober for seven months and these complaints were related to the child's adjustment reaction to her mother's early sobriety.

Family history revealed that Betty was the youngest of five children, four girls and one boy and that her father, an active alcoholic, had divorced the mother, separated and remarried when Betty was 12 years old. The divorce was unfriendly; Betty's mother was enraged at being abandoned and Betty felt caught between two parents who could not communicate with each other.

On intake, Betty, a sensitive, articulate, bright, young woman described feelings of hopelessness and depression. As therapy continued, it became obvious that Betty had been a parent to her mother for some years, had blocked her own feelings, and presented to the world a picture of the perfect family. Since an age appropriate group was not available, Betty was seen for two years in weekly therapy sessions which helped her to begin to work through her impacted feelings precipitated by parental alcoholism and divorce.

Progress has been slowed down by the mother's periodic slips, her denial of an alcohol problem, the ongoing animosity between Betty's parents and her mothers entry into the singles world, complete with overnight absences. As treatment continued, Betty was able to get in touch with an emotionally deprived childhood in which there were not the fond memories of family rituals and caring to use as building blocks for adulthood.

At this time, Betty continues to be seen weekly. She is responsible for her own behavior and has come a long way in detaching from the behavior of her family members. She struggles with perfection, a judgmental approach to friends, and the ongoing fear of abandonment. Betty is fully committed to her own personal growth; her mother continues in treatment as do two of her siblings. It is interesting to note that Betty's progress appears more favorable than that of her two siblings who have only been seen in a non-alcoholism clinic where workers are apparently unaware of the effects of alcoholism on the members of the family.

Summary

There are about 7 million under-aged children of alcoholics in this country. There is an unknown, but substantial number of adult children of alcoholics.

This chapter described the personality characteristics of COA in terms of compulsive and rigid behavior and with a delusional quality of beliefs and values. These characteristics develop because children of alcoholics are forced to deal with the pervasive and destructive problem of alcoholism in one or both parents while denying that any problem exists. They are forced to play roles in the family to protect themselves from the consequences of alcoholism. These roles include *family hero*, *scapegoat*, *lost child*, and *mascot*. They are maladaptations that result in serious psychological impairment and developmental defects.

The principles of treatment for COA are described including a major emphasis on education about the disease of alcoholism. The characteristics of therapists for COA is indicated including the necessity of their training in the mental health of children, family dynamics, and alcoholism. Three case histories utilizing the techniques described are presented.

ACKNOWLEDGMENTS

Gratitude is expressed to the child alcohol treatment specialist in Nassau County, New York, whose insights have helped shape the concepts presented in this chapter. Special gratitude is extended to Caroline Bridges, Coordinator of Children's Services, whose knowledge and love of children are very special. In addition, Miriam Solomon, Alcohol Program Analyst for Nassau County is thanked for her dedication to children and her innovative role in developing services for them.

REFERENCES

Ackerman, R. J. *Children of alcoholics: A guidebook for educators, therapists, and parents*. Holmes Beach, Florida: Learning Publications, 1983.

Al-Anon Family Groups. *Adult children of alcoholics*. Al-Anon Family Group Headquarters, P. O. Box 182, Madison Square Station, New York, New York, 1979.

Allport, G. W. *Pattern and growth in personality*. New York: Holt, Rinehart and Winston, 1961.

Booz-Allen and Hamilton, Inc. *An assessment of the needs of and resources for children of alcoholic parents*. Rockville, Md.: National Institute on Alcohol Abuse and Alcoholics, 1974.

Cantwell, D. P. Psychiatric illness in the families of hyperactive children. *Archives of General Psychiatry*, 1972, 27, 414–417.

Erikson, E. H. *Childhood and society*. 2nd ed. New York: Norton, 1963.

Maslow, A. *Towards a psychology of being* (2nd ed.). Princeton: Van Nostrand, 1968.

Morehouse, E. R., and Richards, T. An examination of dysfunctional latency age children of alcoholic parents and problems in intervention. *Journal of Children in Contemporary Society*, Vol. 15, No. 1, Fall 1982, pp. 21–33.

Pohlisch, K. Soziale und Personliche Bedingungen des Chronischen Alkoholismus. In *Sammulung Psychiatrischer und Nerologischer Einseldarstwedlung*. Leipzig, Germany: G. Thieme Verlad, 1933.

Rosett, H. L. A clinical perspective of the fetal alcohol syndrome. *Alcoholism: Clinical and Experimental Research*, 1980, 4, 119–122.

Skinner, B. F. *Contingencies of reinforcement: A theoretical analysis*. New York: Appleton-Century-Crofts, 1969.

Wegscheider, S. *Another chance: Hope and health for the alcoholic family*. Palo Alto: Science and Behavior Books, 1981.

Woodside, M. *Children of alcoholics*. A report to Hugh L. Carey, Governor, State of New York for Joseph A. Califano, Jr., Special Counselor on Alcoholism and Drug Abuse, July, 1982.

RESOURCE MATERIALS

Cork, Margaret. *The forgotten children*. New York: National Council on Alcoholism, 1969.

Deutsch, Charles. *Broken bottles, broken dreams: Understanding and helping the children of alcoholics*. New York: Teachers College Press, 1982.

National Institute on Alcohol Abuse and Alcoholism. *Services for children of alcoholics*. Research Monograph 4, 1981 (DHHS Publication No. (ADM) 81–1007).

Woititz, Janet. *Adult children of alcoholics*. Holnwood, Florida: Health Communications, 1983.

18

Psychosocial Treatment of Elderly Alcoholics

Sheldon Zimberg

Introduction

In recent years there has been an increasing awareness that alcohol abuse and alcoholism are significant problems among the aged. This awareness has been supported by studies that looked at this problem from a variety of viewpoints including community-based prevalence studies, hospital admissions, arrests for public intoxication, outpatient treatment programs, and interviews with the staff of health, social service, and information and referral agencies.

In the Washington Heights area of Manhattan, a household-prevalence survey was conducted which involved questions related to alcoholism (Bailey, Haberman, and Alksne, 1965). This study noted that for individuals age 20 years and over, a peak prevalence of 23 per 1000 population occurred in the 45–54 age group. The prevalence decreased to 17 per 1000 for the age group 55–65 and then increased to a prevalence of 22 per 1000 at the 65–74 year age group. This study noted that elderly widowers had a rate of 105 per 1000 in contrast to the overall rate of 19 per 1000. In addition to this study, a sample of United Automobile Workers Union members 21 years of age and over was conducted in the Baltimore Metropolitan area (Siassi, Crocetti, and

Sheldon Zimberg • Director of Psychiatry, Joint Diseases, North General Hospital, New York, New York; Associate Professor of Psychiatry, Mount Sinai School of Medicine, New York, New York.

Spiro, 1973). This study found that 10% of the men and 20% of the women age 60 and over were heavy escape drinkers and considered to be alcoholics.

A study conducted on 534 patients over age 60 admitted to a psychiatric observation ward in San Francisco General Hospital noted that 23% were alcoholic (Simon, Epstein, and Reynolds, 1968). Another study conducted at a county psychiatric screening ward in Houston, Texas, noted that 44% of 100 consecutive admissions age 60 and over were alcoholic (Gaitz and Baer, 1971). A prevalence study on alcoholism conducted at Harlem Hospital Center in New York City noted that 60% of the male admissions to the medical service and 43% of the female admissions were alcoholic (McCusker, Cherubin, and Zimberg, 1971); 5 of the male patients (56%) in age group 70 and over were alcoholic but none of the women were. A survey of patients 65 years of age and over admitted to the acute medical ward of a California Veterans Administration Hospital noted that 18% of these patients were alcoholic (Schuckit and Miller, 1975).

In San Francisco it was noted in a study of 722 individuals age 60 and over arrested for minor crimes that 82.3% were charged with drunkenness (Epstein, Mills, and Simon, 1970). This proportion of drunkenness arrests was much higher than in any other age group.

In an outpatient geriatric psychiatry program conducted at Harlem Hospital, 12% of the elderly patients were noted to have a drinking problem (Zimberg, 1969). In a medical home-care program 13% of the elderly patients requiring psychiatric consultation were diagnosed as alcoholic (Zimberg, 1971). The author noted that 17% of patients age 65 and over admitted to a suburban New York community mental health center had alcohol abuse as a problem on admission.

Interviews of the staffs of health, social-service, and criminal-justice agencies were conducted in three communities representing urban, rural, and mixed urban–rural populations regarding the extent of problem drinking among their elderly clients (Carruth, Williams, Mysak, and Boudreaux, 1975). The authors found that 45% of those interviewed had had contact with an elderly problem drinker in the previous year. They also noted that the alcoholism information and referral services surveyed reported that 30% of all calls were for persons over age 55.

It can be seen that a great deal of data has been accumulated from a variety of sources indicating that a significant problem among the elderly has been ignored. It is not possible to determine an actual prevalence of alcoholism among elderly people. However, a reasonable estimate would seem to be 10%–15% with a higher proportion occurring among the hospitalized elderly.

With this recognition of the problem, we must develop a useful classification of problem drinkers among the elderly, questions regarding possible causal factors, and effective treatment approaches. It is clear that elderly alcoholics carry the double stigma in our society of being old as well as alcoholic. This chapter will discuss these questions and describe effective treatment methods with this population of alcoholics in order to dispel stereotyped conceptions that have resulted in the rejection by health-care professionals of alcoholics in general and the elderly alcoholic in particular.

Classification of Elderly Alcoholics

A number of authors have noted that elderly alcoholics can be differentiated into several diagnostic groupings. Simon et al. (1968) and Gaitz and Baer (1971) made distinctions between elderly alcoholics with and without an organic mental syndrome. Such a distinction would imply differing prognoses and treatment approaches. Simon et al. (1968) indicated that alcoholics with an organic mental syndrome had a poor prognosis with respect to dying at an earlier age than elderly alcoholics without an organic mental syndrome. Simon et al. (1968) also noted that of the 23% elderly alcoholic admissions, 7% became alcoholic after age 60 and 16% became alcoholic before age 60 and had long histories of alcohol abuse, thus indicating that about one-third of these patients developed a drinking problem in later life and two-thirds were long-standing alcoholics.

In developing a classification of elderly alcoholics, it would appear that a distinction between late-onset problem drinking and early-onset problem drinking would be a more useful approach than one based on a distinction of psychiatric diagnosis, particularly the presence or absence of an organic mental syndrome. The late- and early-onset problem-drinking classification can permit observations regarding the effects of the stresses of aging that contribute to the onset of other mental health problems in the aged in contrast to factors that existed in alcoholics long before they became elderly and may be unrelated to the developmental problems associated with aging.

Rosin and Glatt (1971) reviewed 103 cases of patients age 65 and over who were seen in psychiatric home consultations or admitted to a regional alcoholism unit or to a hospital's geriatric unit. They also found two distinct groups of alcoholics and noted, as did Simon et al. (1968), that two-thirds of the patients were long-standing alcoholics, with their alcoholism persisting as they grew older, the other one-third representing patients who developed their alcoholism in later life. The long-standing alcoholics had personality characteristics similar to those found among younger alcoholics, but the late-onset alcoholics seemed to have developed their drinking problems associated with depression, bereavement, retirement, loneliness, marital stress, and physical illness. Alcoholism in the late-onset alcoholics seemed related to the stresses of aging.

Based on their data Carruth et al. (1975) reported three distinct types of alcoholics. One type consisted of individuals who had no history of a drinking problem prior to old age and who developed the problem during old age (late onset); a second group consisted of individuals who intermittently experienced problems with alcohol, but in old age developed a more severe and persistent problem of alcohol abuse (late-onset exacerbation); the third group consisted of individuals who had a long history of alcoholism and continued their problem drinking into old age (early onset). The authors did not indicate the relative percentages in the three groups described. It seems possible to conclude, however, that the two former groups could be considered alcoholics of long standing with different drinking patterns in their younger years. The terms *late onset, late-onset exacerbation,* and *early onset* are this author's designations.

The concept of early-onset alcoholism (two-thirds) and late-onset (one-third) among the elderly appears to be a more useful classification. First, it is possible to determine, through the history of the use of alcohol in relation to problems, in which group an elderly alcoholic might be classified. Second, the long-standing alcoholics are more likely to be experiencing medical complications of alcoholism and therefore require medical care. Third, recognizing factors contributing to the development of the problem may make interventions more effective.

Important questions arise, however, if we accept this classification of early and late onset of alcoholism among the elderly. These questions deal with different treatment approaches for these two groups based on differing psychological and social characteristics that may be found among these patients.

PSYCHOSOCIAL FACTORS IN GERIATRIC ALCOHOLISM

Cahalan, Cisin, and Crossley (1974), in their monograph based on a national survey of drinking behavior and attitudes in the United States, discussed some interesting observations concerning the natural history of drinking behavior and problem drinking. They noted that about one-third more individuals had problem drinking in a period before the three-year study period than during the study period itself, suggesting a tendency toward spontaneous remission.

Malzberg (1947), Locke and Duvall (1960), and Gorwitz, Bahn, Warthen, and Cooper (1970) presented data that showed a decline in admissions of elderly alcoholics to psychiatric hospitals and psychiatric clinics. These data, based on admissions to treatment, seem to confirm the epidemiological data developed by Cahalan et al. (1974), and, in fact, have been the major basis for assuming that alcoholism is not a significant problem among the elderly.

Drew (1968) observed that data concerning mortality related to alcoholism and alcoholism treatment outcome could not account for the observed decrease in alcoholics among the older age groups. He suggested that alcoholism is a self-limiting disease with a significant spontaneous remission with advancing age. Imber, Schultz, Funderburk, Allen, and Flamer (1976) described a follow-up of 58 alcoholics who received no treatment for alcoholism. It was noted that the rate of abstinence was 15% at one year and 11% after three years. Vaillant (1983) found that significant numbers of alcoholics give up drinking and experience recovery as they get older and that this course of ultimate remission is the natural history of alcoholism. Therefore, spontaneous remission does seem to occur in alcoholism.

The question arises as to what factors might contribute to a spontaneous remission in elderly alcoholics. It has been established (Salzman, Vander Kolk, and Shader, 1975) that drugs, including alcohol, tend to stay in the body longer and to have more prolonged and more powerful clinical and toxic effect in the body of an aged person. In addition, there is a functional loss of neuronal tissue in the aged which may account for the observed increased sensitivity to drugs of the sedative-hypnotic class (which includes alcohol). It is therefore quite possible that the effects of alcohol on mood and behavior become less pleasant and produce more unpleasant side effects in elderly people. Even long-standing alcoholics are likely to give up alcohol if it has become a noxious substance to them because of their diminished tolerance and its increased toxic effects.

If this explanation is correct, then what factors contribute to the continued problem drinking among some alcoholics into old age and the development of late-onset alcoholism among a significant number of elderly people? The author has noted in his experience with both late-onset and early-onset alcoholics a significant number of social and psychological factors associated with aging that affect these patients. Rosin and Glatt (1971) and Droller (1964) noted in their treatment of elderly alcoholics that depression, bereavement, retirement, loneliness, marital stress, and physical illness were major contributing factors to the drinking problem. Treatment efforts directed at these factors in the elderly, in contrast to treatment efforts directed at the use of alcohol among younger alcoholics, were found to be most beneficial.

Based on these observations it is possible to construct a hypothesis that could account for the spontaneous tendency of alcoholism to remit with advancing age, as well as for the fact that some long-standing alcoholics do continue to have problem drinking and that some elderly individuals develop alcohol problems in later life. Both groups of elderly alcoholics are reacting to the stresses of aging, which, in producing a great deal of anxiety and depression, lead to the use of alcohol in the form of self-medication. Apparently the adverse effects of alcohol use in these aged are less disturbing than facing overwhelming problems, particularly object loss. Therefore the sociopsychological stresses of aging can prolong problem drinking in long-standing alcoholics into old age and can contribute to the development of problem drinking in later life for some elderly individuals. If this hypothesis is correct, treatment approaches will have to consider primarily the sociopsychological stresses of aging as the focus for intervention.

PSYCHOSOCIAL TREATMENT TECHNIQUES

Although awareness of alcoholism among the elderly has developed only recently, there have been reports of successful interventions in relation to elderly alcoholics. Droller (1964) reported on seven cases of elderly alcoholics he visited at home. He found that in addition to medical and supportive treatment, therapy that was primarily social was the most beneficial to these patients. Rosin and Glatt (1971), in their treatment of 103 elderly alcoholics, noted that environmental manipulation and medical services along with day hospital, and home visiting by staff or good neighbors were the services that were most beneficial.

The author, in his experience in an outpatient geriatric psychiatric program (Zimberg, 1969), as a psychiatric consultant to a medical home care program (Zimberg, 1971), and as a psychiatric consultant to a nursing home, noted similar responses to social interventions. The use of group socialization and at times antidepressant medication was effective in eliminating alcohol abuse as a problem among the patients in these programs. The use of disulfiram, AA, or referral to alcoholism treatment programs required by younger alcoholics was not necessary for these patients. It is of even further interest to note that both early-onset and late-onset alcoholics responded equally well to these psychosocial interventions, suggesting common etiological factors for these two groups of elderly alcoholics.

The hypothesis that psychosocial factors are the major contributors to alcoholism among the aged has been supported by the successful use of treatment interventions based on a psychosocial model. In young-adult and middle-aged alcoholics, the first approaches to treatment are directed at the drinking behavior itself, as indicated in Chapter 1, "Principles of Alcoholism Psychotherapy." Only with such directive intervention can the elimination of the use of alcohol be accomplished and an opportunity for learning other coping mechanisms to replace the alcohol be achieved. This direct-intervention approach is designed for the primary alcoholic, that is, in alcoholism that develops as *the* major behavioral disorder that is influenced by sociocultural, psychological, and physiological factors, but remains the main and overwhelmingly severe disorder of addiction.

In contrast, the elderly alcoholic is responding to severe social and psychological stresses associated with aging and is drinking in response to these stresses. If these stresses can be eliminated or attenuated, the secondary use of alcohol is diminished, thus leading to sobriety.

Techniques of Therapy.   The treatment techniques utilized with such patients are based on the author's experience in a geriatric psychiatry outpatient program and involve the use of group therapy. Prior to admission to the group, every patient should have a complete physical and psychiatric evaluation so that physical or psychiatric disorders can be diagnosed and appropriate treatments instituted.

The group therapy can involve up to 15 to 20 patients and should not be insight-oriented or directive as far as alcoholism is concerned. The patients should be elderly persons with a variety of social, psychological, organic mental, and physical disorders, not just alcoholism. The patients with alcoholism should be told that they have a drinking problem and that it is probably related to the difficulties they are having in adjusting to their current life situation.

The group should meet at least once a week and last for one and a half to two hours. Cookies, coffee, and tea should be made available. If meals can be provided, eating together as a group would be helpful. The approach utilized by the group leaders should be supportive and oriented toward problem solving. Drinking problems should be one of the problem areas discussed, but not the only one. Members of the group should be encouraged to discuss other members' problems as well as their own and to give advice and suggestions.

The group sessions could be divided into an informal social and/or eating period during the beginning of sessions, then a discussion and problem-solving period, followed by a socializing period at the end. The socializing period could be expanded through the use of activities therapy involving occupational therapy and/or planning for trips and outings, development of a patient government, and establishment of a patient kitty or dues. Patients requiring medication or medication follow-up can be seen by the physician individually after the group activities are completed.

The staffing of group programs should ideally consist of a psychiatrist knowledgeable about the problems of aging and alcoholism, a nurse or social worker, and one or two paraprofessional workers. These paraprofessional workers can provide a great many services for the patients, who will have many areas of difficulty. Such services should include visiting the homes of patients who miss clinic appointments; accompanying patients to other clinics and community agencies to act as liaison and patient advocates; observing and reporting patient behavior to the professional staff; contacting Department of Social Services to help with patients' economic and housing needs; interviewing patients' friends, relatives, and neighbors to help support the patients living at home; and participating in the group sessions.

Many of the patients treated in such groups will be noted to be clinically depressed. The judicious use of antidepressant medication can be helpful for such patients.

New Developments in Treatment.   With increasing interest in the treatment of elderly alcoholics, some new clinical observations have been made by the author and others interested in this area. Elderly alcoholics who are well-off financially and retired from previously prominent positions seem to experience fewer of the social and economic stresses of aging and respond to more alcoholism specific approaches. They need counseling and support to help them deal with a changed way of life, but the treatment of alcoholism must take priority. Another observation has been that elderly alcoholics who do find their way to alcoholism programs can also be treated in an alcoholism specific way with the addition of psychosocial interventions for the stresses of aging. Most elderly alcoholics, however, still resist referral to alcoholism programs. Also the involvement of home attendants in the group can take the place of paraprofessional workers.

CASE HISTORIES

Late-Onset Alcoholism.   One of the patients with a drinking problem treated in such a group illustrates the value of this psychosocial approach. This case presents a patient with late-onset alcoholism.

The patient was a 64-year-old widower who was a retired railroad mechanic. He was living with his son. He had become quite depressed since his wife's death and had greatly increased his alcohol intake so that it became a serious problem. He was noted to be behaving strangely and was often observed giving money away to strangers. He was referred to the program by a local block association. He had retired from work; his wife's death was a severe blow. Shortly after his referral he became involved in the group and was started on antidepressant medication. He responded quickly to the medication and experienced a significant reduction in depression. He became an enthusiastic participant in the group and soon stopped drinking alcohol. He was visited at home on several occasions by one of the paraprofessional workers, who was able to improve the strained relationship the patient had with his son as a result of his symptoms.

Early-Onset Alcoholism. Another patient treated by this group approach represents a patient with early-onset alcoholism.

This patient was a 70-year-old retired longshoreman who was living alone. He had been divorced from his wife for many years and had no children. He had at least a 40-year history of excessive drinking and had continued to drink heavily since his retirement from work two years prior to his referral to the group geriatric psychiatry program. He was referred by the psychiatric emergency-room staff of the hospital because of the development of hallucinations and confusion. When seen initially, he was in a physically debilitated state and was suffering from urinary incontinence in addition to the psychotic symptoms. He was attempting to get work on the docks and was unable to accept the fact that he was physically unable to do such work. He had several general hospital admissions and was followed in the medical and urology clinics. He was visited by the paraprofessional staff while in the hospital and had his clinic follow-up arranged by them. He was treated with a phenothiazine drug at bedtime and antidepressants during the day. Between admissions to the hospital, he attended many group sessions. Gradually his health improved, his confusion cleared, and he gave up drinking. He made several friends in the group and accepted his retirement.

Alcoholism Specific Therapy in an Elderly Alcoholic. This is a case history about an elderly patient with alcoholism who responded to alcoholism specific therapy in a private practice setting.

The patient was a 65-year-old woman who was married for 33 years. She was from Texas and was a very attractive woman. She married a wealthy man in New York City of a different religion. She found the adjustment to New York City difficult and began to drink more. After the birth of her daughter 32 years ago, her husband became devoted to the child and tended to neglect her. Her drinking increased and reached a level of alcohol addiction about 10 years ago. She drank primarily beer.

She developed serious liver problems due to the drinking and the liver damage reached the stage of early cirrhosis. She had tried numerous attempts at treatment including several hospital detoxifications, AA, and inpatient treatment at several different facilities. She stopped drinking for short periods of time but always resumed the alcoholic drinking in a matter of weeks.

She became increasingly estranged from her husband and her daughter. Her husband was verbally and at times physically abusive to her when she was intoxicated. She had several falls and sustained fractures while intoxicated.

Her internist sent her to the author for alcoholism treatment as a last resort. When first seen, she had been drinking heavily and was in need of detoxification. Detoxification was carried out on an outpatient basis using diazepam. She was quite agitated and tremulous during the first week of detoxification. She completed the detoxification and did not resume drinking. Medical clearance was obtained and she was started on disulfiram 250 mg a day.

The patient appeared quite physically debilitated and unstable on her feet during the first two weeks of treatment. After four weeks of treatment her physical status was somewhat better but she appeared severely depressed. She had a history of previous depression. She had no appetite and showed psychomotor retardation. She was started on desipramine which was gradually increased to 300 mg a day. After two months of treatment she felt much better physically and was less depressed.

The patient began attending AA meetings four to six times a week and her husband went to a few Al-Anon meetings. Since she became sober the relationship between herself and her husband gradually improved.

The desipramine was gradually reduced and then discontinued, but she was maintained on disulfiram. Her liver began to heal and she felt increasingly better. She renewed her activities at her church and became committed to long-term sobriety which has been over two years currently.

This case illustrates an elderly patient with long standing alcoholism who had not responded to many previous attempts at alcoholism treatment. Her seriously deteriorating physical health and the "last chance" referral for alcoholism treatment was successful because the patient had "hit bottom" and the severe coexisting depression was recognized and effectively treated. In this case, alcoholism specific treatment was effective in this elderly alcoholic along with the recognition and treatment of a severe depression.

LOCATION OF TREATMENT PROGRAMS

The question arises as to where these treatments should be provided in order to reach the greatest number of elderly alcoholics. In addition, there is the common question of how one deals with the significant number of elderly unwilling or unable to leave their homes. It has been found that elderly alcoholics perceive their alcoholism in ways different from younger alcoholics. First, older alcoholics generally consume smaller quantities of alcohol because of a lower tolerance, and therefore have fewer *acute* medical problems associated with their alcohol consumption. Many elderly alcoholics are at level 3 of the alcohol-abuse scale (see Table 1, Chapter 1) rather than more severe levels 4 and 5 that are common among younger alcoholics. Some elderly alcoholics who are homeless and on skid-row can be placed at level 6 of severity. For most elderly alcoholics the alcohol that is consumed produces social problems, but less often acute physical problems. Chronic medical problems such as cirrhosis of the liver or peptic ulcer may be present, but the need to detoxify from alcohol and treat alcohol withdrawal manifestations is much less. Therefore, the physical distress associated with alcoholism is seen less in elderly alcoholics which leads to a greater reluctance of the elderly to utilize specialized alcoholism treatment programs.

Denial exists in elderly alcoholics as it does with younger alcoholics, but the confrontation that is required to reach younger alcoholics to get them to recognize that they are alcoholic has not been found to be necessary in most cases. In view of these clinical observations, as well as the responses of elderly alcoholics to sociopsychological approaches related to the stresses of aging and their multiplicity of complex problems (only one of which is problem drinking), it would seem inappropriate to refer such patients to alcoholism treatment programs except when they may have serious medical problems associated with their drinking or because they are more insulated from the stresses of aging due to other circumstances. Treatment interventions will, in general, be much more effective when delivered through facilities serving the aged, such as senior citizen programs, outpatient geriatric medical or psychiatric programs, nursing homes, or home-care programs.

The development of specialized AA programs for elderly alcoholics might be an exception to this suggestion. Such AA programs should utilize elderly alcoholics as speakers to help the participants identify with similar problems. In addition, the group nature of an AA meeting could be enhanced by providing socialization and recreational activities after the formal AA meeting. Conducting such meetings in a senior citizen center would be ideal in regard to location and in regard to the availability of recreational activities.

The Queen Nursing Home in Minneapolis, Minnesota (*Alcohol Health and Research World*, 1975), deals with elderly alcoholics and apparently has had some success. However, the development of such specialized programs may not be the most effective way of delivering services to the elderly alcoholic on a large scale.

The problems associated with delivering services to the elderly in general will also apply to elderly alcoholics. Many people will be unwilling or unable to leave their homes to go to outpatient programs or to participate in groups once they get there. Therefore, the delivery of comprehensive services to the elderly must include outreach and case finding services as well as an effective home-care program. Elderly individuals unwilling to participate in group activities as part of their lifelong life style and personality have to be dealt with individually in an effort to learn what particular interests and competence the elderly person has that might be utilized to catalyze involvement in some aspect of a program. These considerations apply to the elderly alcoholic as well.

APPLYING THE CONCEPTS OF THE THERAPEUTIC COMMUNITY TO THE ELDERLY

Gruenberg (1974) developed the concept of the social-breakdown syndrome to describe and measure the amount of chronic mental disorder existing in a community and in psychiatric institutional settings. The syndrome consists of social and psychological behavioral deterioration resulting from the loss of social supports in the community or the authoritarian and rigid conditions in an institutional setting.

It is possible through the use of the concepts of the therapeutic community (Jones, 1953; Stanton and Schwartz, 1954) to treat effectively manifestations of behavioral disturbances that result from severe social and psychological deprivation and even improve functional capacities in elderly individuals suffering from organic mental impairment. The concepts of a therapeutic community can be applied in ambulatory settings (clinics and day care) as well as institutional settings (psychiatric hospitals and nursing homes).

The principles and practices embodied in the concept of the therapeutic community involve the recognition that an individual patient is part of a social system in which the individual's efforts toward involvement result in positive feedback from the social system as a necessary condition for maintaining feelings of self-worth and the ability to maintain continued cognitive and emotional involvement with the social system. The organization of an institution can either maximize the individual's involvement and provide positive feedback or strip the individual of all responsibilities and self-worth, resulting in a variety of behavioral disturbances. The isolated individual in the community can also be subjected to a state of isolation and helplessness in relation to the community at large.

The practices of the therapeutic community involve the opportunity for patients to have open and direct communication with the staff. Patients are encouraged to participate actively in their own treatment and to make decisions regarding administrative and therapeutic aspects of the treatment program. Patients are encouraged to participate in the decision-making process through patient–staff meetings and the establishment of a system of participatory patient government. Contacts with the community at large are encouraged and built into activities and recreational programs. The relationship between staff and patient is one of mutual respect and cooperation, with the staff providing guidance and direction rather than authoritarian orders and regulations.

The author provided psychiatric consultations to a county nursing home in Rockland County, New York, over a period of two years. Prior to this consultation patients in the nursing home had no say in the various activities that were provided, were often put to bed at 6:30 P.M., and had limited outside activities. All sexual behavior was suppressed. There were several patients with drinking problems, and six to seven patients a year were sent to a nearby state psychiatric hospital because of serious management problems.

The focus of the psychiatric consultation was to establish a therapeutic community at the nursing home, with discussions of various patient problems and the staff rules and attitudes as they related to these problems. The results produced a nursing home where patients made the decisions about the movies they would see and the activities they wanted. Frequent group discussions between staff and patients eliminated some of the areas of patient complaints. Patients' intellectual interests increased so that they asked the local community college to provide courses for them in the nursing home. Behavioral problems including alcohol abuse were eliminated, no longer requiring any patient to be transferred to the state hospital. Married couples who had been placed in separate rooms were permitted to sleep in the same room, and a room was set aside for privacy for patients who had established close relationships. It was apparent that sexual interests in the elderly patients were not really absent, only suppressed. The nursing home became in many respects more like a *home* for the patients since they had a considerable voice in what went on in the facility. The staff benefited by having many fewer management problems to contend with and no longer had to put patients to bed at 6:30 P.M. in order to have a quiet night. All this was accomplished by changing the social system of the nursing home, opening channels of communication between staff and patients, and permitting patients to exercise much greater responsibility for their own care and the care of the other patients.

USE OF ALCOHOL IN INSTITUTIONS

It has been suggested that alcohol be used to improve the management and sociability of the aged in psychiatric hospitals (Becker and Cesar, 1973) and in nursing homes (Chien, Stotsky, and Cole, 1973) because of its mood-changing properties. An extensive review of alcoholism in the elderly and use of alcohol in institutional settings was provided by Mishara and Kastenbaum (1980). The author believes that the principles of the therapeutic community, when applied to nursing homes and psychiatric hospitals, can be more effective in improving patients' feelings and reducing management problems than can the use of alcohol, which carries with it the development of tolerance and therefore the need to use more and more alcohol to achieve the appropriate mood. In addition, elderly people may have more adverse behavioral reactions to alcohol. Alcohol could be used in a nursing home as a beverage on picnics and outings or at meals but has serious risks associated with its use as a mood-changing drug.

Case History: Effect of Social Interventions. A case in a paper on home care psychiatric consultation (Zimberg, 1971) is illustrative of the potent effect of social interventions. A 79-year-old widow of Italian descent, on home care and living in East Harlem, developed severe paranoid ideation, would not leave her house, and avoided social contacts. She had a daughter who lived in the Bronx, but they had little contact. The widow felt isolated and fearful of being robbed. A psychiatric evaluation was conducted in her apartment, and it was felt that she was suffering a psychotic organic mental syndrome due to arteriosclerosis. Recommendations included the use of phenothiazine medication, the assignment of a homemaker to assist in her shopping, cooking, and house cleaning, and the installation of a phone to permit her to call her daughter. The homemaker was assigned and the phone installed, but by mistake the medication was not ordered by the home-care physician. At follow-up discussions several weeks later, it was learned that the medication had never started, but the patient had improved markedly and was no longer paranoid, as a result of the homemaker's presence and the contact with her daughter facilitated by the phone.

This case illustrates the fact that social interventions can improve socially induced behavioral disorders in the elderly. Antidepressant medication and phenothiazine tranquilizers are useful for clearly documented depression and psychosis, but the social and psychological aspects of the treatment are often the most effective for the elderly.

Since elderly individuals in general are more likely to go for help to agencies and programs created for their needs, it is important that such services be knowledgeable about alcoholism and the principles and practices of the therapeutic community. Collaboration and consultation between alcoholism treatment agencies and agencies serving the elderly can provide the pooling of knowledge and experience necessary to carry out effective interventions in the elderly alcoholic population.

SUMMARY

This chapter has presented evidence of the existence of a significant problem of alcohol abuse among the elderly from a variety of sources. The recognition of this problem requires the development of effective treatment interventions for this population of alcoholics.

Elderly alcoholics can be classified into early-onset alcoholics with long histories of alcoholism and late-onset alcoholics, who develop drinking problems in late life. Among elderly alcoholics about two-thirds are early-onset alcoholics, one-third late-onset alcoholics.

The psychosocial stresses of aging, including depression, bereavement, retirement, loneliness, marital stress, economic hardships, and physical illness, are thought to be the major causal factors of alcoholism among the elderly. There is a tendency for alcohol to be consumed less as one ages; however, the alcoholism in early-onset alcoholics and development of alcoholism in late-onset alcoholics can be related to the reaction to the stresses of aging.

The psychosocial treatment techniques of alcoholism among the elderly are described. They include the use of supportive and problem-solving-oriented group therapy, antidepressant medication, group socialization, and recreational activities. Elderly alcoholics are best treated with elderly people who have other problems in programs established for the elderly rather than in separate alcoholism programs, with some exceptions. The use of professional and paraprofessional staff in treatment teams can be the most effective approach to treatment.

Establishing therapeutic communities in nursing homes can improve patient behavior and reduce behavioral and management problems including alcoholism. The use of alcoholic beverages as mood-changing drugs in institutions should be discouraged.

References

Alcohol Health and Research World. Older problem drinker, Spring 1975, 12–17.

Bailey, M. B., Haberman, P. W., and Alksne, H. The epidemiology of alcoholism in an urban residential area. *Quarterly Journal of Studies on Alcohol*, 1965, 26, 19–40.

Becker, P. W., and Cesar, J. A. Use off beer in geriatric patient groups. *Psychological Reports* 1973, 33, 182.

Cahalan, D., Cisin, I. H., and Crossley, H. M. *American drinking practives: A national survey of drinking behavior and attitudes*. New Brunswick, N.J.: Rutgers Center of Alcohol Studies, 1974.

Carruth, B., Williams, E. P., Mysak, P., and Boudreaux, L. Community care providers and the older problem drinker. *Grassroots*, 1975, *July Supplement*, 1–5.

Chien, C., Stotsky, B. A., and Cole, J. O. Psychiatric treatment for nursing home patients: Drugs, alcohol and milieu. *American Journal of Psychiatry*, 1973, 130, 543–548.

Drew, L. R. H. Alcohol as a self-limiting disease. *Quarterly Journal of Studies on Alcohol*, 1968, 29, 956–967.

Droller, H. Some aspects of alcoholism in the elderly. *Lancet*, 1964, 2, 137–139.

Epstein, L. J., Mills, C., and Simon, A. Antisocial behavior of the elderly. *Comprehensive Psychiatry*, 1970, 11, 36–42.

Gaitz, C. M., and Baer, P. E. Characteristics of elderly patients with alcoholism. *Archives of General Psychiatry*, 1971, 24, 327–378.

Gorwitz, K., Bahn, A., Warthen, F. J., and Cooper, M. Some epidemiological data on alcoholism in Maryland based on admissions to psychiatric facilities. *Quarterly Journal of Studies on Alcohol*, 1970, 31, 423–443.

Gruenberg, E. M. The social breakdown syndrome and its prevention. In S. Arieti and G. Caplan (Eds.), *American handbook of psychiatry*. New York: Basic Books, 1974.

Imber, S., Schultz, E., Funderburk, F., Allen, R., and Flamer, R. The fate of the untreated alcoholic. *The Journal of Nervous and Mental Disease*, 1976, 162, 238–247.

Jones, M. *The therapeutic community*, New York: Basic Books, 1953.

Locke, B. Z., and Duvall, H. J. Alcoholism among first admissions to Ohio public mental hospital. *Quarterly Journal of Studies on Alcohol*, 1960, 21, 457–474.

Malzberg, B. A study of first admissions with alcoholic psychoses in New York State. *Quarterly Journal of Studies on Alcohol*, 1947, 8, 274–295.

McCusker, J., Cherubin, C. F., and Zimberg, S. Prevalence of alcoholism in general municipal hospital population. *New York State Journal of Medicine*, 1971, 71, 751–754.

Mishara, B. L., and Kastenbaum, R. *Alcohol and old age*. New York: Grune & Stratton, 1980.

Rosin, A. J., and Glatt, M. M. Alcohol excess in the elderly. *Quarterly Journal of Studies on Alcohol*, 1971, 32, 53–59.

Salzman, C., Vander Kolk, B., and Shader, R. I. Psychopharmacology and the geriatric patient. In R. I. Shader (Ed.), *Manual of psychiatric therapeutics*. Boston: Little, Brown, 1975.

Schuckit, M. A., and Miller, P. L. Alcoholism in elderly men: A survey of a general medical ward. *Annals New York Academy of Science*, 1976, *273*, 558–571.

Siassi, I., Crocetti, G., and Spiro, H. R. Drinking patterns and alcoholism in a blue collar population. *Quarterly Journal of Studies of Alcohol*, 1973, *34*, 917–926.

Simon, A., Epstein, L. J., and Reynolds, L. Alcoholism in the geriatric mentally ill. *Geriatrics*, 1968, *23*, 125–131.

Stanton, A. H., and Schwartz, M. S. *The mental hospital*. New York: Basic Books, 1954.

Vaillant, G. E. *The natural history of alcoholism: Causes, patterns, and paths to recovery*. Cambridge: Harvard University Press, 1983.

Zimberg, S. Outpatient geriatric psychiatry in an urban ghetto with non-professional workers. *American Journal of Psychiatry*, 1969, *125*, 1697–1702.

Zimberg, S. The psychiatrist and medical home care: Geriatric psychiatry in the Harlem community. *American Journal of Psychiatry*, 1971, *127*, 1062–1066.

IV

CLINICAL EVALUATION OF
PATIENT PROGRESS

19

Evaluation of Patient Progress

Douglas K. Chalmers and John Wallace

Introduction

The evaluation of patient progress during the course of treatment is often difficult and characterized by uncertainty. In residential settings, the therapist typically observes behaviors and attitudes that may not generalize to the real world outside of treatment. In outpatient settings, alcoholic patients may comply, minimize, or distort their inner and outer realities.

Despite such difficulties, however, therapists must continuously evaluate patient progress in order that treatment plans may be formulated and revised, referral sources kept informed, and requirements of third-party payers met.

Our purpose in writing this chapter is not to provide the reader with reviews of prediction of relapse studies, program evaluation studies, or patient follow-up studies. Such reviews are available in other sources. Rather, it is our intent to provide a clinical view of patient progress with an emphasis on particular variables that seem of importance to us in arriving at clinical judgments in the clinical setting. Our discussion is in two parts: inpatient evaluation and longer term outpatient evaluation. There is also a discussion of new directions in treatment and evaluation research that can provide a more successful outcome for alcoholics.

Douglas K. Chalmers • Associate Professor of Psychology, School of Social Sciences, University of California, Irvine, California.   John Wallace • Director of Treatment, Edgehill Newport, Newport, Rhode Island.

Inpatient Evaluation

Assessing Physical Health Changes

While the patient's physical health is the responsibility of medical staff, the psychotherapist working with alcoholics cannot ignore these matters. In some programs the therapist may have more continuous contact with the patient than does the attending physician. Along with astute nursing observations, information developed in the therapeutic context may lead to the detection of important changes in the patient's health status. Moreover, information from this context may also suggest additional complexities deserving of further study by medical staff.

Continuous evaluation of the patient's physical health is important to the psychotherapist for still another reason. Alcoholism psychotherapy requires sensitive timing of therapeutic interventions along with accurate judgment of stress levels in the patient. Neither of these can be accomplished when physical health status is ignored. For example, it makes no sense at all to engage an alcoholic freshly out of detoxification in a sharp confrontation about his behavior in a group-therapy setting. Nor is it appropriate at that time to encourage the patient to conduct a detailed examination of his future plans.

Continued Withdrawal Signs. Withdrawal signs do not automatically cease with the end of the formal period of detoxification. These may continue in subtle form for even lengthy periods. In lay terms the alcoholic is said to be not yet "physically sober." During this period he is also said to be "thirsty," meaning that bodily demands for alcohol are still present. This is a time of much uncertainty for both patient and therapist. Care must be taken to make the patient as comfortable as possible in the therapeutic context since any additional stress may force him to withdraw completely from the program or leave the hospital temporarily in search of alcohol.

Continued withdrawal is evidenced by such signs as tremor, agitation, sweating, illogical thinking, depressed mood, anxiety, and, on occasion, a sudden and unexpected delayed seizure.

The therapist should be alert for such symptoms as persistent headache, dizziness, difficulty in breathing, cardiac arrhythmias, flushing, sudden drops in energy, slurring of speech, difficulty in walking, memory deficits, complaints of abdominal pain, and poor appetite. These may reflect continued withdrawal, but they may also indicate chronic conditions and diseases of increased likelihood in alcoholics (e.g., hypertension, liver disease, gastritis, ulcer, carbohydrate-metabolism disorders, brain dysfunction, anemia, heart disease, polyneuropathy, emphysema, and stroke).

Serious Mental Illness. The therapist working with alcoholics, as with any patient population, must be aware of the possibility of undetected serious mental illness in certain of his patients. Establishing the existence of severe psychopathology in alcoholics is not difficult *if* judgment is suspended until detoxification has been completed. Intoxicated alcoholics and patients in the early stages of withdrawal present a complex and confusing diagnostic picture. Many signs of frank psychopathology are evident. Hallucinations, loosening of associations, flight of ideas, paranoid delusions, psychopathic behaviors, depression, suicidal ideation, and manic acting-out are commonly observed in drinking alcoholics and alcoholics in the first stages of withdrawal. The therapist should fix firmly in mind that reliable diagnoses cannot be made on the basis of *chemical behavior*. Rather, the patient's status should be evaluated as progress through the program proceeds. In the event that signs of severe psychopathology persist as treatment progresses, therapeutic plans must be altered, since alcoholism complicated by psychosis requires specialized treatments. In the presence of clear indications of serious mental illness, prognosis should be guarded.

Evaluating Psychological Factors

Certain psychological factors seem to be related to both relapse and adjustment to sobriety. These are separate issues since sobriety and psychological well-being are partially related but not perfectly correlated. A patient may achieve and maintain sobriety but continue to show numerous problems of personal and social adjustment. And, on the other hand, patients with few apparent psychological difficulties may relapse.

Evaluating the Drinking Attitude. Perhaps the most critical factor in assessing the patient's progress is that of drinking attitude. In evaluating the drinking attitude, it is useful to bear in mind the components of attitudes in general. Attitudes are made up of three component parts: belief, affect, and action. Each of these components stands in either positive or negative relation to some object or activity. Hence, drinking attitudes may be categorized as follows:

1. Positively congruent
2. Negatively congruent
3. Incongruity among components
4. Incongruity within components

For example, a patient may state that he believes that drinking makes him creative (+), that it makes him feel good (+), and that he intends to hang out with people who drink once he leaves the hospital (+). In this case the relations among belief, affect, and action components are congruent and the overall attitude toward drinking is positive. Hence, this is categorized as a positively congruent attitude toward drinking.

A negatively congruent attitude would be as follows: a patient states that he believes drinking reduces the quality of his work (−), that he feels depressed when drinking (−), and that he intends to take Antabuse (−).

Incongruity among the components of the attitude would be indicated in the following: a patient states that he believes drinking makes him more creative (+), but it makes him depressed (−) and he does intend to take Antabuse (−).

Incongruity within the components occurs when a patient states that he believes drinking makes him creative (+) but he also believes it makes him irresponsible (−); he states that he feels good after the first few drinks (+), but as the drinking continues he feels depressed (−); he also states that he will continue to see friends who drink (+) but also intends to go to AA meetings (−).

This analysis of drinking attitudes allows certain nonobvious predictions. Positively congruent attitudes toward drinking are indicators of poor progress in treatment and a high likelihood of relapse afterwards.

Negatively congruent attitudes toward drinking are, in and of themselves, ambiguous. Overly compliant patients, patients who have something to gain from pretending to be highly motivated in treatment, sociopaths, and malingerers, along with a portion of the sincerely motivated, tend to verbalize negatively congruent attitudes. Moreover, negatively congruent attitudes toward drinking may signal an intense underlying conflict over whether or not to drink. In certain patients the more rigid the attitude organization becomes, the more intense the impulse to drink can be assumed to be. As a consequence of these many considerations, negatively congruent attitudes toward drinking are not necessarily good indicators of progress, nor are they valid predictors of continued sobriety.

Attitudes that reflect incongruity among the various components are varied indicators of progress. There are six possible variants, three with two negative components and three with two positive ones.

The set of *predominantly negative incongruent attitudes* are as follows:

(a) Belief (−), Action (−), Affect (+). The patient may believe that drinking has negative consequences for him and he shows actions that are inconsistent with drinking. Progress in this case is good with moderate predictions of maintenance of sobriety.

(b) Belief (−), Affect (−), Action (+). The patient may believe that drinking has negative consequences for him and he has negative feelings associated with drinking. However, he refuses to take actions inconsistent with drinking and displays actions consistent with drinking (e.g., refuses to go to AA and plans to live with a drinking alcoholic upon release from the hospital). Progress in this case is only fair and the probability of maintenance of sobriety moderate in the short run and poor in the long run.

(c) Affect (−), Action (−), Belief (+). The patient has negative feelings associated with drinking and shows actions inconsistent with drinking. However, he believes that drinking does lead to some set of positive, important consequences for him. Progress in this case is fair with slightly less than moderate predictions of maintenance of sobriety.

Predominantly positive incongruent attitudes are those in which the incongruency between components is characterized by two positive components and one negative. For the most part, all of these three cases suggest poor progress and high probability of relapse. In the case of positive beliefs and feelings associated with drinking while actions are negative for drinking, probability of relapse is decreased slightly. This is precisely the situation that exists when an alcoholic is coerced into treatment or to attending AA meetings.

The most interesting attitude organization is that which shows *incongruity within each of the components*. In this case both positive and negative positions are represented in each attitude component. Hence, the attitude organization is as follows:

Belief (+), (−); Action (+), (−); Affect (+), (−). The patient may believe that drinking has some positive outcome for him, but he also believes it has some negative outcome. He shows some actions consistent with drinking, but some that are inconsistent. In addition, he has mixed feelings associated with drinking.

Incongruity within the components is a sign of excellent progress and suggests a high probability of maintenance of sobriety. This is a nonobvious hypothesis. However, such incongruity within components indicates awareness of the reality of the drinking–not drinking conflict, realistic acceptance of it, and willingness to discuss it openly. Moreover, the tension generated by conscious awareness of the conflict produces sustained motivation in treatment and a level of vigilance ideal for the maintenance of sobriety outside the treatment context.

Belief in the Possibility of Controlled Drinking. Despite anecdotal evidence for spontaneous remission of unknown frequency and duration in alcoholism, the possibility of a stable pattern of drinking for the vast majority of alcoholics in treatment is an exceedingly dangerous hypothesis. Nor is this hypothesis rendered any less dangerous by recent methodologically inadequate studies of controlled drinking, ecologically irrelevant laboratory studies of drinking behavior, and enthusiastic reports of drinking alcoholics themselves.

The persistence of the belief in controlled drinking as a possibility for oneself as treatment proceeds is a very poor prognostic sign. In clinical experience, it is not only an almost perfect predictor of relapse in the long run but it frequently predicts relapse in the short run as well. Patients in group-therapy contexts who stubbornly refuse to abandon this hypothesis usually return to patterns of destructive drinking, either dropping out of treatment to do so or drinking shortly after release from the hospital. Recent claims that this predictable outcome occurs largely because of expectations communicated to the patient by the therapist, other patients, and members of Alcoholics Anonymous are absurd. Typically, the patient believed in the controlled drinking hypothesis *before* he entered treatment or Alcoholics Anonymous and encountered contrary communications. His belief in his ability to control alcohol *prior* to treatment obviously did not protect him from dangerous drinking. In fact the persistence of this belief in the face of massive evidence to the contrary lies at the very heart of alcoholism. It is diagnostic of the disease in its active form.

Resistance to Help from Others. Progress is poor and the probability of relapse high in patients who continue to insist that they can stay sober by themselves. These patients typically resist suggestions, ideas, and recommendations made by the therapist, counselors, and other patients. Such resistance is a sure sign of the continuance of certain common alcoholic characteristics—grandiosity, extreme self-centeredness, and denial. Invariably, such patients will insist on doing things their way despite the fact that their own ideas, plans, and actions never worked in the past.

Refusal to Participate Openly. Patients who actively resist sharing in the group context and deliberately isolate themselves during treatment are poor risks for continued sobriety. These must, of course, be differentiated from *passively participating patients.* The patient who actively resists and isolates himself reveals nothing about himself, verbally or nonverbally. Patients who passively participate show many signs of nonverbal involvement. Moreover, they will contribute when asked directly to do so by the therapist. In contrast to actively resistant and self-isolating patients, passively participating patients are better risks for continued sobriety.

Resistant and self-isolating patients have not accepted their alcoholism, nor do they usually intend to stay sober once released from the hospital.

Continued Guilt over the Alcoholic Past. As treatment progresses, the psychotherapist must evaluate changes in his patient's level of guilt over past drinking and drinking behaviors. A continued high level of guilt is evidence of poor progress and a definite indicator of high probability of relapse. On the other hand, however, a complete absence of guilt and lack of concern over past behaviors may indicate a deeply ingrained sociopathic orientation to life, which may not bode well for recovery either. Realistic acceptance of past behaviors in the conceptual framework of the disease of alcoholism coupled with clear evidence of willingness to assume responsibility for present and future behaviors constitutes excellent progress and increases the probability of continued sobriety.

Hostility toward Treatment Staff and Generalized Hostility. Continued hostility toward treatment staff as therapy progresses may, in some instances, be justified. Not all alcoholism treatment programs are intelligently conceived or adequately staffed. It is more often the case, however, that a continued high level of hostility directed at treatment personnel is not justified and, hence, is an indicator of poor progress and predictive of relapse. When this occurs one may assume that the patient perceives treatment staff not as his allies in achieving sobriety, but as controlling agents preventing him from acting on strong motivation to drink. Such patient attitudes may also indicate generalized hostile attitudes toward perceived authority figures of all kinds.

While specific hostility evidenced in the treatment context indicates very poor progress, anger, hostility, and resentments directed at persons *outside* the treatment context are quite common in the early periods of alcoholism therapy. While these must always be taken seriously by treating staff and while they do increase the probability of relapse if not reduced, they do not invariably result in relapse. Sustained hostility and continued resentment toward another do indeed make the alcoholic uncomfortable but do not inevitably result in drinking. Paradoxically, *justified* resentments toward another are more difficult for the alcoholic patient to deal with and, hence, are more predictive of relapse than unjustified or irrational resentments. Unjustified resentments can be exposed for what they are in the course of therapy and either reduced in intensity or eliminated entirely. Justified resentments, however, are far more difficult to deal with therapeutically. In the case of the alcoholic who is looking for an excuse for continued drinking, justified resentments are easily invoked as reasons. Moreover, justified resentments are often perceived as sufficient reason for drinking by misinformed significant others. The alcoholic is often aware that drinking out of such motivations will not eventuate in social disapproval. In some instances it will be not only condoned but encouraged.

Generalized hostility toward others both within and outside of the treatment context is a very poor sign of progress and holds an associated high probability of relapse. The continuously angry, generally resentful alcoholic embroiled in one interpersonal conflict after another is not likely to stay sober.

Specific and Generalized Denial. Denial specifically associated with drinking matters is an indicator of poor progress in treatment. The alcoholic who continues to deny the impact of drinking on his health, mental and emotional functioning, and social relations is not likely to stay sober. Paradoxically, however, denial of other serious life problems early in sobriety is a good sign of progress. This tactical use of generalized denial early in sobriety is an effective means for the recently sober alcoholic to reduce intolerable stress, contain anxiety, and achieve the positive attitude necessary to move ahead with his recovery program.

Self-Centeredness Early in Treatment. While self-centeredness might be thought of as a negative factor, it is actually a positive sign early in treatment. The alcoholic who persists in showing preoccupation with the welfare of others to the point of jeopardizing his own sobriety is not progressing in therapy. Preoccupation with others, especially significant others such as mothers, spouses, children, and lovers, is particularly hazardous for the alcoholic early in treatment. In some cases such preoccupation is little more than guilt-motivated behavior. But whatever its motivation, excessive concern with the welfare of others sets the alcoholic up for drinking in several ways. First, it distracts him from his own program of recovery. Second, it exposes him to the fears, anxieties, and emotional problems of other people at a time when he can barely deal with his own. Third, preoccupation with others frequently results in frustration and disappointment with them, and these are emotions the newly sober alcoholic does not handle well. In this sense, then, a healthy degree of self-centeredness in the early period of sobriety is an indicator of good progress and a factor in favor of continued sobriety.

Acceptance of a Physiological Factor. In my experience, alcoholics who come to construe their alcoholism as a physiological disorder complicated by psychological, sociological, and cultural factors show the best chances of recovery. This is not to say that the patient must come to believe in a simplistic and naive disease concept of alcoholism. Nor must he ignore the many psychological, social, and cultural factors that are associated with the disease and complicate it further. But if the patient construes his drinking problem as a purely psychological disorder, his chances of continued recovery are greatly reduced. There are reasons for this. If the patient construes his problem in purely psychological terms, he is likely to test his ability to drink again once he begins to feel better after a period of abstinence. Many patients report that once their personal and social lives returned to normal, they felt their psychological problems had been resolved and they could drink without hazard. Unfortunately, the vast majority of such patients quickly found themselves in difficulty with alcohol once again. A second consequence of construing his problem in purely psychological terms is that the patient is more likely to keep alive the controlled-drinking hypothesis for himself. And as I have already indicated, this hypothesis concerning self is an excellent predictor of relapse.

While acceptance of a physiological factor in alcoholism is not in and of itself sufficient for the maintenance of sobriety, it is a sign of progress in therapy and is positively associated with continued abstinence.

Acceptance of a Realistic Continuing Recovery Program. The patient who recognizes the need for and is accepting of a postdischarge continuing recovery program has made excellent progress in his inpatient program. If he seriously intends to go to meetings of Alcoholics Anonymous and shows realistic, detailed plans for doing so, that is a very good sign indeed. Both experience and research have demonstrated that attendance at AA meetings and a sincere effort to work in that program are excellent predictors of continued sobriety after discharge. While it is true that some patients are able to maintain sobriety without postdischarge involvement in Alcoholics Anonymous, it is also true that for the majority this does not appear to be the case.

Patient plans concerning educational, employment, marital, and vocational rehabilitation goals constitute another important factor to be evaluated in assessing progress. Unfortunately, there is no general statement that can be made. In some instances such plans are clearly premature and efforts to actualize them are likely to result in a return to drinking. In other cases realistic plans leading to appropriate efforts to actualize such plans may be important in maintaining sobriety. For some patients a job will help keep them sober. For others it will contribute to relapse.

Changes in Self-Esteem. The patient's attitude toward himself is an important factor to be considered in evaluating progress. Expressions of self-dislike and frank self-hatred are not uncommon among alcoholics. As treatment progresses, these should be replaced by positive self-regarding attitudes. Of course, the typical picture of chronic low self-esteem evident in many alcoholics will take many months and possibly years of continuous sobriety to alter completely. Some degree of positive change in self-regard should be evident, however, if sobriety is to be maintained.

Depression, Anxiety, and Frustration Level. The psychotherapist must continuously evaluate a host of possible emotional reactions to abstinence and other general changes in the life circumstances of his patient. Depression is an important factor to be assessed, since it can operate as a trigger to initiate drinking. Anxiety, frustration, and stress in general can also serve to trigger drinking episodes. Insomnia is a particularly difficult problem for many recovering alcoholics. Many report resorting finally to drinking in order to deal with the stress of insomnia. As a consequence, sleeping patterns should be evaluated carefully in inhospital programs and, if necessary, therapeutic interventions to deal with insomnia should be made.

Quality of Sobriety: General Adjustment to Abstinence

Much of this discussion of inpatient evaluation of progress has been devoted to probability of relapse. Our concerns with abstinence and matters directly related to drinking are not intended to minimize the important question of general adjustment to abstinence; nor do we wish to maintain that abstinence is sufficient for psychological and social adjustment in sobriety. In the context of short-term inpatient programs, however, the priorities are clear: the drinking problem must be dealt with first if further changes are to be expected in personal and social functioning. While we are aware of opinions and some evidence to the contrary, it seems to us that most observations suggest that very little improvement can be expected in the general life adjustment of the person if alcoholic drinking persists.

To be sure, while abstinence is necessary, it is not a sufficient condition for effective psychosocial adjustment. As sobriety deepens, issues related directly to drinking recede into the background and problems of psychosocial adjustment—problems in living—become critical. In the next section of this chapter, some of these problems of long-term adjustment to sobriety will be considered. Moreover, factors other than patient psychological characteristics will be considered in predicting relapse.

OUTPATIENT AND FOLLOW-UP EVALUATION

The Problem of Alcoholic Relapse

Although we know a great deal about alcoholism treatment in terms of the short-term problems of physical rehabilitation while the patient is under medical care, our knowledge of treatment in relation to long-term alcoholic rehabilitation is extremely limited. This disparity in knowledge is often reflected in the comment: "We can get an alcoholic sober, but how do we get him to stay sober?" The rate of drinking relapse following inpatient treatment is discouragingly high, and of those who relapse, more than 80% do so within two months after discharge. Furthermore, the dropout rate from outpatient treatment is typically greater than 50%. On the other hand, it is known that if an alcoholic can remain abstinent for one year, his chances of remaining abstinent are excellent.

The phenomenon of relapse into alcoholism is clearly the most baffling feature of this disorder. As a result, clinicians have routinely attributed return to alcoholic drinking to characteristics of the alcoholic, rather than to shortcomings of the treatment process. Thus, relapse has been attributed to such features as low motivation, unconscious behavior patterns triggered by release of stimuli, and personality or moral deficits. This situation is not likely to change until alcoholism therapists begin assuming some of the treatment responsibility for the maintenance of sobriety and begin developing systematic knowledge of relapse factors. At this time, research on alcoholic relapse has taken the form only of follow-up evaluation. This research has centered around descriptive and demographic characteristics of patients as prognostic factors. The most prominent finding here is that patients of high social stability (maintenance of job, residence, and an intact family) have a better prognosis than do patients of low social stability. These characteristics, while accounting for differences in follow-up rates at different kinds of treatment facilities, are nonetheless the same characteristics that would predict differences in adjustments of alcoholics who participated in no treatment at all.

In the remainder of this chapter, we will first describe kinds of patient outcome at follow-up. We will then discuss factors that contribute to alcoholic relapse. Finally, we will discuss some of the implications of obtaining feedback from clients after discharge for improving treatment practices.

Varieties of Outcome States

Three dimensions or criteria will be used to describe the variety of outcome states of treated alcoholics in the community. Knowing where the client lies on these three dimensions can help the clinician both to evaluate the current state of the client and to predict the next outcome state he is likely to be in. The first criterion is whether or not the client is currently *drinking* (now or within the last month).

The evidence indicates consistently that for alcoholics, drinking is a significant correlate of physical, social, mental, and emotional distress. Any attempt to progress with treatment while an alcoholic client is drinking is doomed to failure, and both experience and empirical evidence indicate that the client's drinking will only become worse in the process. This latter effect is likely due to the increased stress generated by being in treatment. Resumption of drinking by a client who has been treated for alcoholism constitutes "alcoholic relapse" and is a sign of further morbidity in his or her health.

Another outcome dimension we will employ is *craving*. Here we are talking not about physical craving concomitant upon alcoholic withdrawal, but rather psychological craving—characterized as a "subclinical withdrawal syndrome"—which can be set off by a persistent exposure to cues associated with the absence of alcohol or by persistent dysphoric mood states. Put simply, whether the alcoholic client is drinking or not, he can be in a state either of continually wanting to drink or of having "lost the desire" for a drink. For a client who continually craves alcohol, whether drinking or not, alcohol remains the central and unifying symbol of his life.

Associated with the craving state is a constant recognition of the *need to control alcohol*. This overconcern for control reveals itself in the abstinent alcoholic as an agonizing battle against the first drink, and in the drinking alcoholic in the cluster of high-tension endeavors called "controlled drinking." Both of these are characterized by a preoccupation or obsession with the control of one's alcoholic impulses. In contrast, the client who does not show the craving/control syndrome does not show this obsessive overconcern with control and has integrated his life around new, more positive symbols.

The two dimensions described thus far together generate four distinct outcome states. The sober client is considered an *arrested alcoholic* if he still exhibits the craving/control syndrome. He can be considered a *recovered alcoholic* if he no longer exhibits this syndrome. Arrested alcoholism is associated with a high likelihood of alcoholic relapse.

The drinking alcoholic client can be considered to be in a "controlled" drinking state if he is showing craving/control, and he can be considered in a "normal" drinking state if he does not show the craving/control phenomenon. Of the four states, controlled drinking can be considered the most predictive of relapse into alcoholism, inasmuch as the overconcern for control may readily produce the commonly observed flip from overcontrol to loss of control. Normal drinking in a treated alcoholic is best considered, in clinical experience, a transitory phenomenon that appears whenever the pathognomic control symptom has temporarily abated.

The final outcome dimension is called *life-style pathology*. A client who maintains the same pathological life style as he had prior to treatment for alcoholism continues to accrue negative life–health consequences. That is to say, he continues to suffer negative consequences in the vocational, interpersonal, legal, psychological, and/or emotional domains. An alcoholic who is both drinking and engaging in a pathological life style is considered to be in a "pathological-drinking" state. At this point, his relapse into drinking can be considered a relapse into alcoholism. A state which is commonly neglected by clinicians but which has high prognostic relevance for pathological drinking is one in which the alcoholic exhibits a high degree of pathology in his life style, despite the fact that he is maintaining abstinence. That is to say, his life style replicates in many aspects his life style while in a pathological-drinking state, except for the drinking, *per se*.

We have delineated six different outcome states of an alcoholic in the community, each of which has different relevance both for predicting relapse into alcoholism and for treatment guidelines. In the next section we will examine in more detail factors predictive of relapse, particularly those which come into play following a relatively extended period of abstinence. During this discussion the term *relapse* will apply to relapse into drinking following a period of abstinence, inasmuch as the drinking state under these circumstances is clearly the most pathognomic indicator of eventual, if not immediate, relapse into the pathological-drinking state.

Factors in Alcoholic Relapse

Short-Term versus Life-Style Abstinence.   We have emphasized the necessity for abstinence on the part of the client during the treatment phase if any positive results of treatment are to occur. As has been pointed out previously, however, those factors fostering short-term abstinence are not necessarily the same factors fostering long-term abstinence or an abstinent life style. Among the reasons for this disparity is that the defense structure of the newly sober alcoholic client is susceptible to a somewhat different rationale for sobriety than is the case for the alcoholic with a longer period of abstinence.

In the initial section of this chapter, we discussed psychological factors predictive primarily of short-term abstinence. In this section we shall briefly describe some of the modifications in these factors necessary for producing motivation for life-style abstinence. It was pointed out earlier that positive congruity among the belief, affect, and action components of the drinking attitude, along with congruity within each component, was an unrealistic posture for producing short-term sobriety in the newly sober alcoholic. That is, in the early stages such congruity within the drinking attitude is clearly an indicator of superficial compliance with the treatment staff as opposed to representing internalized change. By contrast, with continuing sobriety the reverse prediction gains primacy. In order to maintain an abstinent life style that is comfortable, it will eventually be necessary for the client to integrate, and make positively congruent, his beliefs, feelings, and intentions with regard to his own use of alcohol.

While belief in controlled drinking will remain a significant predictor of relapse for alcoholics of longer-term sobriety, the meaning behind this belief will change. With longer-term sobriety, the alcoholic becomes aware that the recognition of his need to control his drinking is in fact a premorbid *sign* of his alcoholism and not, as he earlier believed, a *goal* to be valued.

While the alcoholic's preferred defense mechanisms of denial and repression can be usefully deployed to produce short-term abstinence, the continued use of these mechanisms in handling his everyday life stresses later in sobriety becomes counterproductive to the maintenance of sobriety. In other words, eventually the alcoholic is going to have to employ the same openness by which he altered his drinking attitudes to begin to find new ways to deal with his other life problems, lest he return to the life style that sowed the seeds of his pathological drinking in the first place. It is for this reason that the use of continuing outpatient treatment and/or a continuing recovery program is essential for the maintenance of a sober life style. Such a commitment is dependent critically on the alcoholic's perception of his *need* for continuing self-scrutiny. The increase in self-esteem so necessary for the alcoholic's recovery must be clearly and continuously tied in to the fact of his abstinence. If this is not the case, the increase in self-esteem will give way to the belief that he can now drink without consequence and thus to an almost complete negation of treatment efforts to that point.

It was earlier stated that, in achieving short-term sobriety, failure to recognize a physiological basis for his alcoholism was predictive of relapse. Although this remains the case for *maintaining* abstinence, the belief must be modified in the following way: The alcoholic recognizes that as long as he is not drinking—that is, as long as he is maintaining an abstinent life style—he will not have any specific ill-effects of the drug, alcohol. However, he must eventually recognize his ingrained propensity to cope with life via drug use, together with the concomitant psychological side effects of continued drinking as a method of coping. Thus, during his abstinence his relationship to his disease is almost entirely mental and emotional. The capacity of both internal cues (such as mood changes and craving) and external cues (such as life stresses, which have long been previously associated with alcohol intake) to trigger the drinking response, and hence the physiological component of his disease, must be recognized as a psychological phenomenon to be dealt with accordingly.

In the early stages of sobriety, because guilt is counterproductive to treatment and the acceptance of his alcoholism, the client is not encouraged to delve deeply, beyond superficial drinking experiences, into his life problems prior to treatment. For the maintenance of long-term sobriety, however, the alcoholic must be gradually encouraged to look at, but not live in, his drinking past in order to become aware of those pathological mechanisms and ways of behaving that reinforced his earlier life style. Similarly, while the alcoholic's hostility cannot be dealt with in any great depth during the initial stages of treatment, the maintenance of an abstinent life style requires that the alcoholic gain skills in expressing his hostility in a productive way. Such inability to express hostility has been cited as the most common factor given by alcoholics themselves for relapse.

Finally, self-centeredness, a useful state of early sobriety and a precursor of the development of self-esteem, must eventually give way to acquiring modes for preventing the focus on self from becoming unrealistic and obsessive—a state that is counterproductive to the maintenance of sobriety. The alcoholic will eventually find that altruistic behavior oriented toward helping another alcoholic, beyond the initial motivation of keeping himself sober, will allow him to relieve obsessive self-focus, to gain the capacity for reliable feedback about himself from others, and to see and compare the self-changes that have taken place during his sobriety.

We emphasize that activities oriented to life-style abstinence do not begin until at least several months of continuous abstinence, and often only after one year of abstinence. The first few months of treatment must concentrate solely on deploying the alcoholic's given defense mechanisms for achieving freedom from immediate relapse following detoxification. Almost all therapeutic intervention at this point is oriented toward education about drinking attitudes and practical techniques for staying away from the first drink and gaining physical comfort. *It is only after several months that the alcoholic can even begin with self-change issues.*

The alcoholic's rationale for life without alcohol grows in unison with a comfortable life style based upon the commitment for lifelong sobriety. Thus, drinking at the later stages must be viewed as an act inconsistent with one's new life style. Here rests the distinction earlier made between the arrested and the recovered (more accurately, "recovering") alcoholic. While the arrested alcoholic does not drink, the most favorable position that he can maintain is one of resignation to a life without alcohol, peppered by a great deal of resistance and occasional rebellion. The recovered alcoholic, on the other hand, not only accepts his condition as a realistic limitation, but, moreover makes a positive commitment to a life style free of alcohol. Thus, rather than seeing the absence of alcohol as a limitation on his freedom and resigning himself to not drinking, he actively *chooses* freely not to drink.

Interpersonal Factors. Far and away the most likely triggering incident for the alcoholic's seeking treatment occurs within the client's family. If the client is married, leverage for seeking treatment most commonly rests with the spouse. There is evidence to indicate that longer-term sobriety in the alcoholic is just as strongly related to life change and attitude change of the spouse as it is to his own change.

As mentioned above, the most common reason given by alcoholics themselves for their relapse is inability to express hostility. Hence, for the married alcoholic it is critical that an outpatient program involve the spouse and, if at all possible, other members of the family. We are aware of at least one study in which personality change of the spouse of the alcoholic client was the strongest predictor of the client's maintaining abstinence following treatment (Rae and Drewery, 1972).

Other Environmental Factors. During the alcoholic client's drinking career, certain objects, persons, and events became highly associated with the *intoxication state,* a positive affective state, while certain other objects, persons, and events became firmly associated with the *withdrawal state,* a negative affective state. These events not only served and continue to serve as cues to signal their associated states, but also have served as powerful reinforcers for drinking behavior and behaviors linked to drinking behavior.

Cues for the "high" state or intoxication state include passing an old drinking haunt, going to a social gathering where alcohol is served, associating with drinking friends, talking about the past use of alcohol, and the sight of alcohol itself in its various manifestations. Drinking in these situations may have become almost instinctive, and avoidance of these situations is clearly indicated in the early part of sobriety.

On the other hand, it is also true that participating in these situations can *substitute* for the intoxication state without the actual use of alcohol. In other words, an alcoholic client who is not drinking can participate in a conditioned "high" in these or similar situations if he can manage to avoid using alcohol. Endless conversation about past drinking experiences in meetings of Alcoholics Anonymous often clearly serves this function. There is, however, a problem with this kind of substitution. Just as a high produced by alcohol will eventually produce the aversive withdrawal state, a conditioned high (or substitute high) will also yield to the opposed aversive state. The informal institution of the "meeting after the meeting" in Alcoholics Anonymous is probably the best kind of antidote for this aftereffect.

It is the situations that cue off the *aversive* withdrawal types of experiences that are clearly the most dangerous for the alcoholic in any stage of recovery. It is these "low" states that the alcoholic was strongly motivated to avoid during the latter part of his drinking career. These are cues associated with the *absence* of alcohol. These conditioned aversive cues produced the craving (psychological, in this case) and agonizing abstinence experiences that led to escapist drinking bouts. Examples of conditioned aversive cues that evoke these "lows" are associates who do not drink, separation from a partner or loved one who served as a drinking companion, the bed in which the client went through withdrawal, and the absence of money used previously to finance the alcohol habit.

In this context it is easier to see why relapse is such a widespread phenomenon in the alcoholic client. His behavior is tightly hemmed in by *both* situations that remind him of drinking and situations that remind him of the absence of alcohol. During the earlier phases of sobriety, when he cannot as easily handle the conditioned withdrawal or craving stage, he should avoid activities that get him into too "high" a state. Only after he has learned to handle the aversive states with progressively more confidence can he safely indulge in positive, euphoric states.

Thus far we have been considering states that are produced because they are similar in quality to the mood states evoked by the use of alcohol or by its termination. A related set of problems is encountered when we consider the variety of other positive and negative mood states not directly related to drinking. For example, the sudden termination of a host of erstwhile stable, everyday situations can produce negative affective states that may easily *generalize* to the alcohol-craving state. These may include major events such as being fired at work, death of a close family member, marital separation, or loss of financial security.

Not only must changes in major life events be considered, but there is some evidence to indicate that alcoholics may be even more affected by smaller, less significant life changes, such as a change in work hours, trouble with the boss, change in responsibilities at work, or change in recreation. In other words, any event that produces a negative dysphoric state is capable, in early sobriety, of producing relapse by virtue of the generalization of that state to the craving state. This failure to differentiate between distinct dysphoric states was brought about largely by the alcoholic's long-standing habit of drinking in order to avoid any semblance of discomfort.

By the same token, any event that produces a strong euphoric state can also cue a relapse by virtue of its similarity to the intoxication state. It is occasions such as getting married, marital reconciliation, or getting a bonus at work that were previously positive occasions for drinking that become readily assimilated to the "high" intoxication state.

During outpatient treatment, then, the clinician must monitor both the positive and negative events occurring in the alcoholic's life which are capable of producing life stress and must work both to lower their affective intensity and to distinguish for the client these affective states from the similar intoxication and withdrawal states. Eventually, with long-term sobriety, the alcoholic's attitude toward these stressful events begins to take on a less threatening form and to become discriminated from the alcohol-related affective states.

Attitude Changes.   The recovered alcoholic of long-term sobriety has *altered the meanings* of events and their relationship to him. As long as the alcoholic maintains a *dysynchronous* or competitive stance vis-à-vis the world about him, he is in constant danger of being susceptible to relapse. As this attitude gradually becomes displaced by a *synchronous* or complementary perceptual/cognitive mode, the alcoholic becomes much less vulnerable to the vicissitudes of his everyday life situations. That is to say, the events and people in his life no longer have the power to produce the psychological craving states that lead to alcohol relapse. This change in attitude toward a more synchronous mode appears to be, in our experience, essential to long-term sobriety. In the remainder of this section, we will describe a number of the implications of this attitude change.

The alcoholic's general feeling of his place in the world, which is a feeling of separateness or isolation, must give way to the feeling of being a *part of*, and in some kind of harmony with, what is going on around him. A *perception of self* that formerly was vulnerable and tenuous gives way to a feeling of safety and security. Self-centeredness gives way to a *sense of worth*, whereby the client no longer feels victimized. A boring, alien, hostile world becomes one that is friendly and interesting. While other people were viewed as deceitful, opportunistic, threatening, they are now perceived as similar, friendly, and unthreatening. Whereas previously he overreacted to trivial situations, he is now capable of *reorienting his attention* away from these trivia.

In the later stages of sobriety, the alcoholic client is relaxed, accepting, and able to *let things happen*, in contrast to his earlier behavioral orientation of vigilance, manipulation, and competitiveness. He now *accepts responsibility* for his actions and reactions, which at the earlier stage he was intent on avoiding. He no longer perceives the future in terms of impending doom and constant worry. A relaxed internal environment and sense of well-being displace his earlier state of continuous fear and anxiety.

Primary versus Secondary Alcoholism. "Primary" alcoholism is said to be pure alcoholism with no psychiatric genesis. The rationale here is that any psychiatric dysfunction that occurs with the primary alcoholic is essentially an *effect* of his excessive drinking. The "secondary" alcoholic, by contrast, is said to be one whose alcoholism is essentially a symptom of a more fundamental psychiatric disorder. In the latter case, outpatient treatment obviously must eventually be tailored to dealing with the primary diagnosis if relapse is to be avoided.

Alcoholism has been found to be associated with affective disorders, cyclothymic personality disorders, schizophrenic reactions, chronic depressive reactions, paranoia, psychoneurosis, and sociopathy. It is not clinically uncommon to find that the client's alcoholism has functioned effectively to cover up one or more deeper emotional disorders. However, it is clearly counterproductive to treatment to attempt to deal with these disorders *until the client has achieved at least several months of continuous abstinence.* Of course, gross debilitating symptoms such as psychotic episodes and suicidal depressions must be managed, but, as a rule, attempts to move too quickly in uncovering ingrained personality disorders will almost certainly result in relapse.

Alcoholic Craving. Probably the surest sign of imminent relapse is a psychological craving for alcohol. That is, after a period of sobriety, at which time physical craving (craving during withdrawal) is not a factor, a *dysynchronous internal state (as defined above), together with the appropriate environmental cues, will set off the craving phenomenon.* Psychological craving can be conceptualized as a state of hyperarousal that is related to anxiety and depression. It is a very dangerous state in terms of relapse because of its similarity for the alcoholic to the familiar state of abstinence agony occurring during actual alcohol withdrawal.

Psychological or symbolic craving can take the form of actual physical manifestations, such as the sweats, shakiness, jumpy nerves, and/or upset stomach. Phenomenological craving will be simply the fantasy or awareness of an intense desire for a drink. Therapy at these times is oriented toward reshaping the alcoholic's threshold levels, such that when the normal cues that excite craving are perceived, they will not be *labeled* in such a way that craving inevitably results. The gradual change from a dysynchronous (a continuously threatened and vulnerable internal state) to a synchronous state will, as discussed above, work toward this relabeling process.

Behavioral Antidotes to Relapse. If we think of alcoholic behavior in terms of ethology, all of the behaviors that combine to produce drinking (getting the money for liquor, buying it, finding a place to drink, and drinking) become a kind of *fixed action pattern* that is released by a sign stimulus, which is the drinking cue in the environment to which the alcoholic is susceptible. All of the ways, at least in early sobriety, in which alcoholics "don't take that first drink" become, in these terms, *displacement activity.* Examples of such displacement activity for arrested alcoholics include compulsive overwork, constant talking about alcohol, compulsive overeating or sexual activity, and obsession with a love relationship. Such behavioral displacement activities, while counterproductive for long-term sobriety, are probably essential for producing the necessary *initial* sobriety following detoxification.

Following successful displacement activity, in behavioral terms the task confronting the alcoholic client is to develop and refine a response hierarchy to the internal and external drinking cues *that places the drinking response at a progressively lower position in the hierarchy.* But how do you suppress a response—the drinking response—that has been prepotent for such a long time and has had such a long history of reinforcement that it has almost become a fixed action pattern?

The answer is that you cannot—without a strong support group. Having family or friends attend Al-Anon or attend joint sessions with the client is highly beneficial in terms of confronting the client with some of the interaction patterns that trigger craving and eventual drinking. In addition, support groups like Alcoholics Anonymous are highly effective in performing the function of teaching the alcoholic client alternative modes of response to stress. AA presents to the alcoholic client a myriad of behavior-therapeutic activities, involving substitution of other behaviors, mostly interpersonal, for the drinking response.

For the recovered alcoholic of long-term sobriety, continued involvement in Alcoholics Anonymous activities not only presents a constant reminder of his previous life style, but, by fostering explicitly the goals of maintaining a synchronous internal state, also assures him a degree of harmony and comfort within an abstinent life style.

Feedback from Follow-Up Contacts

Whether or not the alcoholic client pursues outpatient treatment beyond the initial treatment contact, it is extremely useful to obtain information at regular intervals, preferably monthly, regarding his current outcome state. There are two reasons for obtaining systematic follow-up in this way.

The first reason is that by seeing the *pattern of outcome states* for the alcoholic client over a several-month period, the clinician is better able to predict the *next* outcome state and thereby to provide *preventive* treatment for relapse. In addition, if the clinician finds he can no longer be of direct help, he can still be a useful source of referral for the client.

If the patient has a relapse, this is obviously cause for concern, but is by no means cause for despair on the part of the clinician. Many alcoholics with long-term sobriety have had several periods of relapse while in the early phases. Sobriety appears to be progressive inasmuch as many of the tools acquired during periods of sobriety do not have to be relearned in the next period of sobriety. Moreover, many alcoholics appear to require a *variety of different kinds of treatment modes* before achieving permanent sobriety. The alcoholic's readiness to work for permanent sobriety in most cases increases despite what appears to be a hopeless case of continuous relapse. The clinician must be able to make informed decisions about reentry to the helping system for a relapsed alcoholic.

The second reason for obtaining reliable feedback at follow-up is to further the clinician's longer-term goal of being able to provide intelligent client screening and to provide *alternative modes of treatment* for alcoholics of different backgrounds and descriptions. Keeping systematic records of outcome at six months for clients at a given facility

NAME OF PATIENT_____ HOSPITAL:_____

                                                                       DISCHARGE DATE:_____

DATE OF INTERVIEW:_____

NAME OF INTERVIEWER:_____

<u>PLEASE DO NOT OMIT ANY QUESTIONS</u>

1. Have you been in a hospital again or in a halfway house for a problem related to alcohol since you left the hospital? Yes____ No____. If YES, which one and how many times?
_____

2. Have you been arrested at all for any alcohol-related offense since you left the hospital? Yes_____ No____. If YES, how many times?_____

3. Have you had anything (any alcohol) to drink during the past month? Yes____ No____

4. About how many days in the last 6 months since you left the hospital have you been drinking?_____ IF PATIENT NEVER DRANK AT ALL SINCE DISCHARGE, SKIP #5 & 6.

5. About how many days after leaving the hospital did you take your first drink?_____

6. About how many days ago did you have your last drink?_____

7. Have you returned to the hospital for any counseling or therapy since you left the hospital? Yes_____ No_____

8. Have you attended any meetings of Alcoholics Anonymous during the past month? Yes_____ No_____

9. Have you attended AA meetings at all since you left the hospital? Yes_____ No_____

10. Have you had any other forms of counseling or therapy since you left the hospital? Yes_____ No_____

11. Has anyone in your family attended Al-Anon? Yes_____ No_____

12. Have you used ANTABUSE at all since you left the hospital? Yes_____ No_____

13. When you were in the hospital what experiences were most helpful to you? I will read off some of the experiences and then you tell me which <u>two</u> you believe were <u>most</u> helpful to you: (CHECK TWO)

     The Doctor _____   Group Therapy _____   Contact with other patients_____
     The Nurses _____   Family Therapy_____   AA Meetings _____
     The Lectures_____   Films _____   AA Volunteers _____
                                                 Occupational Therapy _____

14. I will read off a list of possible things that might have happened in your life since you left the hospital. After I read each one, please simply answer YES if it happened to you, and NO if it didn't happen to you. (CHECK IF YES)

     Death of spouse_____   Mortgage over $10,000_____
     Divorce_____   Change in responsibilities at work _____
     Marital separation_____   Son or daughter leaving home_____
     Jail term_____   Trouble with in-laws_____
     Death of close family member_____   Outstanding personal achievement_____
     Personal injury or illness_____   Change in living conditions_____
     Getting married_____   Change in personal habits_____
     Fired at work_____   Trouble with boss_____
     Marital reconciliation_____   Change in work hours_____
     Retirement_____   Change in residence _____
     Change in health of family member_____   Change in recreation_____
     Pregnancy in family_____   Change in church activities_____
     Sex difficulties_____   Mortgage or loan less than $10,000_____
     Gain of new family member_____   Change in sleeping habits_____
     Business readjustment_____   Change in number of family get-togethers_____
     Change in financial situation_____   Change in eating habits_____
     Death of close friend_____   Vacation_____
     Change to a different line of work_____   Minor violations of the law_____
                                                 Change in social activities_____

COMMENTS OF THE INTERVIEWER _____

Figure 1. Telephone Follow-Up Form

will inform the staff of which kinds of clients are being helped most by their regimen and which are helped least. The latter alcoholics can then be referred to other facilities that specialize in that variety of client, thus maximizing the cost-effectiveness of the original facility in helping the alcoholic client. Moreover, the benefits of follow-up feedback for tailoring treatment modes to different kinds of clients are of critical interest in avoiding waste of valuable resources.

The simplest kind of systematic feedback is the *telephone follow-up* during which the staff member checks, on a short form, answers to questions that can be asked within a ten-minute conversation. This form can also be administered face to face. An example of such a form is presented in Figure 1. The form was designed for telephone follow-up of clients following discharge from an inpatient facility, although it can be modified slightly to be further appropriate for outpatient clients. The form assesses additional kinds of treatment obtained, arrests, information about relapse and timing of relapse, continuing use of support groups, the client's perception of helpfulness to him of different modes of treatment, and a checklist of stressful environmental events (Holmes and Rahe, 1967).

DIRECTIONS IN EVALUATION RESEARCH

Studies of treatment outcome have shown variable results. Both very high and very low recovery rates have been reported. As might be expected, neither extreme is representative of the field. Deviantly high recovery rates are usually confounded by a host of methodological problems including such things as sample bias, inadequate measurement operations, failure to control investigator bias, improper handling of patient dropouts from treatment, and so forth.

On the other hand, exceedingly pessimistic views of the effectiveness of alcoholism treatment (e.g., Emrick, 1982; Miller and Hester, 1980) may be attributable to the effort to generate a single number, or "average," to describe a range of outcomes from a large collection of treatment programs that vary considerably in quality, populations served, and comprehensiveness. Moreover, care must be taken that results from studies of the natural history of alcoholism (e.g., Polich, Armor, and Braiker, 1981) not be mistakenly promulgated as *treatment outcome* findings.

In approaching the question of the effectiveness of alcoholic treatment, investigators need to differentiate populations carefully. It is not appropriate to focus outcome studies exclusively on populations in which alcoholism is complicated by pervasive and complex negative extratreatment factors such as extreme poverty, mental illness, social instability, and so forth. Whereas these populations do, of course, require continuing study, it is not reasonable to expect studies of them to yield much reliable information about alcoholism treatment *per se*. In effect, positive effects of alcoholism treatment are likely to be obscured by these powerful, negative extratreatment factors that treatment alone could not be expected to overcome.

Studies of alcoholism treatment effectiveness are most appropriately conducted on treatment populations in which negative extratreatment factors are minimal or absent and treatment effects can be observed more clearly. In fact, when socially stable populations are studied, positive treatment outcome rates of 50% to 60% are not unusual (e.g., Patton, 1979).

Among clients who relapse, the great majority do so within the first month or two following discharge (Chalmers, 1974). The importance of clients' life situations following treatment in determining abstinence, as discussed below, underscores the inadequacy of the traditional unitary model whereby clients are given intensive treatment followed by occasional aftercare or check-up visits.

A few general trends within evaluation research indicate a more hopeful turn of events for alcoholism treatment. There are (1) a systems view of the alcoholism treatment process; (2) an emphasis on lifestyle change processes; and (3) differential diagnosis and treatment planning.

A Systems Orientation. A systems view of the treatment process assumes that there are a number of different categories of variables that determine treatment outcome; the problem is to discern how they separately and jointly contribute to recovery. The methodology of this approach is based on multivariate regression analysis. According to one systems model, components of the treatment process are broken down into pretreatment, treatment, and posttreatment categories and the relative contributions of these components to outcome at follow-up are compared (Moos and Finney, 1983; Costello, 1980; Chalmers, 1974). Pretreatment and posttreatment components include both client factors (demographic, personality, intake functioning) and lifestyle factors (life stress, family and vocational coping, additional treatment, etc.).

Pretreatment knowledge of client factors, such as social stability, are known to have a strong effect on abstinence at follow-up. Results with the systems model have shown, however, that the effects of client factors on abstinence are primarily indirect, exerting their influence by way of treatment response and posttreatment coping responses. This kind of result implies that more attention be paid to matching clients to treatment components.

Another finding of the systems approach to evaluation concerns the overwhelming influence of posttreatment factors, relative to treatment factors, in maintaining abstinence at follow-up. That is, life stressors encountered by clients after discharge, and the means of coping with these life situations are the most important predictors of recovery. Treatment effects appear to exert primarily an indirect effect on outcome by way of their impact on coping responses after treatment (Cronkite and Moos, 1980).

Lifestyle Change. The systems model's findings regarding the inordinate influence of lifestyle factors on abstinence has led to the suggestion that alcoholism treatment may be more effective when oriented toward clients' individual life situations. Discharged inpatient clients undergoing outpatient treatment, for example, are twice as likely to maintain abstinence by frequent participation in Alcoholics Anonymous, a lifestyle support system (Chalmers, 1979).

New trends in behavioral medicine involve a biopsychosocial, interdisciplinary perspective, which stresses the links between the client and his environment (see the volume entitled *Behavioral Medicine: Changing Health Lifestyles*, edited by Davidson and Davidson, 1980).

One promising approach to a treatment philosophy oriented toward life circumstances involves teaching clients tools for relapse prevention. Such an approach follows from research documenting the kinds of conditions under which relapse occurs, such as interpersonal conflict, social pressure, and negative emotional states (Marlatt and Gordon, 1980). Documenting individual stressors and teaching specific relapse prevention strategies for life circumstances during alcoholism treatment may well optimize the generalization of treatment gains to the client's posttreatment environment. One of the missing links in alcoholism treatment may well be an adequate analysis of individual precipitants to relapse.

Assessing Clients' Personality and Intake Status. A final promising direction in evaluation research concerns the matching of clients to treatment components. Unfortunately, a large number of alcoholism treatment staff hold to a unitary, stereotyped view of the addicted client, thereby ignoring clients' needs and disabilities, and resisting program intents at differential diagnosis and needs assessments (e.g., Hadley and Hadley, 1972). There is evidence that the more specific and individualized the treatment, the lower the dropout rate and the higher the success rate. Awareness by treatment staff of patient personality needs and lifestyle characteristics permits critical knowledge of clients' potential responses to treatment modalities and life situations.

Client characteristics demonstrated to affect treatment response and outcome differentially include degree of alcohol dependence, age, marital status, interpersonal conceptual level, depression, psychiatric disturbance, and cognitive deficit. Treatment aspects whose effectiveness has been shown to depend on client characteristics include drug therapy versus milieu therapy versus psychotherapy, structured versus unstructured treatment settings, and institutional versus informal residential settings.

Diagnostic testing would likely be more useful to treatment staff if it included lifestyle functioning and "wellness" scales in addition to pathology scales. Traditional psychiatric jargon should be operationalized into behavioral referents relevant to relapse potential, rather than reified as permanent client dispositions.

References

Chalmers, D. K. *A multivariate outcome study of alcoholics and their spouses.* CORE Report #2, School of Social Sciences, University of California, Irvine, 1974.

Chalmers, D. K. The alcoholic's controlled drinking time. *World Alcohol Project,* 1979, 2, 19–32.

Costello, R. M. Alcoholism treatment effectiveness: Slicing the outcome variance pie. In G. Edwards and M. Grant (Eds.), *Alcoholism treatment in transition.* Baltimore: University Park Press, 1980.

Cronkite, R. C. and Moos, R. H. Determinants of the post-treatment functioning of alcoholic patients: A conceptual framework. *Journal of Consulting and Clinical Psychology,* 1980, 48, 305–316.

Davidson, P. O. and S. M. Davidson (Eds.). *Behavioral medicine: Changing health lifestyles.* New York: Brunner/Mazel, 1980.

Emrick, C. D. Evaluation of alcoholism psychotherapy methods. In E. M. Pattison and E. Kaufman (Eds.), *Encyclopedic handbook of alcoholism.* New York: Gardner Press, 1982.

Hadley, P. A. and Hadley, R. G. Treatment practices and philosophies in rehabilitation facilities for alcoholics. *Proceedings of the American Psychological Association.* 1972, 80, 779–780.

Holmes, T. H. and Rahe, R. H. The social readjustment rating scale. *Journal of Psychosometric Research,* 1967, 11, 108–130.

Marlatt, G. A. and Gordon, J. R. Determinants of relapse: Implications for the maintenance of behavior change. In P. Davidson and S. M. Davidson (Eds.), *Behavioral medicine: Changing health lifestyles.* New York: Brunner/Mazel, 1979.

Miller, W. R. and Hester, R. K. Treating the problem drinker: Modern approaches. In W. R. Miller (Ed.), *The addictive behavior: Treatment of alcoholism, drug abuse, smoking, and obesity.* New York: Pergamon Press, 1980.

Moos, R. H. and Finney, J. W. The expanding scope of alcoholism treatment evaluation. *American Psychologist,* 1983, 38, 1036–1044.

Patton, M. *Validity and reliability of Hazelden treatment follow-up data.* Center City, Minn.: Hazelden Educational Services, 1979.

Polich, J. M., Armor, D. J., and Braiker, H. B. *The course of alcoholism: four years after treatment.* New York: Wiley, 1981.

Rae, J. B. and Drewery, J. Interpersonal patterns in alcoholic marriages. *British Journal of Psychiatry,* 1972, 120, 615–621.

SUGGESTED READINGS

Alcoholics Anonymous World Services. *Living sober.* New York, 1975.

Baekeland, F., Lundwall, L., and Kissin, B. Methods for the treatment of chronic alcoholism: A critical appraisal. In R. J. Gibbins, Y. Israel, H. Kalant, R. E. Popham, W. Schmidt, and R. G. Smart (Eds.), *Research advances in alcohol and drug problems.* Vol. 2. New York: Wiley, 1975.

Bateson, G. The cybernetics of "self": A theory of alcoholism. *Psychiatry,* 1971, *34,* 1–18.

Dohrenwend, B. S., and Dohrenwend, B. P. (Eds.). *Stressful life events: Their nature and effects.* New York: Wiley, 1974.

Deikman, A. F. Bimodal consciousness. *Archives of General Psychiatry,* 1971, *25,* 481–489.

Estes, N. J., and Hanson, K. J. Sobriety: Problems, challenges, and solutions. In N. J. Estes and M. E. Heinemann (Eds.), *Alcoholism: Development, consequences, and interventions.* St. Louis: C. V. Mosby, 1977.

Ludwig, A. M., and Wikler, A. "Craving" and relapse to drink. *Quarterly Journal of Studies on Alcohol,* 1974, *35,* 108–130.

Madsen, W. *The American alcoholic: The nature-nurture controversy in alcoholic research and therapy.* Springfield: Charles C Thomas, 1974.

Solomon, R., and Corbit, J. An opponent-process theory of motivation. *Psychological Review,* 1974, *81,* 119–145.

Index